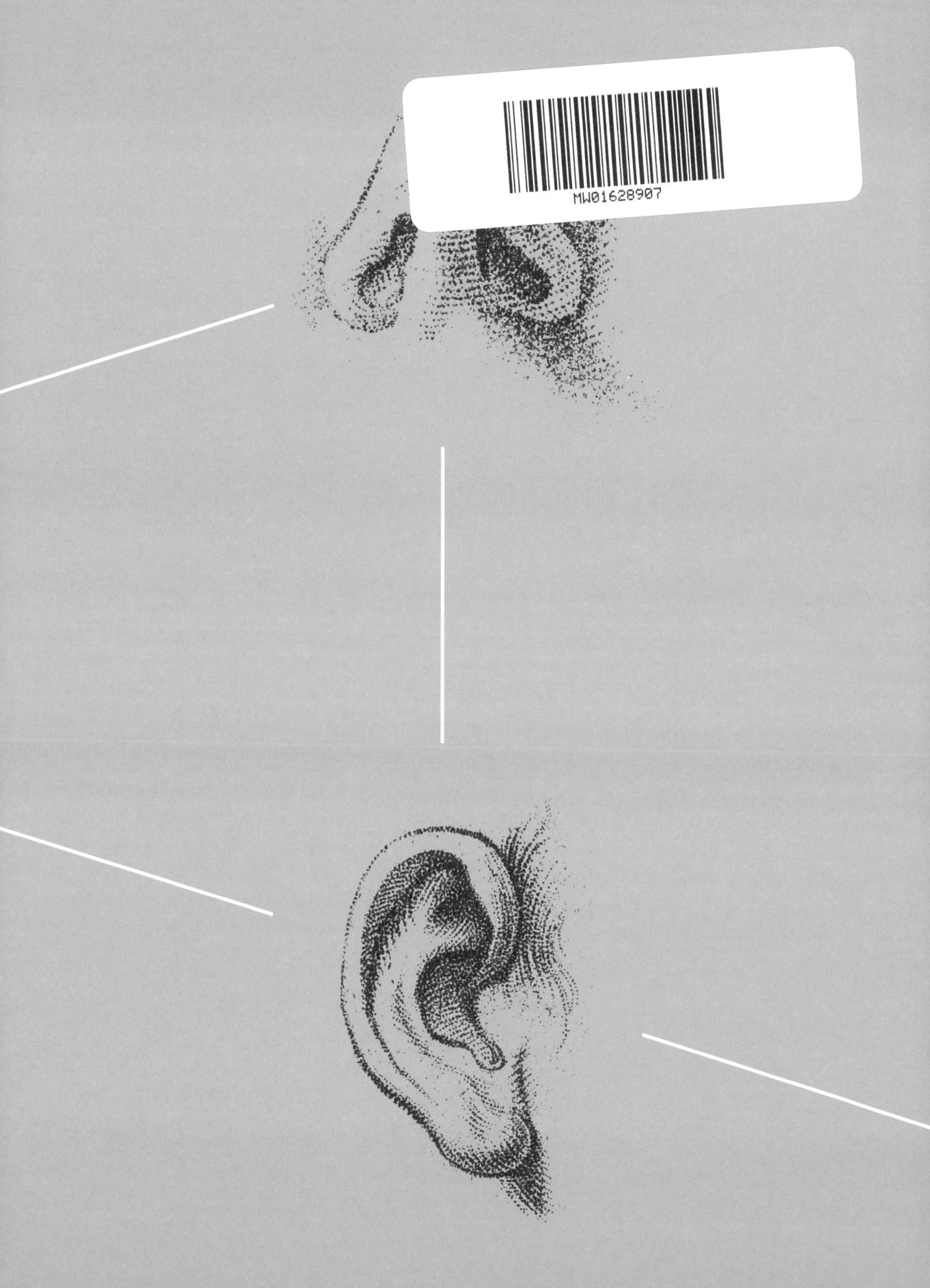

abrasive,
buttery, clammy, doughy,
effervescent,
foamy, gurgling, hissing,
icky, jangling, knotty,
lemony, minty, nubby, oily,
pungent, quiet,
rank, silky, tart, unctuous,
viscous, waxy, xilinous,
yeasty, zingy

The Senses: Design Beyond Vision

Ellen Lupton & Andrea Lipps

COOPER HEWITT, SMITHSONIAN DESIGN MUSEUM
& PRINCETON ARCHITECTURAL PRESS
NEW YORK

Published by
PRINCETON ARCHITECTURAL PRESS
202 Warren Street
Hudson, NY 12534
Visit our website at www.papress.com

In association with Cooper Hewitt,
Smithsonian Design Museum
2 East 91st Street
New York, NY 10128
www.cooperhewitt.org

Published in conjunction with the exhibition *The Senses: Design Beyond Vision* at Cooper Hewitt, Smithsonian Design Museum, April 13–October 22, 2018.

22 21 20 5 4 3

Director of Cross-Platform Publishing, Cooper Hewitt, Smithsonian Design Museum PAMELA HORN
Cross-Platform Publishing Associate MATTHEW KENNEDY
Production Editor, Princeton Architectural Press SARA STEMEN
Art Direction DAVID GENCO
Book Design & Layout DAVID GENCO & ELLEN LUPTON
Cover Design DAVID GENCO
Typefaces MAISON NEUE, Timo Gaessner, Milieu Grotesque | TIEMPOS, Kris Sowersby, Klim Type | CHAP, Schick toika

Special thanks to Ryan Alcazar, Janet Behning, Abby Bussel, Benjamin English, Jan Cigliano Hartman, Susan Hershberg, Kristen Hewitt, Lia Hunt, Valerie Kamen, Jennifer Lippert, Sara McKay, Eliana Miller, Nina Pick, Wes Seeley, Rob Shaeffer, Marisa Tesoro, Paul Wagner, and Joseph Weston of Princeton Architectural Press—KEVIN C. LIPPERT, PUBLISHER

Library of Congress Cataloging-in-Publication Data
Names: Lupton, Ellen, editor. | Lipps, Andrea, editor.
Title: *The Senses: Design Beyond Vision* [edited by] Ellen Lupton & Andrea Lipps.
Other titles: Senses (Princeton Architectural Press)
Description: First edition | Hudson, NY: Princeton Architectural Press, 2018 "This book is published in conjunction with the exhibition *The Senses: Design Beyond Vision* at Cooper Hewitt, Smithsonian Design Museum, April 13–October 22, 2018." Includes bibliographical references and index.
Identifiers: LCCN 2017049544 | ISBN 9781616897109 (hardback)
Subjects: LCSH: Design—Human factors—Exhibiitons | Senses and Sensation—Exhibitions | BISAC: DESIGN / Graphic Arts / General | ART / Collections, Catalogs, Exhibitions. / General | DESIGN / Essays
Classification: LCC NK1520 .S445 2018 | DDC 745.4—dc23

The Senses: Design Beyond Vision is made possible in part by support from Barbara and Morton Mandel Design Gallery Endowment Fund, Ehrenkranz Fund, Amita and Purnendu Chatterjee, and New York State Council on the Arts with the support of Governor Andrew M. Cuomo and the New York State Legislature.

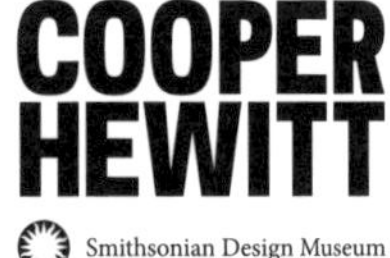

Foreword

Caroline Baumann, Director
Cooper Hewitt, Smithsonian Design Museum

Design is extending the realm of the senses. Experimenting with new and familiar materials, customizing products, and embracing the differing needs and experiences of users, contemporary designers are realizing newfound sensations and capitalizing on our extraordinary powers of perception to enrich and improve daily life. *The Senses: Design Beyond Vision*—the book and exhibition of the same name—explores the fertile territory of multisensory design and deepens understanding of its value. When we use our creative insights into the senses to expand access to information, products, and environments, we also expand the discourse on inclusive design.

Conceived and curated as an interactive environment alive with scientific fascination and aesthetic wonder, *The Senses* amplifies the intimate link between design and sensory experience. Accessible to visitors of all abilities and backgrounds, the exhibition invites visitors to see, hear, touch, and smell design. Inventive projects, products, and installations—created by a global roster of designers and thinkers—range from the practical to the playful, with each encounter activating the creative synergy of brain and body. A digital animation translates bird songs into bursts of color and motion. A light installation changes from cool to warm in response to visitors' movements. Vessels explore the sonic and tactile properties of glass. When designers open up to multiple sensory dimensions, products and services reach a greater diversity of users. Maps that can be touched as well as seen facilitate mobility and knowledge for sighted and non-sighted users. Audio devices translate sound into vibrations that can be felt on the skin. Tableware uses color and form to guide people living with dementia.

Beautifully written and a compelling journey in and of itself through the senses, this book does far more than document the contents of an exhibition. It is a provocative manifesto for inclusive design. Cutting-edge methodologies and emerging design guidelines appear alongside insights drawn from scientific research. Essays by Sina Bahram, Hansel Bauman, National Design Award winner Bruce Mau, and others explain how sensory design can help build more rewarding and inclusive experiences.

The Senses joins with Cooper Hewitt's campus initiatives to broaden access to the museum and engage the public in design's contribution to expanding accessibility. Toward that end, we are iterating to make Cooper Hewitt's exhibitions and resources as broadly available as possible. Partnerships with leading organizations, including New York University's Ability Project, New York City's Mayor's Office for People with Disabilities, Columbia University Digital Storytelling Lab, Mark Morris Dance for Parkinson's, and Google, are helping us build out our network of knowledge and expertise. In our galleries, we are exhibiting the latest developments in adaptive and universal design products and organizing collaborative spaces for experimentation and learning, emphasizing that—in every discipline of design—accessibility is essential for innovation.

The Senses: Design Beyond Vision is made possible in part by support from Barbara and Morton Mandel Design Gallery Endowment Fund, Ehrenkranz Fund, Amita and Purnendu Chatterjee, and New York State Council on the Arts with the support of Governor Andrew M. Cuomo and the New York State Legislature. Special thanks to Wendy Evans Joseph and her Studio Joseph team for their wondrous, immersive exhibition design and David Genco for his thoughtful design of the book and the exhibition's graphics. Senior Curator of Contemporary Design Ellen Lupton and Assistant Curator of Contemporary Design Andrea Lipps—an unbeatable creative team—forged fresh ways to interact with museum content and extended the exhibition's impact through their evocative texts. Harnessing the power of the senses, we heighten our abilities to further design's reach and influence.

Acknowledgments

Ellen Lupton & Andrea Lipps

This book celebrates sensory design from cover to cover. Its form and content were overseen by Pamela Horn, Cooper Hewitt's Director of Cross-Platform Publishing. She was assisted by the exacting and attentive Cross-Platform Publishing Associate Matthew Kennedy, who also provided essential curatorial assistance. Julia Pastor delivered integral support, joining us as Curatorial Assistant during the project's home stretch. Wordsmith Alix Finkelstein brought polish and depth to key texts. Graphic designer David Genco created this book's inventive design. Jennifer Tobias provided charming and personable illustrations. Fiona Hallowell applied her scrupulous editorial eye to every page. We are grateful to our colleagues at Princeton Architectural Press for their careful attention to the craft of publishing; special thanks to Sara Stemen, Jennifer Lippert, and Kevin Lippert. As authors and curators, we truly cherish the creative teamwork that is publishing.

Over sixty-five projects are represented in *The Senses: Design Beyond Vision* exhibition, with even more projects included in this book. This body of research highlights the inspiring, tireless, and inventive work of hundreds of designers, architects, scientists, engineers, manufacturers, and users engaging in sensory design practice. Moreover, communities of stakeholders provided their expertise, insights, and guidance throughout the process of organizing the exhibition and book. We thank all of these contributors for their generosity in sharing their work, process, and experiences with us.

The exhibition was designed by Studio Joseph, whose creativity, keen eye, and sensitivity have ensured that the exhibition design reflects the spectrum of sensory design objects on view. It has been a pleasure to work with this outstanding firm, especially Wendy Evans Joseph, Monica Coghlan, Jose Luis Vidalon, Derek Lee, and Emma Chen. David Genco's design for the exhibition graphics and identity inspired the design of this book. Audio description was sponsored by Woman of Her Word, voiced by Michele Spitz; Michele's generous contribution made the exhibition's multimedia content accessible to visitors who are blind or visually impaired.

We had invaluable conversations with experts working in diverse areas of inclusive design and culture, including Sina Bahram, Hansel Bauman, Susan Chun, Ann Cunningham, Chris Downey, Chancey Fleet, Stephen Gorman, Cliff Hahn, Lucia Hasty, Karen Kraskow, Steven Landau, Annie Leist, Ansel Lurio, Amy Mason, Joshua Miele, Ellen Ringlein, Debbie Kent Stein, and Lindsay Yazzolino.

Dozens of professionals at Cooper Hewitt made *The Senses: Design Beyond Vision*—the book and exhibition—possible, including our production team, registrars, conservators, educators, development staff, and more. We are particularly grateful to Caroline Baumann, Director, who embraced the exhibition's theme and pushed us to be rigorous and ambitious. We thank Cara McCarty, Curatorial Director, for championing the exhibition from the start and inspiring the exhibition staff to act creatively. We are indebted to the collegiality, creativity, and professionalism of Yvonne Gomez-Durand, Acting Head of Exhibitions, whose excelled at managing a complex, creative process. Additional thanks to everyone on the museum's staff, including Shamus Adams, Julie Barnes, Cat Birch, Laurie Bohlk, Perry Choe, Mary Fe da Silva, Kira Eng-Wilmot, Deborah Fitzgerald, Matt Flynn, Chris Gauthier, Gregory Gestner, Michiko Grasso, Greg Herringshaw, Janice Hussain, Halima Johnson, Kathleen Kane, Steve Langehough, Laura Meli, Matthew O'Connor, Wendi Parson, Ruki Ravikumar, Kim Robledo-Diga, Donnalyn Robles, Wendy Rogers, Ruth Starr, Ann Sunwoo, Jessica Walthew, and Mathew Weaver. Cooper Hewitt's expert art handlers and installers realized the exhibition and ensured the safety of the objects on view: Peter Baryshnikov, Joel Bacon, Jennifer Dennis, Sam Dollenmayer, Richard Fett, Grady Gerbracht, Paul Goss, Joel Holub, Rick Jones, Nathaniel Joslin, Jen Kuipers, Warwick McLeod, Chris Moody, Milo Mottola, Larry Silver, Michael Sypulski, and J. B. Wilson.

We were joined by two dedicated Curatorial Capstone Fellows—Adèle Bourbonne and Binglei Yan—from the Masters Program in History of Design and Curatorial Studies at Parsons The New School and Cooper Hewitt, Smithsonian Design Museum. Their attention to detail, organization, and untiring support kept the project running smoothly; as contributors, they each share a voice in this book. Maya Friedman, strategist at Man Made Music, provided expert research early in the project.

Finally, we extend our deepest gratitude to our families. To Ellen's husband, Abbott Miller, and wonderful children, Jay and Ruby Miller, much thanks for your love and endurance. To Andrea's husband, Ryan Heiferman, and young children, Luca and Liv Heiferman, thank you endlessly for your patience, support, and love.

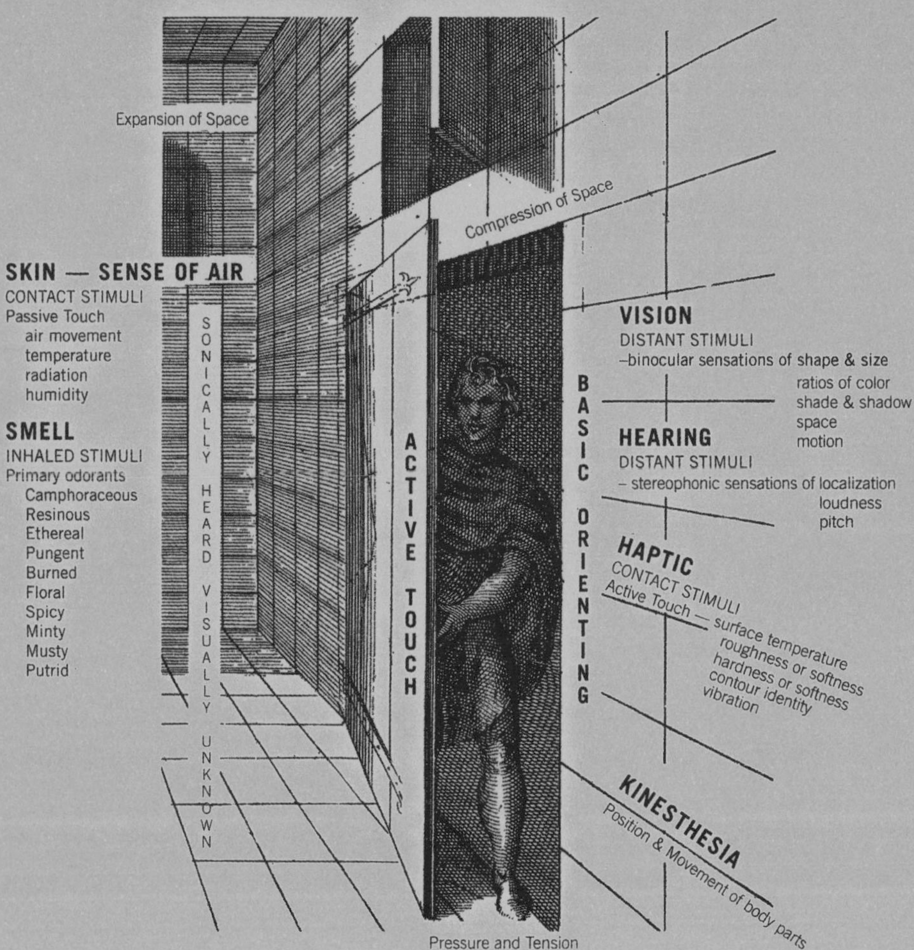

Joy Monice Malnar and Frank Vodvarka,
Ranges of the Senses, from *Sensory Design*,
University of Minnesota Press; © 2004 by
Joy Monice Malnar and Frank Vodvarka

Ellen Lupton & Andrea Lipps

Why Sensory Design?

Reaching beyond vision, this book is a manifesto for an inclusive, multisensory design practice. Sensory design activates touch, sound, smell, taste, and the wisdom of the body. Sensory design supports everyone's opportunity to receive information, explore the world, and experience joy, wonder, and social connections, regardless of our sensory abilities. This book documents extraordinary work by some of the world's most creative thinkers, and it gathers together ideas and principles for extending the sensory richness of products, environments, and media.

This book accompanies the exhibition *The Senses: Design Beyond Vision*. As curators at Cooper Hewitt, Smithsonian Design Museum, we sought out work and insights from designers, researchers, and users. We searched for artifacts that could be directly experienced by the museum's visitors. We learned about the fusion of mind, body, and sensation.

The senses mix with memory. From infancy, human creatures engage in countless acts of lifting, licking, touching, sniffing, throwing, dropping, hearing, balancing, and more, constantly testing the edges of physics to understand (or "make sense of") the world we were born to discover. The brain fires neurons, prunes synapses, and forges pathways. Thus meaning and memory take form. When we encounter an oddly shaped coffee cup or an updated operating system, we don't see it as completely alien but focus our attention on disparities between what's new and what we've encountered in the past. What would this page taste like if you licked it? What sound would this book make if you dropped it? We can imagine these sensations without needing to enact them. Prior experience tells our brains what to expect.

The senses move us through space. The eye or ear is not a fixed camera or a microphone wired to a wall; our sense organs are connected to a head that turns, arms that reach, and bodies that wander and seek.[1] The sounds, smells, and shifting shadows of a room or a streetscape help orient this knowledge-hungry body. Sensory experience hits us from all directions. Traditionally, designers focused on creating static artifacts—the monument, the vessel, the elegant monogram, or the essential logotype. Today, designers think about how people interact over time with a product or place.

The senses merge and mingle. As kids, we learn to think of the five senses as separate channels, like five radio stations playing at once. Some stations buzz along in the background, while others dominate. The real picture is more complex. As the brain combines different modes of information, the senses mutually change one another. A cold, fizzy soda tastes better than a warm, flat one. A bar of chocolate wrapped in richly patterned paper primes our desire for the bittersweet goodness within. Golden light makes a room feel peaceful and warm, while cool daylight hues charge it with energy. Designers consider interaction of bodies and things. What sound does a chair make when it scrapes along the floor? How hard does a button need to be pressed to register a response? How much does a surface flex when we push against it?

The senses are unique to every person. Some people have smell receptors that make broccoli taste appallingly bitter; to others, cilantro tastes like soap. Some people have a diminished sense of smell. This condition, called *anosmia*, vastly diminishes the pleasure of eating and of otherwise exploring the world; it affects six million Americans. Christine Kelly, who became anosmic after a sinus infection, creates smell wheels that illustrate how her sense of smell has been distorted—smells that should pique the appetite or calm the nerves became noxious and muddy. People with color blindness see red and green or blue and yellow as similar hues. Individuals with multiple sclerosis, leprosy, neuropathy, or severe burns can lose sensitivity to touch. Individuals with SPD (sensory processing disorder) can feel unbearable distress

Anosmia smell wheel showing the monotony of smell loss, 2015; Christine Kelly (American and British, b. 1959); Watercolor and ink; Courtesy of Christine Kelly

Anosmia smell wheel nine months after onset showing more intense but still not pleasant smell experiences, 2015; Christine Kelly (American and British, b. 1959); Watercolor and ink; Courtesy of Christine Kelly

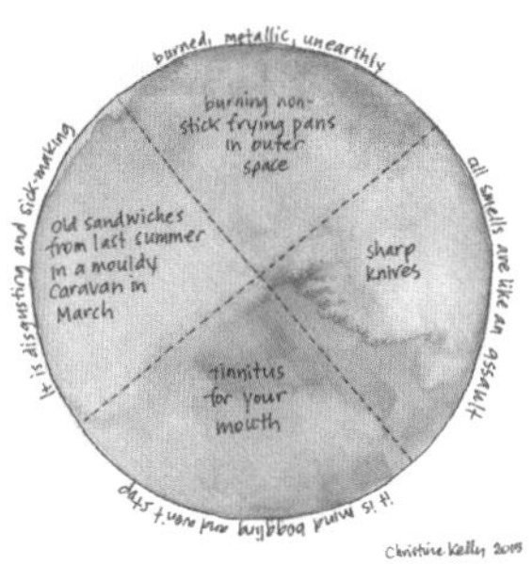

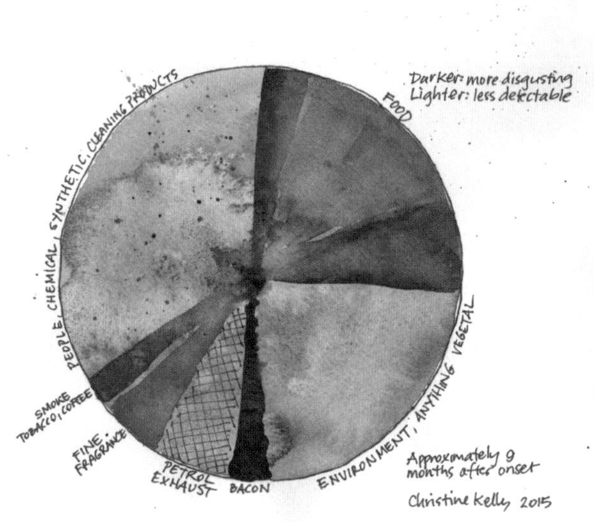

from tags and seams in clothing or crave constant bodily motion. Some sensory differences yield extreme pleasure. ASMR (autonomous sensory meridian response) is a delicious tingling in the scalp and spine triggered in some people by sounds such as crunching, crackling, or rubbing. In videos popular with the ASMR community, manicured hands gently crush plastic-wrapped pastries or rustle crisp sheets of paper, narrated by whispering voiceovers.

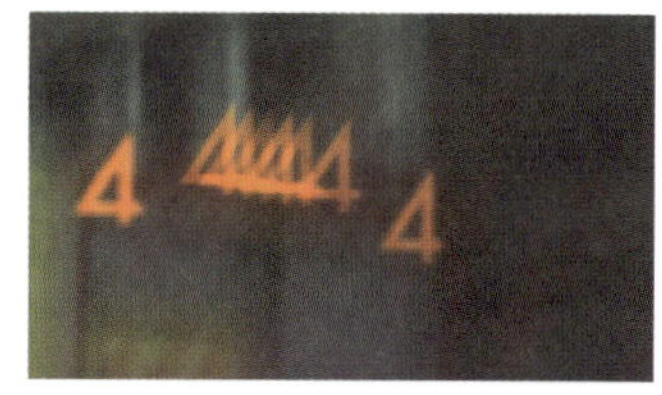

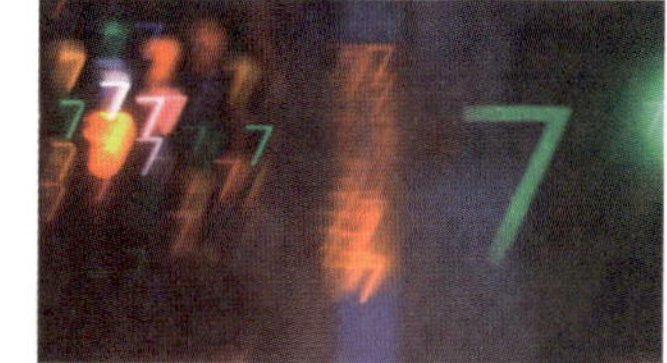

The senses trigger and amplify other senses. For people with synesthesia, the brain makes cross-connections between the senses. Music can play in color, while letters can conjure sounds or textures. Neurologist Richard E. Cytowic has devoted his career to studying synesthesia. Once seen as a rare disorder, synesthesia is now known to be a widespread condition with dozens of variations, affecting one out of every twenty-three individuals. A child with synesthesia begins establishing cross-sensory connections early in life. When learning the alphabet, a child might link the color green with words that start with *g*. Such associations become fixed for life, cemented both by nurture and nature.[2] David Genco, a graphic designer with synesthesia, assigns color, gender, and personality to numbers. In his interactive video project *Synesthetic Calculus*, video clips visualize unique ways of remembering numbers via sensory connections.

The senses are plastic. Cytowic compares synesthesia to fireworks—a sudden spray of color is triggered by a word, letter, or sound. While synesthesia is a specific neurological condition, some degree of sensory alchemy permeates daily life. "Inwardly, we are all synesthetes," Cytowic told us. "We just don't notice how our senses interact." The human mind has a gift for connecting sensations—we link tastes and colors, sounds and spaces. Some people who are deaf or blind become acutely attuned to multiple senses, using areas of the brain typically devoted to sight or sound to process other inputs. People perceive objects and spaces with sound and touch as well as with vision. People experience sound by feeling vibrations and seeing movements as well as hearing by ear.

Synesthetic Calculus (stills), 2012;
David Genco (Luxembourgian, b. 1985);
Video; Courtesy of David Genco

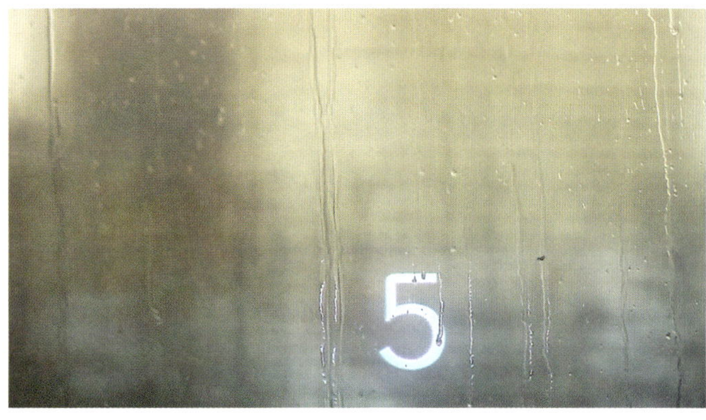

Scientists are creating sensory substitution devices that enable a blind person to convert audio signals into low-resolution mental images, or that allow a deaf person to convert a grid of vibrations felt against the skin into recognizable speech. "Lingual vision" is the ability to understand features of an object via electrical stimulation of the tongue. A lollipop-shaped stimulator placed inside the mouth can help a soldier traverse a dark night, or a diver navigate a murky sea, or a blind person perceive the outlines of objects and their locations in space. Cytowic told us, "The brain doesn't care where the signals come from—your eyes or your big toe. Send in anything, and the brain will figure it out. Reality takes shape in the dark theater of the brain."[3]

The senses chatter constantly with one another. Indeed, it takes serious mental effort to pull our sensations apart. It is tough to separate the sweet, sour taste of a mango from its bright, caramel-tinged aroma. Do you sometimes close your eyes when trying to decipher a faint sound or an odd aftertaste? That's why the lights go down before a concert begins. Darkness helps us hear more clearly. Shutting out visual signals can help bring other senses into focus. In his essay "Designing LIVE," Bruce Mau tells sighted designers, "To design for all the senses: start with a blindfold."

The senses have long been dominated by vision. In the Western tradition, the eye symbolizes knowledge and enlightenment. Visual observation is the bedrock of modern science. Today, digital devices pump out an endless feed of graphics and text, stoking demand for quick hits of visual energy—often at the expense of our other senses. Smell sits at the bottom of the pyramid, in part because it resists attempts to be visually diagrammed, as Adam Jasper and Nadia Wagner point out in their essay "Smell."

Sensory design rebels against the tyranny of the eye. When Finnish architect Juhani Pallasmaa published his book *Eyes of the Skin* in 1996, many architects began to question the dominance of visual form and the Western obsession with "ocularcentrism." The overbearing eye fosters detachment and isolation, breeding the harsh atmosphere of modern schools and hospitals.[4] Architecture, says Pallasmaa, should embrace and envelop the body with authentic materials and tactile forms. Sensory design slows space down, making it feel thick rather than thin. An intimate room reverberates with shifting shadows and surfaces wrought from wood, wool, or stone. An atrium changes with the sun. Rough walls and dense fabrics absorb clatter and din.

Sensory design enhances health and well-being. A scent player for Alzheimer's patients stimulates the appetite by releasing the smell of grapefruit, curry, or chocolate cake at mealtimes. Tactile graphics are used to communicate ideas through the sense of touch. Buildings with spacious hallways and vibrant materials accommodate everyone, including people experiencing blindness, deafness, or memory loss.

Sensory design is inclusive. Each person's sensory abilities change over the course of a lifetime. By addressing multiple senses, designers support the diversity of the human condition. In his essay "The Inclusive Museum," Sina Bahram points out that museums have long used ramps and elevators to ensure that visitors with disabilities can enter the building, but museums often fail to offer these visitors a rich experience once they get inside. Universal design expert Karen Kraskow conducted interviews with singers, an artist, a tech consultant, an architect, a former jewelry designer, and others who are blind or visually impaired, learning how they live and flourish.

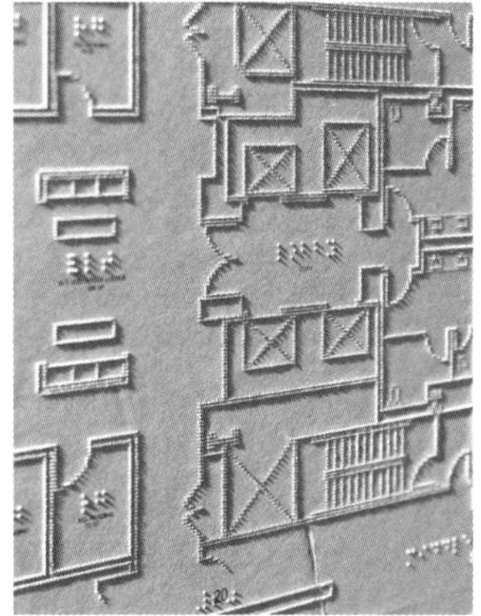

Tactile Architectural Drawing (detail), San Francisco LightHouse for the Blind and Visually Impaired, 2015; Chris Downey (American, b. 1962); Embossed digital print with ink, raised lines, and braille; Printed by San Francisco LightHouse for the Blind and Visually Impaired; Photo by Don Fogg

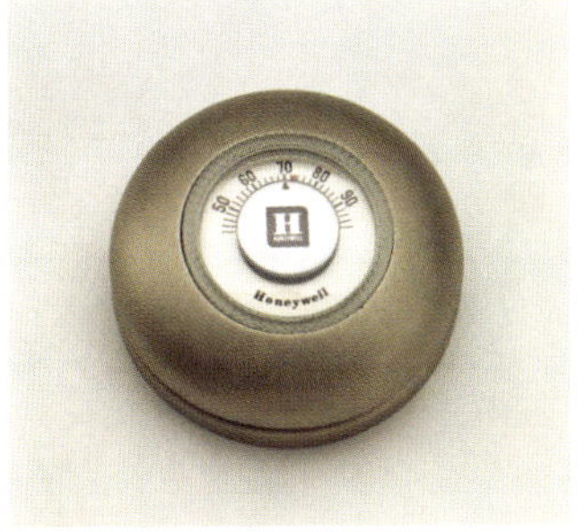

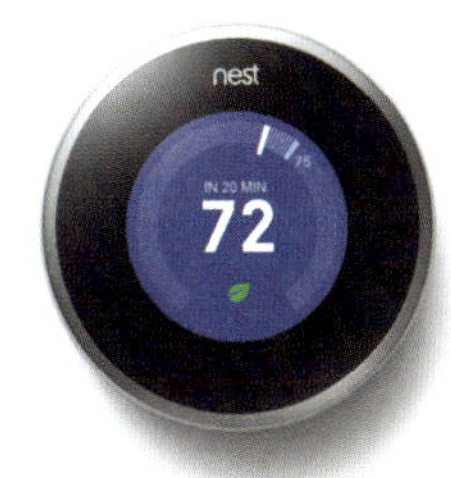

T-86 Round Thermostat, 1953; Henry Dreyfuss (American, 1904–1972); Manufactured by Honeywell, Inc. (Minneapolis, Minnesota, USA, founded 1906); Metal, molded plastic; 4.5 × 8 cm diam. (1 ¾ × 3 ⅛ in.); Gift of Honeywell Inc., 1994-37-1; Photo by Hiro Ihara © Smithsonian Institution

Nest Learning Thermostat, 2012; Tony Fadell (American, b. 1969); Manufactured by Nest Labs, Inc.; Forged stainless steel, glass, injection-molded plastic, electronic components; 4.1 × 8.1 cm diam. (1 ⅝ × 3 3⁄16 in.); Gift of Nest Labs, Inc., 2013-19-2-a,b; Photo by Ellen McDermott © Smithsonian Institution

Sensory design embraces human diversity. According to the New York City Mayor's Office for People with Disabilities, inclusive design creates a "multisensory enhanced environment that accommodates a wide range of physical and mental abilities for people of all ages."[5] People sense the movement of objects, air, and bodies through touch, sound, and smell as well as vision. Acoustic designer Shane Myrbeck (Arup) notes that the classic Honeywell thermostat is an accessible design that offers an eyes-free tactile interface, while operating the digital touch screen of the Nest requires vision. Smartphone interfaces promote accessibility for blind and low-vision users by combining audio and haptic signals with touch-screen technology. Apple's iPhone has a built-in screen reader and an array of accessibility modes—available to every user of every device. Steven Landau and Joshua Miele are creating tactile models, maps, and diagrams, while Liron Gino has designed a music player that translates sound into tangible vibrations.

Sensory design considers not just the shape of things but how things shape us—our behavior, our emotions, our truth. Sensations respond to an insistent, ever-changing environment. When our body presses into the cushioned surface of a chair, both body and chair give and react. We grab objects in order to use them as tools for breaking, bending, mashing, or joining together other objects and materials. Tools are active extensions of our sense of touch. Tasting food is more than a chemical response—it involves the muscular, skeletal action of crushing and transforming matter. We use our senses to change our world.[6]

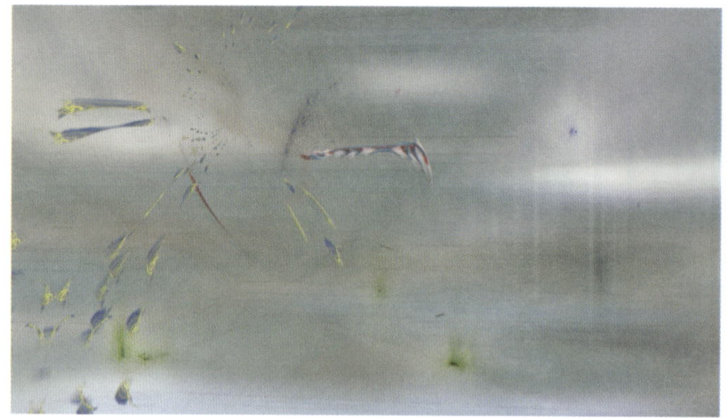

New York Soundscape: New York Public Library (still), 2015; Karen van Lengen (American, b. 1951) and James Welty (American, b. 1950); Animated film; Collection of the Museum of the City of New York; Courtesy of the designers

Sensory design honors the pulse of living, breathing spaces. The loudest car on a train is the "quiet car." The carriage shakes along the tracks and shudders against the damaged infrastructure. Talking is forbidden, but you can hear the clink of ice, the crackle of food wrappers, and the whir of people slurping, sipping, breathing, and snoring. Libraries, too, are quiet places filled with sound. Karen van Lengen and James Welty explored the sounds of the New York Public Library, the Seagram Building, and other iconic interiors for their 2015 project *Soundscape New York*. Van Lengen created drawings inspired by sounds in space, from a rolling cart to books opening and closing. Welty created a temporal animation of van Lengen's drawings.

Sensory design is grounded in phenomenology. This field of thought explores how humans and other creatures perceive the world. Philosophers in the early twentieth century brought new attention to bodily perception. Scientists and philosophers since the Renaissance had separated mind and body, distrusting sensation as mere illusion and favoring instead objective mathematical laws. Phenomenology situates knowledge in the body: sensual encounters enable consciousness.[7] The human organism is an open, breathing membrane in continual contact with its surroundings. The earth moves as we move along it. Dust swirls, leaves crush, and molecules shiver into waves of sound. As other creatures cross our path, we ripple into action to create sounds and gestures.

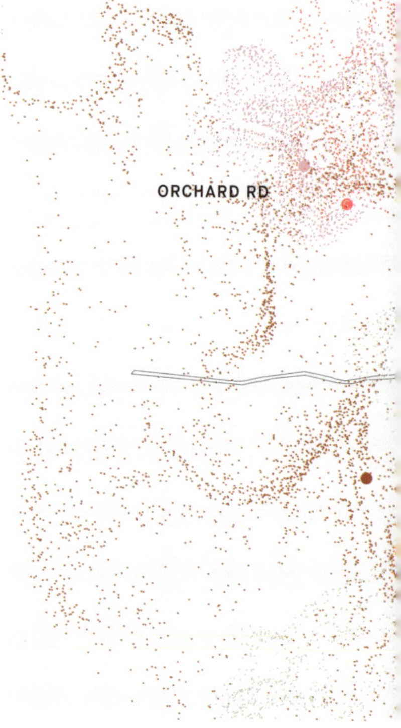

Sensory design knits together time and space. When we look at a building, our gaze darts from its small details to its larger volumes to create an understanding of the whole. In their landmark book *Sensory Design*, Joy Monice Malnar and Frank Vodvarka describe the different ways we encounter architecture.[8] We judge the scale of a building in relation to our own limbs and torsos. As we pass through a doorway, space hugs us tight and then lets us go. Air mutters through the HVAC system and ripples over our skin. Our feet pound against a building's floor, and our hands grasp its railings and knobs. Our daily routines—cooking, cleaning, smoking, bathing—produce an embedded brew of smells that make interiors memorable. Windows puncture walls and expand space. Hansel Bauman, author of "DeafSpace," notes that people who are deaf or hard of hearing use reflective surfaces to see what is happening behind them. Reflections duplicate space, creating visual echoes.

Scentscape 06. 2015 – City of Singapore (detail), 2015; Kate McLean (British, b. 1965); 118.9 × 84.1 cm (46 13⁄16 × 33 7⁄64 in.); Courtesy of Kate McLean

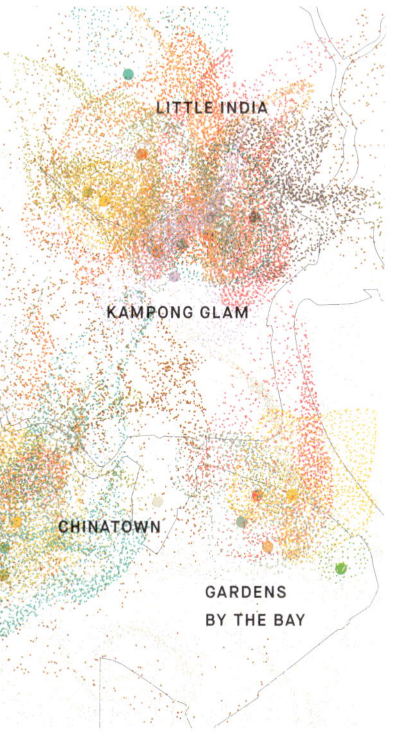

Sensory design celebrates the qualities of place. Graphic designer Kate McLean created a sensory map of Singapore using experiential data generated by over two hundred residents who went with her on "smellwalks." Suspended in the humid air of this island city are the smells of curry, jasmine, and Manila rope. Little India and Kampong Glam are districts especially dense with scent. McLean's map locates distinctive smells and visualizes their trajectories. Smell cannot be abstracted from bodily experience: "Using humans as sensors is a method that aggregates personal insight.... It is about the acceptance of the subjective as worthy and useful data."[9]

Designers often find themselves at odds with the body. Modernism tended to favor hygiene and control over organic processes. Beatriz Colomina and Mark Wigley chronicle the war between cool abstraction and the hot messy senses in their book *Are We Human?* Modern design served as an optical painkiller, an anesthetic that dulled the body by massaging the eye. Our modern obsession with smooth, slippery objects arose alongside the drugs invented to blunt pain in the age of modern medicine.[10] Whether banning ornament from architecture or barring friction from interfaces, designers often aim to make people feel less, not more. Don't worry. Be happy. Teflon will calm your nerves and smooth your edges.

Body-numbing visuals saturate design culture. News feeds serve up glossy images of products and buildings that most readers will never meet up close. Museums embalm artifacts in climate-controlled pods of glass and plastic.[11] Design students learn to worship visual form and abstain from touching, smelling, and tasting. Vision crowds out the other senses. Looking trumps making. Digital artists Wang & Söderström create strange still lives populated with glistening, hyperreal artifacts simulated with digital tools.

Touch borders on all the senses. Skin, the body's largest organ, flows from the outside in at every port of entry: ears, eyes, nose, mouth, anus, and genitals.[12] The mouth and tongue embrace the chewy heat of charred meat or the buttery chill of ice cream. Filmmaker David McDouggal writes, "I can touch with my eyes because my experience of surfaces involves both touching and seeing."[13] The eye strokes the contours of distant glistening bodies the hand can't reach.

Sensory design confronts the body. Designer Jinhyun Jeon's wooden dinner spoon embraces sensory knowing. Our hands measure the object's weight and length. Our skin registers the material's temperature and smoothness. Our fingers navigate changes in form, finding nuance in the bumps along the spoon's edge and at the handle's tip. Our ears prick at the muted clank when the spoon is placed on a tabletop. Our nose picks up the faint glow of lightly stained maple. Objects gain meaning and value in our embodied experience of them.

Sensory design has the power to forge new languages. In 2017 and 2018, IFF (International Flavors & Fragrances Inc.) partnered with Dutch design collective Polymorf to explore the role of scent in human interaction. They collaborated with Professor of Language, Culture, and Cognition Asifa Majid and senior perfumer Laurent Le Guernec to imagine an "invisible dictionary" of nuanced emotional states reflecting the complexity of modern life. Inspired by Majid's research

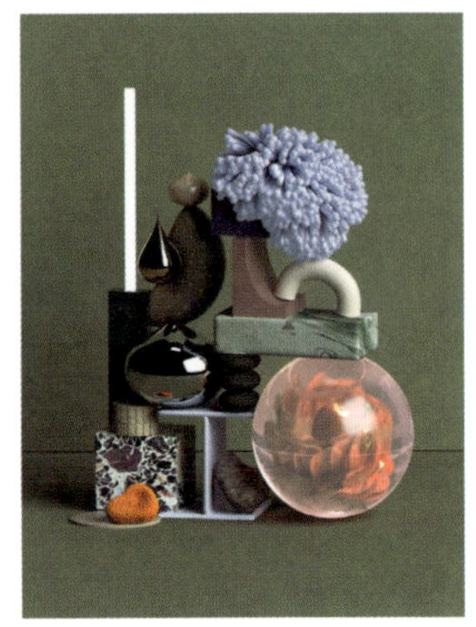

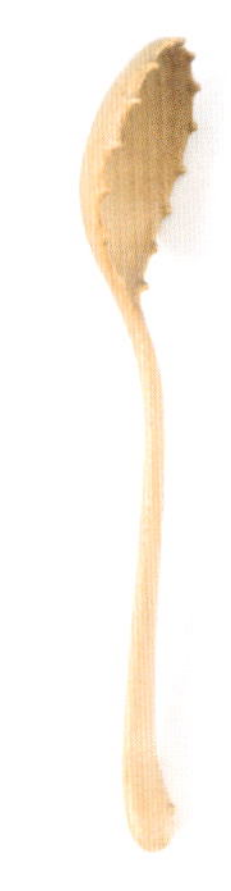

Treasures 3, 2016; Anny Wang (Swedish, b. 1990) and Tim Söderström (Swedish, b. 1988), Wang & Söderström (Copenhagen, Denmark, founded 2016); 3D software: 3Ds Max, Vray, Modo; Courtesy of Wang & Söderström

TSS II Spoon, from the Sensory Dinner Spoon collection, 2016; Jinhyun Jeon (South Korean, b. 1981), Studio Jinhyun Jeon (Eindhoven, Netherlands, founded 2012); Maple; 2.5 × 2.6 × 13.2 cm (1 × 1 × 5 3/16 in.); Courtesy of Jinhyun Jeon

with indigenous communities such as the Jahai, who have developed an elaborate smell vocabulary, the project presents such uniquely contemorary emotional states as "a moment of collective *déjà vu*," "the torment caused by the inability to act," and "being perfectly entangled with another." Le Guernec composed original scents using IFF-designed molecules to represent the feelings on display. Rather than offer literal or figurative depictions of these emotions, Le Guernec's olfactory creations are abstract and sensorial—like language itself. In the installation, a series of translucent pedestals are softly lit from within. When activated by a visitor, each pillar diffuses a scent through a line of laser-cut text. Visitors, by connecting each named emotion with a special smell, begin to assimilate a new dialect.

Sensory design rubs up against the living-thingness of the world. A room is not just a cube punctured with windows and doors. It is a sensing creature with deep pockets and velvet shadows. It curves like an eyeball and bends like an elbow. The wool canyons of a blanket trap warmth. The folds of a curtain seize light and sound. A rug inhales noise; floorboards sigh with grief. Sensory design tweaks our skin, bones, and muscles. It tickles, pinches, and pops. It plays rough. It touches us, and we touch back.

Dialect for A New Era, Installation, 2017; Artistic Concept and Interface Design: Frederik Duerinck (Dutch, b. 1976) and Marcel Van Brakel (Dutch, b. 1970), Polymorf (founded Netherlands, 2003); Perfumer: Laurent Le Guernec (IFF); Scientist: Asifa Majid; Creative Direction: Jean-Christophe Legreves and Anahita Mekanik (IFF); Scientific Advisor: Sissel Tolaas; Plexiglass, metal interior, LED lighting, scent diffusion; Courtesy of IFF

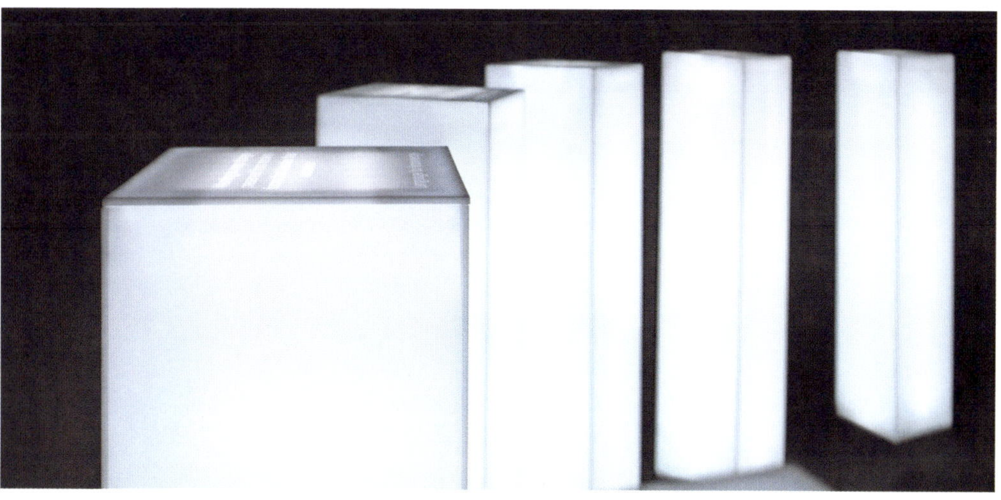

Bruce Mau

Designing LIVE: A New Medium for the Senses

We have allowed two of our sensory domains—sight and sound—to dominate our design imagination. In fact, when it comes to the culture of architecture and design, we create and produce almost exclusively for one sense—the visual.

Most design is caged by the image. We "look" at design, we don't "feel," "experience," or "sense" it. In fact, most design is non-sense design—cold, technical, formal, and inhuman—engineered to serve business or technical functions rather than to surprise, inspire, and delight. Such examples include products that work in the computer program where they were developed, but fail in real life; environments that look good in renderings, but are soulless to live in; processes that make sense in theory, but not in practice. So much of our daily experience is an assault on our senses. Our senses are forced to serve as the interface for unrelenting friction and conflict instead of the pathway to inspiration, coherence, and beauty. We are designing the invention of a new medium—the medium of LIVE—all senses design. Like the early days of photography or television, there is no road map, there are no standard formats, there is no existing methodology for the medium of LIVE. We need to explore, experiment, and invent new formats and combinations of sensory experience, new ways of telling stories. We need to design the LIVE design process to open the medium for full immersive experience.

LIVE experience has the bandwidth of reality—it is fully immersive, and the visitor's body and mind are alive and available for full engagement of all the senses. (Notice we do not use the term "viewer," which would only reinforce our existing cultural bias.) However, designers do not have an established creative process for the integration and synthesis of design for all the senses. Our design practice is built for the image. If we are to develop an all-senses design method, we will need to consciously focus on the senses and build a process of synthesis.

BRUCE MAU serves as chief design officer of Freeman, a company that designs and produces experiences and events for organizations worldwide. He is cofounder and chief executive officer of Massive Change Network (MCN) in Chicago.

To design for all the senses: start with a blindfold.

Begin the work from something other than the visual. The visual so dominates our imagination that we need to shut it down to allow our brain to explore other channels and possibilities. Composer John Cage made a work of silence to help us hear that everything we do is music. We have only one center of attention. The blindfold helps us to focus and move it around to our other senses.

Design the feeling of the idea.

Neuroscience tells us that we are emotional decision makers, not rational spreadsheets. Most of our decisions are made live—in real time without our awareness. Use the language of passion to translate the intellectual into the emotional. Crying is a measuring stick for the quality of your work.

Focus on the visitors' experience, not our message.

We take responsibility for the delivery of the visitors' experience—the story, the tone, the feeling, the cadence, the beginning, middle, and end, the nuance—everything. Our responsibility is not to deliver our message—it is to inspire their feeling, to experience something they have never felt and thought before.

Orchestration is the big idea, the challenge, and the practice.

The greatest value of design thinking and the culture of architecture is the capacity for complex synthesis. The great challenge of our time is synthesis—coherence, intelligence, clarity, beauty. Not discrete solutions to isolated problems, but systematic design ecologies. The ability to understand and synthesize complex, diverse inputs across many disciplines into one compelling, immersive experience is the magic and meaning of design. It is also the underlying method of designing LIVE.

"What is for the eye must not duplicate what is for the ear."

—Robert Bresson, filmmaker

Every sense experience produces expectation in the other senses. If it looks cold we expect it to feel cold. Our work lies in the play between the senses. In conventional media we see what we hear. We hear what we see. We do what we are told. Open the space between the senses to inspire freedom and imagination and demonstrate the power of human creativity.

Design for each of the senses then synthesize.

Our work is the orchestration of LIVE experience, not a singular image or object. Design the experience for each of the senses independently before you synthesize. Think of each sense as a track in a complex polyphonic composition. You control the mixing board, moving the focus and designing the overlap and interaction of sensory experience for maximum emotional impact.

Design for our sense of time.

LIVE immersive experience happens in time. We know we are alive because we experience time. Therefore, our work is not a fixed object or space. It is a controlled release of ideas and information over time. It is a dramatic experience that evolves and builds in the mind of the visitor. Time is a plastic dimension. We can stretch it or compress it. Think theater, opera, performance art, and happenings. Use storyboards (or whatever it takes) to understand and design the time.

Design for our sense of touch.

Touch is our first language, the first sense that we acquire. Touch is our silent interface with the material world. Touch is the third dimension of surface that speaks to our emotions. Unconsciously, touch tells us whether to trust, whether to pull away or lean in and embrace. Think about how much time Apple spends getting the texture, the touch of every product just right. We know from neuroscience that human touch changes our experience in profound ways. We open up, cooperate more, and feel more connected when we are touched.

Design for our sense of movement.

Our visitors are not static points of view. They are alive and mobile, constantly shifting, exploring, and discovering. Design for discovery and allow them to participate in the story. They move at different speeds. Design for a range of engagement that is the reality of LIVE. Design something brilliant for the visitor who is not going to give you the time of day, and design a reward for those who are inspired and want to go deep into your world. In the words of architect Morris Lapidus, "More is never enough."

Design sound for emotional impact.

Turn the sound off on any Hollywood film and it will be immediately evident how powerfully the sound colors our emotional experience. Sound can trigger fear and violent response or gentle intimacy. It can draw us together into joyful collective expression, or provide spiritual solace and respite. Most experience is noise, not music. Noise is chaos. Music is design. Remember, everything we do is music—once again, John Cage—or at least has the potential for music.

Design for our sense of taste.

Food is a deep and defining part of our culture. At every major experience of our lives—birthdays, weddings, anniversaries, accomplishments, and transitions—food plays a central role in bringing us together for our celebrations and sacraments. Whenever we spend extended periods of time together, food and drink will be part of sustaining our energy and our ability to focus and participate. Design the potential for taste to be an inspirational social experience, to draw people together to learn and share.

Design for our sense of smell.

The sense of smell is only a few synapses away from the brain. Smell is the most direct pathway to memory. That is why we can remember smells four times more accurately than images, and for a much longer time. We respond to smell in the most visceral way—directly, unconsciously, like the animals that we are. Designing scents is as much art as science and can be profoundly powerful in its emotional impact. Remember that we become "nose blind" very quickly, so part of designing for our sense of smell is creating a way to refresh our ability to wake up and smell the roses.

Design for our sense of connection.

The more digital and distant our world becomes, the more we crave a sense of meaningful connection. This is the power of LIVE. Designing for our sense of social contact, allowing for human connection and the serendipity that happens when we experience one another, is perhaps the greatest opportunity and beauty of LIVE experience.

Design for synesthesia.

Color changes what we feel. Sound transforms what we see. Smell determines what we taste. Synesthesia—the experience of one sense evoking another—is more common than we realize. To design for LIVE we need to design the overlaps and intersections of the senses.

Design for the intersection of digital and physical.

The future of the new medium of LIVE is the synthesis of digital and physical. Every year, new digital technologies change what is possible and transform the expectations of our audience. Visitors arrive with new possibilities and ways of engaging in stories and ideas, and those technologies change their ambitions and expectations.

Finally, open your eyes and compete with beauty.

Nothing moves us more than beauty. We move to the light of genius and joy. We fall in love with it. We pay more for it. We will not win without it. No matter how smart your LIVE design solution, without beauty it will fail. Use all the formal dimensions of design—color, contrast, proportion, texture, image, material—to compete with beauty and win. Extend the idea of beauty beyond the visual to all the senses to fully master the design of LIVE.

Sina Bahram

The Inclusive Museum

My first memory of visiting a museum is from elementary school. I remember trooping onto a bus full of children and the two-hour ride to the museum. When we arrived, I was separated from the rest of the kids and placed in the charge of an older gentleman. He gave me a pair of headphones and a cassette player with an audio tour of the museum on tape.

The reason for this special treatment was because I am blind. Though I have some light perception, it is not enough to appreciate museum exhibits from a purely visual point of view. The kind man spent several hours walking me through the museum, letting me touch things that most visitors weren't allowed to. He found exhibits with audio, olfactory, or tactile components (though more often he was forced to simply verbally describe something that I could not touch or interact with). All the while, he answered—or tried to answer—each and every one of the unending questions that were a hallmark of my childhood. This was a school trip that I'll never forget.

It is important for us to ask why this experience was necessary. Why couldn't I participate with my nondisabled peers? Why were the museum's exhibits and other activities not designed with inclusion and accessibility in mind? After all, museums have made their physical spaces accessible for decades with automatic door openers, ramps, and other affordances for those with mobility impairments. Yet there

SINA BAHRAM is an accessibility consultant, researcher, and entrepreneur. He is the founder of Prime Access Consulting (PAC), an accessibility firm whose clients include technology startups, research labs, Fortune-1000 companies, and both private and nationally-funded museums. He holds graduate and undergraduate degrees in computer science. In 2012, he was recognized as a White House Champion of Change by President Barack Obama.

seems to be a collective failure to recognize that the job is not complete just because those with disabilities can enter the building. Once inside a museum, disabled visitors often find that the level of effort, resources, consideration, and study dedicated to providing equal access for all visitors is disappointingly low.

Attempting to answer the above questions, as well as improve this situation for future generations, drives the work that I do. As an adult, I became a computer scientist with a strong passion for using technology as an equalizer. Today, I have the amazing job of working and playing with museums daily. I started a company, Prime Access Consulting, to help museums make their digital interactives, websites, mobile apps, exhibits, and environments accessible to and inclusive of the widest possible audience. One of the primary philosophies that we bring to this work is that of universal design, sometimes called inclusive design.

Universal design is the act of considering all audiences, or as many as we can, at the beginning of a project, and iterating upon this consideration until we arrive at a solution that is usable by far more people than if we had not taken such a design tact. "Inclusive design" is a newer term, used by many contemporary designers and advocates. While "universal" implies a potentially unattainable burden for designers and developers, "inclusive" is an invitation. It's warm, and it aligns with most people's basic values. We include our friends, our loved ones, and so on. Inclusive design recognizes that people have multiple forms of identity and difference, including age, ability, language fluency, socioeconomic status, and cultural background. Accounting for those differences doesn't mean making everyone the same.

Whichever term you prefer, universal design and inclusive design address the big picture. Accessibility, on the other hand, consists of those things we do specifically for those with functional differences. Consider an automatic door opener. We may think it to be a pure accessibility accommodation because it is for those with mobility impairments, yet anyone can use it, from those with a temporary sore leg to someone carrying packages in both arms, and so on. Alternatively, a sign language tour tends to be more of a pure accessibility accommodation as it is most critical for those with a hearing impairment. If, by now, it seems that there is a lot of overlap between accessibility and inclusive design, even to the point where accessibility may be thought of as a subset of universal design, that is because that's exactly the case. Such a realization is key to understanding the emergent benefits of thinking about all visitors.

This issue of accessibility and including the widest possible audience has been considered not only by the museum community, but by every sector one can imagine. In the design and development of technology, home appliances, consumer goods, and education, just to name a few, universal design has been widely adopted as the strategy that yields the greatest possible accessibility to the highest number of people.

In 1997, the Center for Universal Design at North Carolina State University in Raleigh published seven principles of universal design for buildings, outdoor environments, and products. Each principle inspires me to ask a question that should be considered at the design phase of any digital or physical object with which museum visitors might interact. Let us examine each of these seven principles as well as a museum-inspired question around each. I've shared a few answers that my clients and I have come up with, but these examples are by no means the only right solutions to these critical inquiries. For some of these principles, the example provided does not come directly from the museum world. I use the lack of such an abundance of museum-based examples as a clear reminder of how much work is left to be done.

1. Equitable Use

Can visitors with different functional limitations get a similar, or equitable, experience?

In the image, we can see a large multi-person, multi-touch interface composed of three vertical touch screens put side-to-side to form a touchable wall of art in the San Francisco Museum of Modern Art. It is easy to write off an experience so rooted in the visual as inaccessible—even uninteresting or inappropriate—for a blind or low-vision audience. Yet this wall of art has a braille and large-print label inviting visitors to plug headphones into it and to activate an accessibility button. Upon being pressed, the accessibility button toggles on a voice layer that walks the user through the experience. The images of art on-screen are all beautifully described. The videos have audio description and captioning, and any text is enlarged. The gestures to control this interface have been specifically influenced by the industry-leading solution for touch-screen accessibility for the blind, Apple's iPhone. This touch-based digital exploration of modern art requires only the use of a single finger to be fully controlled, thus allowing those with reduced dexterity to participate. By gliding a finger across the screen, a vision-impaired visitor can explore the artworks on display, listen to their visual descriptions, interact with multimedia such as videos, and in short, enjoy the same experience as their sighted peers.

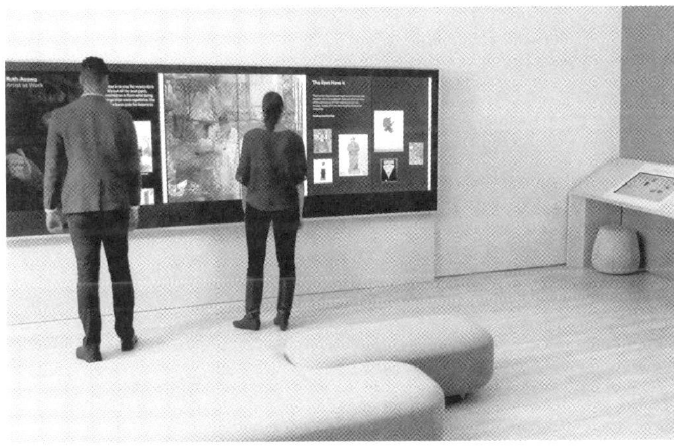

Painting & Sculpture Interpretive Gallery at the San Francisco Museum of Modern Art; Photo © Belle & Wissell, Co.

2. Flexibility in Use
Can visitors interact with the information in a variety of different ways?

If we think of visitors who cannot see or hear perfectly, the ideas of multimedia-based content, digital text being displayed, or a touch-screen interactive may appear to be quite problematic, but they do not have to be! In the image below, we see a photo of one of many digital interactives at the Canadian Museum for Human Rights. This interactive is one of dozens at the museum equipped with a universal keypad, speech output, captioning, tactilely differentiable buttons, and many other design considerations. The digital interactive is usable by someone who is blind or low vision, deaf or hard of hearing, or has trouble performing complex physical gestures—and to a myriad of individuals that have limitations we cannot, nor try to, predict.

The universal keypad with its rubberized large buttons and clear markings is not the only solution for making such interactives accessible. Other approaches such as that from SFMoMA, discussed previously, allow for making the touch screen natively accessible without a keypad. This diversity of choice is essential to devising inclusively designed experiences. There is no one-size-fits-all solution in any technical field. Inclusive design is no exception.

Turning our attention to a non-technology approach, the Museum of Contemporary Art in Chicago recently held a relaxed performance for one of its public events. This performance allowed those with autism, those who have trouble sitting for a long time, those who may not be comfortable sitting in the dark, and many others to enjoy a show, but with some drastically relaxed expectations around audience behavior. As is the case with so many of these examples, while those with disabilities may have been the impetus of such an approach, it proved helpful to so many more visitors. For example, think of a woman who is pregnant and needs more frequent restroom breaks, or a family attending with babies or very young children.

Holding a relaxed performance is not the only way of including those with sensory impairments. Some museums, for example, periodically open their institution an hour earlier to invite those on the spectrum or anyone with a sensory sensitivity to crowds and loud noises to enjoy the museum in a more peaceful way.

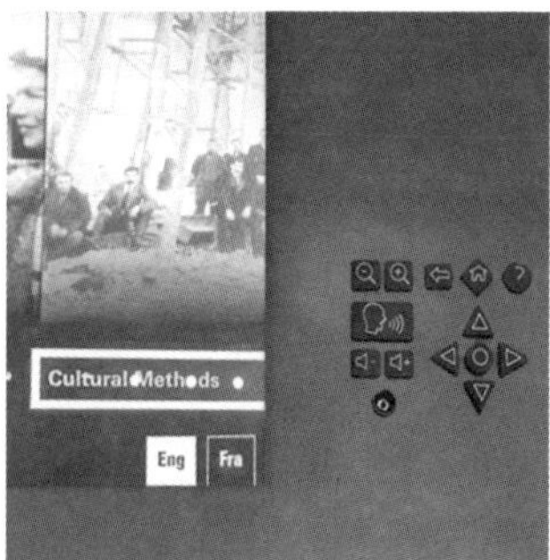

Digital interactive at the Canadian Museum for Human Rights; © CMHR / Ian McCausland

3. Simple and Intuitive Use

Can visitors with different experiences or knowledge benefit from the information being presented?

In this image, we can see a bathroom sign that indicates gender in multiple languages. In English, it says "Women." In Spanish, it says "Mujeres." The information is also presented by way of a pictogram and replicated in braille. This redundant display of information is helpful to a wide variety of visitors. Persons with disabilities, those who speak a different language, and visitors who are native speakers can all utilize this inclusive sign. Furthermore, there are overlaps in terms of the pictogram's audience. Yes, the pictogram is critical for someone who does not read English or Spanish, but it is also helpful to those with a reading disability, children, and other individuals who may simply be in a hurry.

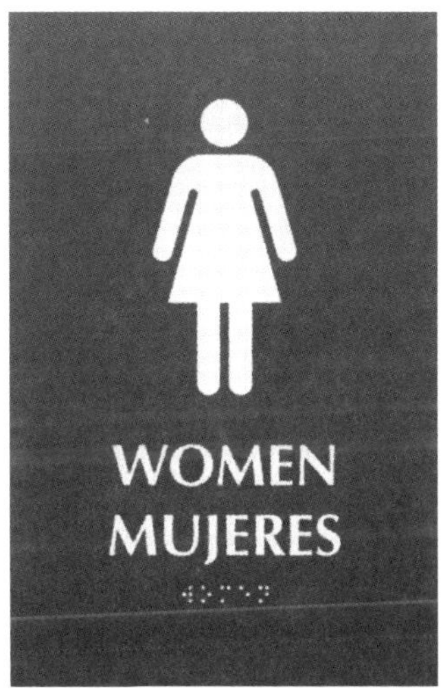

4. Perceptible Information

Can visitors access and interact with the information being presented, independent of a sensory disability and disturbances in the environment?

If we are to be pedantic, there are really two questions embedded in this principle. The first deals with equal access despite a sensory disability; the second revolves around disturbances in the environment.

Let's take the second query first: disturbances in the environment. For acoustic disturbances, such as crowd noise or distracting sounds from surrounding exhibits, a simple volume knob can work wonders. Such a knob allows visitors to turn up the volume of any audio if the surrounding environment is noisy, but it can also facilitate augmented volume for deaf or hard-of-hearing visitors and lower volume for those with audio sensitivities. Again, simply giving users a choice and control over the way they wish to consume the information being presented massively elevates their experience.

Turning our attention to the first query, consider information taken from the Coyote system. Coyote is an online platform that streamlines the creation and distribution of visual descriptions. Originally a project that my firm developed with the Museum of Contemporary Art in Chicago, it is now being used by multiple institutions to drastically revolutionize the pipeline that institutions, and individuals, use to create and convey the visual description of art. At the core of Coyote is the belief that visual description is not throwaway copy. It is a content-creation task deserving of a mature workflow. Such a workflow tool was absent, and so we invented Coyote to fill this deep unresolved need. Coyote also expanded the premise of visual description, especially around images on the web: for instance, rather than having one official description for a given image, in Coyote multiple descriptions can exist for a single visual object. In fact, these descriptions can be of different forms, some short and some long, and in different languages. We do this because of our fundamental thesis that no single description is most appropriate, or correct, for any given object. Instead, we strive for a multiplicity of voices. Much like everything else in inclusive design, this way of thinking and implementing not only helps persons with disabilities but has many other far-reaching benefits. One such benefit is to return agency back to the visitor at an art museum. By surfacing these visual descriptions for everyone, not just those who have trouble seeing, Coyote allows visitors to feel okay consuming information about what is visually going on, instead of promulgating that unfortunately common experience within an art museum that leaves visitors asking, "What am I looking at, and why is it important?"

5. Tolerance for Error

Can visitors always return to a consistent, known starting point so that, for example, they don't cause systems to crash or behave unexpectedly, regardless of the actions they take?

Museums generally do a good job with this concept. We are used to having digital interactives that always return to a known starting point upon request or after a time-out. Almost all digital interactives follow a firm rule that software should fail gracefully and quietly in visitor-facing interfaces. But what happens when there is an accessibility mode that can be toggled on or off?

An accessibility mode may be available, which changes the way an interactive exhibit behaves. Perhaps it simplifies the gestures that can be used, allows for a keypad instead of a touch screen, or enlarges text. If such a feature is available, then we must be sure to make clear how to turn such a mode off for visitors who may not require such an interface.

In this image, we can see the on-screen prompt notifying users that an accessibility mode is on and how to turn it off. This message serves two purposes. It allows visitors to turn off a feature that they do not need, and it notifies anyone able to see the message of the availability of such features in the first place. It is important to keep in mind that accessibility features should not be hidden away, but instead embraced and advertised. We should be proud of the increased number of people we are trying to welcome into our institutions.

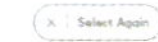

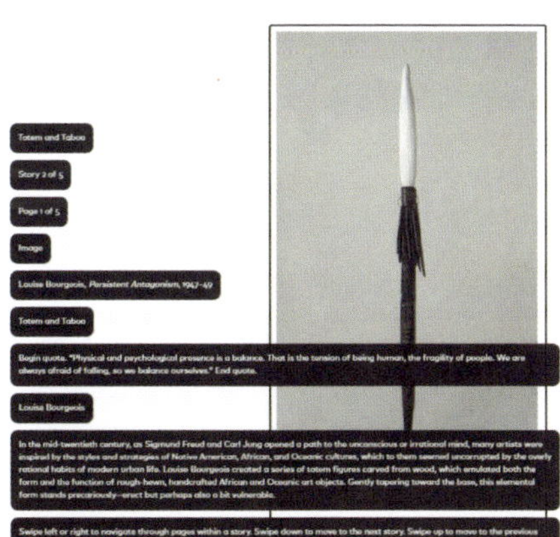

Captions provide eyes-free commentary as a story is read aloud. Painting & Sculpture Interpretive Gallery "Table Experience," San Francisco Museum of Modern Art. Courtesy SFMoMA. Project partner: Belle & Wissell, Co.

6. Low Physical Effort
Can visitors fully appreciate the given information without needing much physical effort or dexterity?

In this image, we see a beautiful ramp at the aforementioned Canadian Museum for Human Rights. Notice that the handrails on this ramp are placed in two positions, one several inches lower than the other. This thoughtful design decision has many implications. It can assist wheelchair users, children walking with their parents, or individuals of small stature. Speaking of wheelchair users, the ramp, combined with elevators, is obviously a critical affordance for making the museum physically accessible, but it is hardly for wheelchair users alone. By adopting this ramp as a central mechanism of traveling between floors, the museum achieves better audience flows (no crowded stairwells), makes it easy for those with roller bags or other wheeled accessories, allows large groups to travel together more easily (critical for the school groups that frequent the museum), removes the social awkwardness of one member of the party splitting off to use an elevator, and allows visitors to enjoy a beautiful journey through the building's unique architecture.

Ramp with dual handrails at the Canadian Museum for Human Rights; © CMHR / Ian McCausland

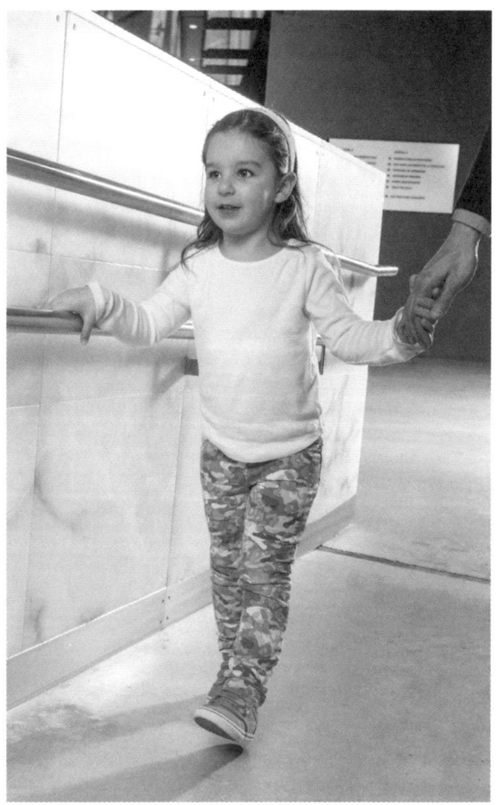

7. Size and Space for Approach and Use

Can visitors get close to the exhibit, have enough space in which to move around—even with a wheelchair, walker, or crutches—and manipulate it, independent of posture or other physical limitations?

In this image, we see tactile replicas of Andy Warhol's work at the Andy Warhol Museum. These have been placed on tables such that a wheelchair user can approach from three different sides. Some of the replicas (not visible here) are also on turntables so that one can turn the object being felt instead of turning one's own body. The important takeaway here is that we should not model our visitors as just one persona. Most of the time, a person is not only blind or only a wheelchair user, but has multiple functional differences from their fellow visitors. Sometimes, these functional differences are temporary, such as a broken arm or forgetting one's glasses. By building up our approach in layers, and considering the experience holistically, we can strive for the most inclusively designed experience possible.

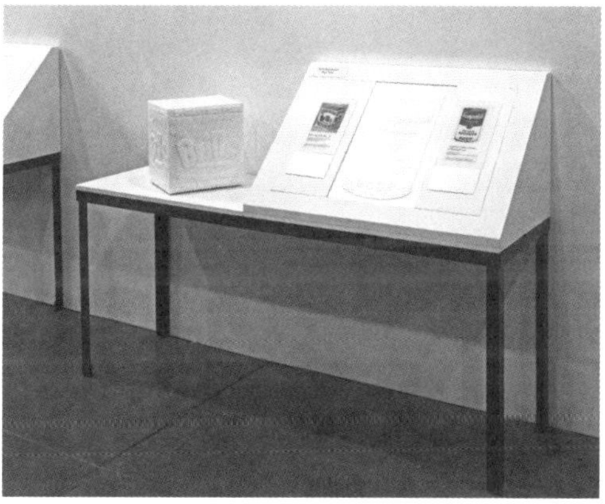

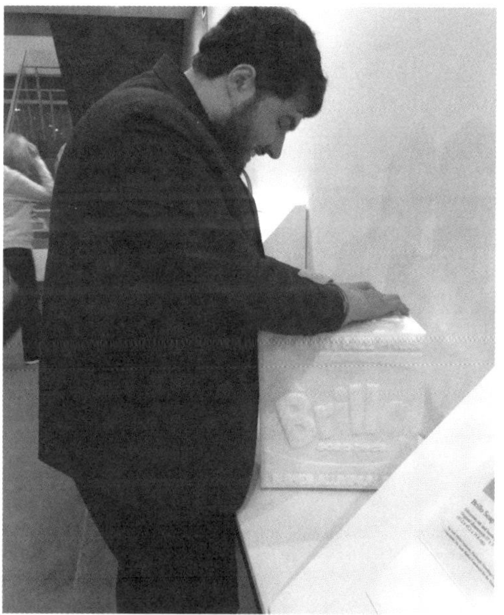

LEFT: Tactile panel installation at The Andy Warhol Museum, Pittsburgh. RIGHT: Sina Bahram explores tactile installation at The Andy Warhol Museum, Pittsburgh; photo by Pamela Horn

Conclusion

Social inclusion and interaction are among the many benefits of following universal design. While I greatly enjoyed my first museum experience as a child, I wished that I could have interacted more with my classmates, felt part of the group, and been able to participate in the same activities. This element of inclusion should be a central motivating factor when designing exhibits. Inclusive design facilitates this social inclusion and interaction among visitors by allowing us all to interact with and enjoy the offerings of an institution together and in similar ways, instead of providing a well-meaning but still isolating experience.

We will not get these solutions 100 percent correct the first, second, or tenth time, but we cannot allow fear of the lack of perfection to continue being used as a justification for doing very little. Inclusion is not a binary pursuit with a finite destination. Inclusion is a state of thinking and acting toward a shared purpose based on a commitment to iteration, refinement, and self-improvement.

Reflecting further upon my museum experience as a young child, I am reminded of the words of American author and poet Maya Angelou, "I've learned that people will forget what you said, people will forget what you did, but people will never forget how you made them feel." Exhibits following universal design principles can facilitate a powerful feeling of inspiration, awe, wonder, and excitement for all visitors, not just those who meet an idealized persona. More important, following such best practices can help prevent many visitors from feeling excluded, unwelcome, or ignored—something that has been true for far too long. I hope that you, dear reader, will join me and my colleagues in our journey to make all users feel welcome and accepted.

Tactile Map, National Mall, Smithsonian Institution (detail), 2017; Steven Landau (American, b. 1960), Touch Graphics (Elkton, Maryland, USA, founded 1997); Digital print with ink and raised graphics

This tactile map is designed to be beautiful and useful to many people, including those who are sighted, blind, and low vision.

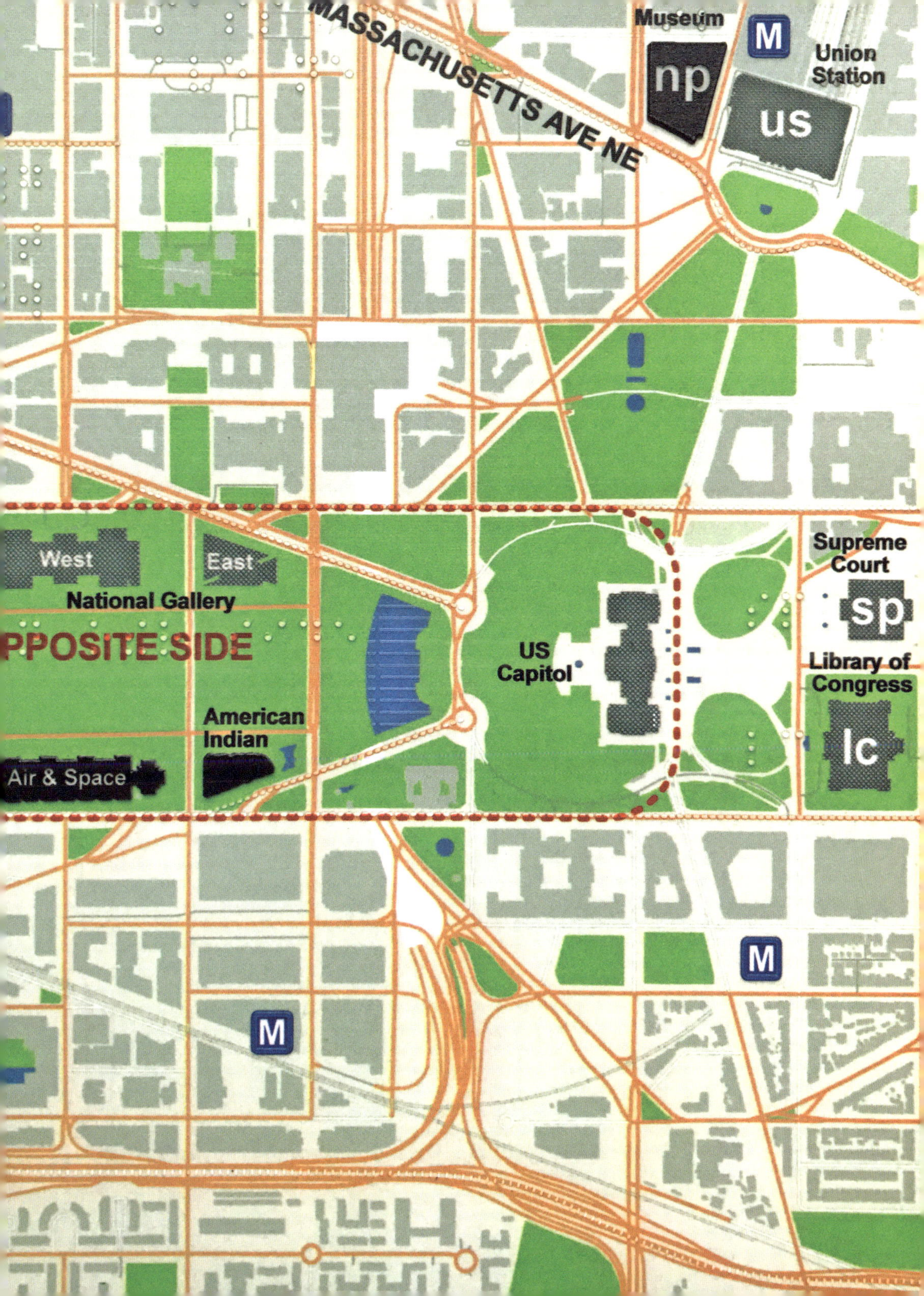
MASSACHUSETTS AVE NE
Museum
np
M
Union Station
us
West
East
National Gallery
PPOSITE SIDE
US Capitol
Supreme Court
sp
Library of Congress
lc
American Indian
Air & Space
M
M

Notes on Touch, Sound, Smell, and Flavor

What are the senses and what are they for? The senses assemble reality from vibrant morsels of stimulation—odor molecules meet the mucous membrane, light falls upon the retina, vibrations pulse against the eardrum. The senses are protective mechanisms. A foul smell, a bitter taste, or a rustling in the grass—each sign of danger puts the organism on alert. Our hairs raise, our throats clench, our muscles tense, our eyes dilate, our body odor turns sour. The senses deliver joy as well as warnings, lighting up the body from head to toe and from inside out. From the tang of strawberries to the crinkle of satin, many of life's pleasures come from sensory experience. Beauty arrives in a rush of light, warmth, texture, and vibration.

Touch delivers full-bodied impressions of places and things. Touch penetrates the body. It brings pain and pleasure, warnings and delight. It can calm us, alarm us, connect us, and overwhelm us. Our hands and fingers wield stones and sticks, slings and arrows, brushes and pens. Our feet and limbs scuttle up rocky paths and blunder down slithery slopes. Our tongues probe hot gobs of oatmeal and the polished underbelly of a spoon. Our bodies feel the weight of a wool blanket, a rough embrace, or a hot day in August.

Touch is specialized

Skin, the main instrument of touch, is more than an exterior envelope. This varied surface—thick or thin, hairy or smooth—wraps inside the mouth, nose, ears, and genitalia. The receptors in our fingertips gather hyper-detailed data about the things we touch, while other regions of the skin convey impressions in lower resolution.[1] Try studying the face of a coin first with your index finger and then with your elbow. Was that heads or tails? Your elbow will never know. The edges of coins are designed to be legible to the fingertips. Reach into a purse or pocket and see if you can tell a dime from a nickel by its size, thickness, and patterned edges.

Touch is layered

A chunk of wood or a blob of silicone delivers tangled impressions of temperature, texture, pressure, and resistance. What is the feeling of wetness? Splash some water on your face. Wetness is a "touch blend" that includes the coolness of evaporation and the weight or pressure of the moisture on your skin.[2] Intellectually, one can pick apart the ingredients that make up how something feels, but the embodied brain swirls those elements together into a unified perceptual Gestalt.

Frogspawn Typography, 2014;
Monique Goossens (Dutch, b. 1971);
Courtesy of Monique Goossens

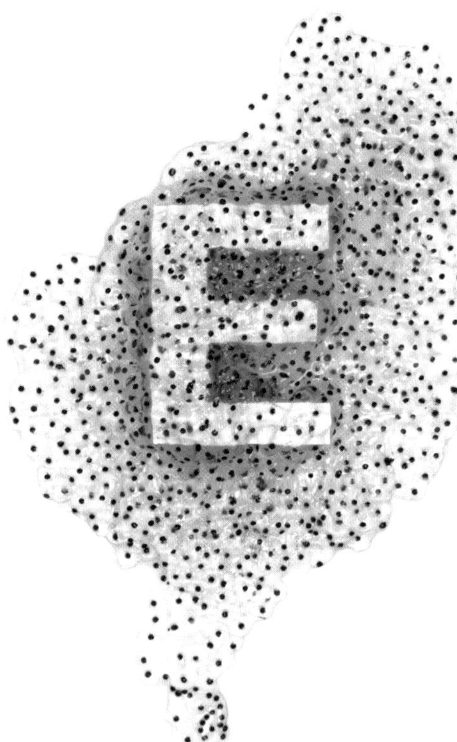

Touch is social

From a pat on the arm to a slap on the face, touch communicates love, trust, or dominance. All people crave touch. Infants deprived of touch fail to thrive. Care facilities for the elderly have begun to employ robotic pets—known as "socially assistive robots"—to satisfy this need for living contact by way of artificial beings.[3] Equipped with digital sensors and a purring heart, these uncanny creatures respond to touch. Stroke the kitty's head and it nuzzles against your hand; pet the back of its head until it rolls over for a belly rub and eventually falls asleep.

People who are deaf-blind communicate through touch-based processes, from finger spelling to exploring objects with their hands or feet. Diagramming the elements of a room on the back of a deaf-blind person's hand helps them picture the environment. Some people who are deaf-blind use a grammar of touch that includes pressure, location, speed, hand shape, and motion. For example, a gesture's pressure can be firm or light, while moving in circles or taps. Expressing the sign for "yes" with increased speed and pressure makes the message more emphatic ("Oh, yes!").[4]

Touch is spatial

Proprioception is the awareness of a body's location, posture, and movement, enabled by receptors distributed throughout the skin, muscles, tendons, and joints. Vision and hearing further contribute to this sense of movement and orientation. Try touching your nose. The ability to instinctively move your arm, hand, and fingertip to this exact, invisible location requires an integrated understanding of the body's parts and motions. Now, try picturing each joint in your body—from knees and elbows down to each segment of each finger or toe. This act of focusing on the skeleton's areas of articulation creates a fleeting geometric schema of your posture in space—a fragile constellation of points. Environmental psychologist James J. Gibson calls this awareness "subjective skeletal space."[5]

Touch is active

When your soft body bears down against a hard chair (or, if luck will have it, your hard body sinks into a soft chair), you are experiencing passive perception. In contrast, the process of touching your nose or grasping an object requires active perception.

Sitting doesn't need to be passive, however. Chairs designed for active sitting may help people burn energy, build core strength, and feel alert. The Tip Ton chair was designed by Edward Barber and Jay Osgerby for use in schools. Manufactured by Vitra following several years of research, the Tip Ton chair tilts forward on a blade-like base. The forward position, designed for working at a desk, helps users sit with their spines straight rather than slumped. The back-leaning position supports resting during a lecture or break. The ability to change position frequently helps students stay focused during long periods of desk time.[6] The designers considered other sensory factors as well. Lightweight plastic makes Tip Ton chairs easy to stack and move around and also limits noise. According to Barber, "Clattering chairs are a big problem in large numbers."[7]

Active seating can be useful to people with sensory processing disorder (SPD). People with SPD can feel overwhelmed by bright lights, the sound of people eating, or the texture of clothing. Other people with SPD need intense stimulation—physical, auditory, or tactile. Products created for children and adults who are calmed by bodily motion include inflated "wiggle cushions" and therapy balls. Springy surfaces allow users to shift, bounce, and move about while seated. Seats covered with spiky, furry, or bumpy textures offer further stimulation.[8] Compression garments use weights and stretchy fabrics to exert reassuring pressure on the torso.[9]

Touch is haptic

When sitting in a chair, you feel pressure against the surface of your skin as well as within your muscles and other tissues. Body-based touch and skin-based touch work together to create haptic perception, defined by Gibson as the system by which the individual "feels an object relative to his body and the body relative to an object." Receptors located in the muscles and the skin relay signals to the brain about feelings of motion, pressure, pain, heat, and resistance. Every human hair—wrapped around its base with nerve fibrils—is a feeler reaching into the environment. Likewise, the fur, horns, and antennae of animals have remote sensing functions. Humans use sticks and other tools to extend the sensory grasp of their limbs. A pencil, paintbrush, or walking stick is an antenna exploring the environment.[10]

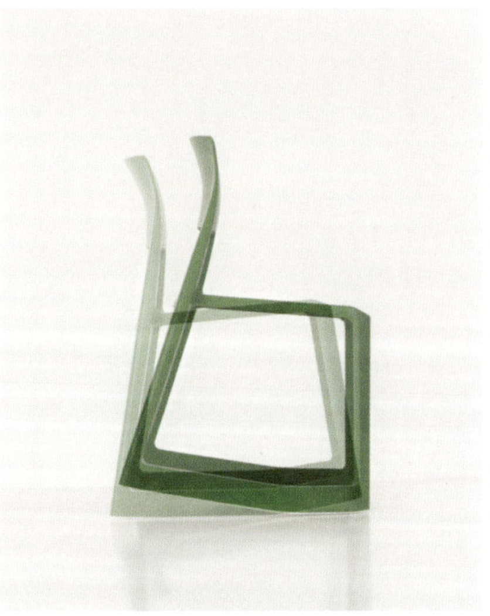

Tip Ton Chair, 2011; Edward Barber (British, b. 1969), Jay Osgerby (British, b. 1969), Barber & Osgerby (London, UK, founded 1996), Vitra (Birsfelden, Switzerland, founded 1950); Polypropylene, polyethylene; 78.6 × 50.9 × 55.5 cm (30 15⁄16 × 20 1⁄16 × 21 7⁄8 in.); Photo © Peer Lindgreen

The act of pushing a button or swiping a screen engages motion and pressure. Digital buttons and menu bars use drop shadows, beveled edges, translucent layers, and juicy highlights to invite action from users. Interaction designer Josh Clark explains, "We now touch information itself: we stretch, crumple, drag, flick it aside. This illusion of direct interaction changes the way we experience the digital world."[11] Designers use sounds, vibrations, textured surfaces, responsive animations, and gesture-based interactions to make digital interfaces become more physical. Alas, the replacement of tangible controls with seamless touch screens renders many products useless to people with blindness or low vision.

Touch is visceral

We feel with our skin, our limbs, and our inner organs. Dwelling deep within the gut are sense receptors that regulate appetite and digestion, alerting the brain when the stomach is stretched and indicating which nutrients need to be broken down and absorbed.[12] These nutrient-based receptors are similar to taste buds—responding to chemicals in food—but are distributed beyond the reach of consciousness. Gut-level sensors also respond to danger and desire. In her book *The Tactile Eye*, film critic Jennifer M. Barker explains that a "gut response" or a "visceral reaction" jolts the body at its core. When sex or violence portrayed on screen stirs desire or make us recoil in shock or revulsion, we are responding physically to what we see and hear.[13]

Monique Goossens, a graphic artist from the Netherlands, has created letterforms from hairnets, strands of hair, and clumps of frog eggs. Meticulously photographed and printed, her images are both elegant and alarming, provoking feelings of disgust as well as awe and fascination.

Section of human skin. The base of each hair is wrapped with nerve fibrils.

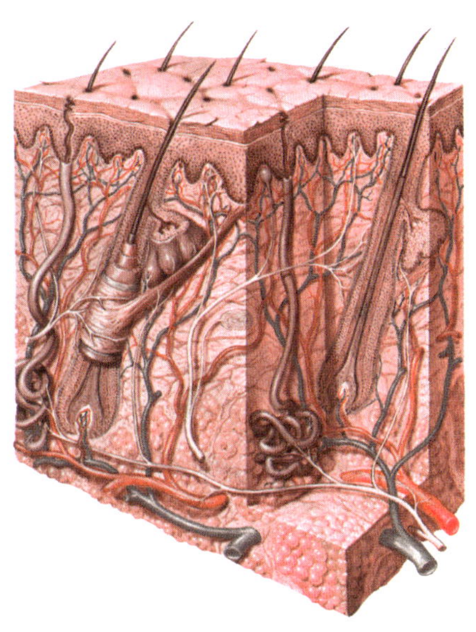

Touch is emotional

In a well-known study, participants encounter a researcher in a hallway on their way to the session. This investigator, who happens to be carrying a stack of papers and a drink, stops and asks the participant to briefly hold the beverage cup. (Unknown to the human subject, this cup is a star player in the study.) In some instances the cup is warm, and in others it is cold. Soon after, subjects are asked to evaluate a job candidate. Subjects who had been holding the warm drink tend to feel more favorably toward the candidate than those who had held the cold one. Physical warmth translates into positive emotions.[14]

Touch is visual

The eye is a surrogate for the skin. We can look at things and see if they are sticky or slick, nubby or smooth, sharp or blunt, before we ever touch them. Glance around and find a surface that looks soft—a cushion or a drape, a dog or a cat, or the pattern printed on this page. Scientists describe softness as the "compliance" of a surface, its ability to deform in response to pressure. Surface compliance is often visible. We see softness. We notice how a surface behaves when it's prodded or poked. The nubby grain of a fleece jacket and the dullness of a rubber tire help us predict how a surface will feel and behave.[15] We hear softness, too—a wineglass or a murder weapon won't smash or clatter when it falls upon a thick carpet. Designer Petra Blaisse is known for creating large-scale curtains that move and breathe across the expanse of a stage or an architectural facade. Blaisse's Touch series of wallcoverings (commissioned by Wolf-Gordon) feature detailed photographs of wool, felt, fur, and knitted or woven fabrics. Printed at large scale, each wallcovering appears soft and fuzzy, even though it's flat.

Sidewall, Cord #1, 2013; Petra Blaisse (British, b. 1955); Made by Wolf-Gordon Inc. (New York, New York, USA, founded 1967); Rotogravure-printed on vinyl; 293.4 × 137.2 cm (9 ft. 7 ½ in. × 54 in.); Collection of Cooper Hewitt, Smithsonian Design Museum, Gift of Wolf-Gordon, 2004-26-1; Photo by Matt Flynn © Smithsonian Institution

Touch unites the senses

Visible textures add depth to printed pages and flickering screens. Sounds and colors that seem warm or cool, dull or sharp change the emotional valence of a product or place. Well-shaped tools feel good in the hand. Textured surfaces enhance the sound of a room. Objects designed for touch enable people with impaired vision to use everything from kitchen tools and bathroom faucets to books, maps, and currency. Designing for touch creates a humane and inclusive world.

Net Typography (TOP), 2013; Hair Typography (BOTTOM), 2013; Monique Goossens (Dutch, b. 1971); Courtesy of Monique Goossens

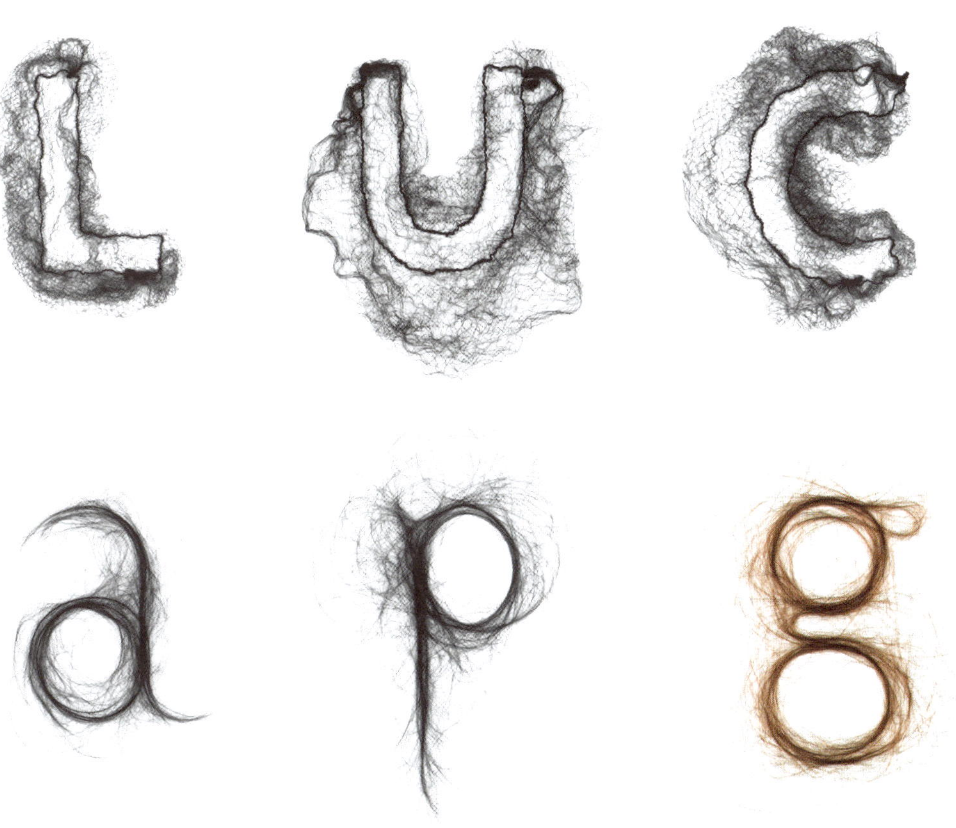

Every sound originates in a disturbance. A glass shatters, a shoe falls, a bell tolls. The disturbance makes molecules bounce against other molecules. This chain of motion takes the form of a wave, spreading outward from the initial disturbance in a pulsing pattern of alternating compression and decompression. The wave moves through air, water, wood, and glass, through flesh and bone, through earth and rock. When the wave causes mechanisms inside the ear of a human or other creature to vibrate, the brain processes the wave as sound.[1]

Sound is not the same as hearing

Hearing happens when sound waves cause a creature's eardrums to vibrate, passing signals to the auditory nerve and the brain. Hearing aids are designed to amplify sound waves. Cochlear implants, also created for people with damaged hearing, turn sound waves into electrical impulses that stimulate the auditory nerve; the brain interprets these signals as sound. Mastering this process takes time and isn't successful or desirable for all people. Hearing is not the only way to experience sound. At a concert, drums beat against the chest and pulse up through the feet. In a park, wind rattles the trees and cools the skin. On the street, the pavement shakes when a truck rumbles by.

Sound is personal

Individuals have their own hearing ranges, just as people have differences in vision. These differences change over time. People in developed societies routinely correct their vision with eyeglasses and contact lenses, but they are less likely to use hearing aids. Hearing aids are expensive, and some users attach a stigma to them. Others find them uncomfortable, obtrusive, or difficult to use.

The loudness of sound is measured in decibels, and its frequency is measured in Hertz (Hz). A whistle or siren creates high-frequency sound waves, while a drum or truck engine produces waves at a low frequency. Sounds lower than 20Hz are experienced as vibrations. A person's ability to hear soft or loud sounds varies depending on the frequency. Many people can more easily understand words spoken in a low-pitched voice than a high-pitched one.

Sound is haptic

Many digital devices employ interfaces that communicate through tactile vibration and physical movement or resistance. These haptic signals can convey degrees of intensity or they can assign unique patterns to different types of message. A vibration can tap the skin with a precise pattern, or it can blur into an overall texture. Vibrations localized on one part of a touch screen can give users the impression that they are manipulating mechanical controls, not just stroking a glassy surface. Ultrahaptic technologies cause air itself to vibrate and change pressure, creating a tangible illusion of objects and actions.

Designing how a phone or watch vibrates is concurrent with designing how it sounds. Conor O'Sullivan, Sound Design Lead for Google, says, "Haptics and sound are both waveforms, so I treat them together."[2] Vibrations and audible signals combine into a unified experience. Have you ever felt an earthquake? The sound and the vibration merge into a wave of audible motion. When a smartphone rings, the device itself resonates—its materials vibrate to amplify the sound emitted through the speaker. The device interacts with its environment as well. Its vibration sounds different when the phone rattles against a glass tabletop than when it nuzzles into a warm, soft palm.

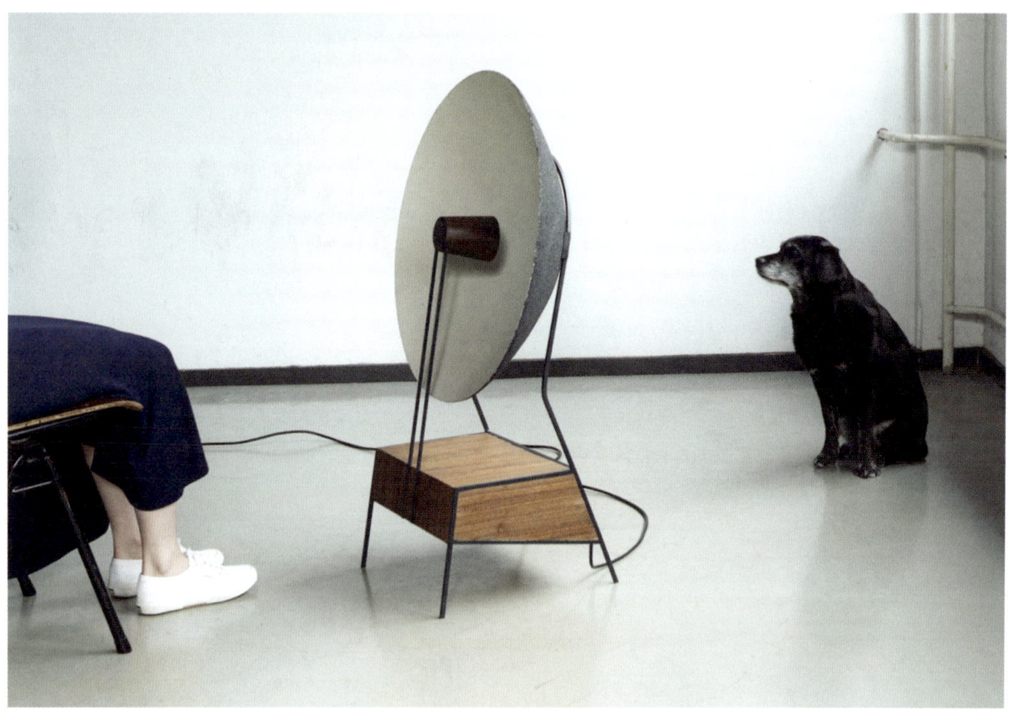

Sound Scene, 2016; Sanne Gelissen (Dutch, b. 1988), Sanne Geeft Vorm (Eindhoven, Netherlands, founded 2016); Glass fiber laminate, wood, metal; 110 × 40 × 65 cm (43 5/16 × 15 3/4 × 25 9/16 in.); © Design Academy Eindhoven Photographs. Photo by Femke Rijerman; Courtesy of Sanne Gelissen

Sound is spatial

Although sound enters the ears in a single wave, a hearing person walking through a park can make out children laughing, gravel crunching, and engines whirring in the distance. The direction of sound helps listeners untangle these different sources and build a picture of places and events. Just as binocular human vision creates a sense of depth by combining two images (one picture from each eye), binaural hearing creates depth by combining input from the left and right ears. Sitting at a dinner table, a person with normal hearing can tell two voices apart, not only because the sounds have different frequencies but because they have unique locations. It's harder to distinguish the same voices coming from a radio or television. Binaural recording is a technique for creating three-dimensional sound by recording sound with two microphones positioned apart from each other a distance equivalent to a human head. Listeners using headphones or occupying

a controlled environment will feel the experience of live sound.[3] Bats and whales use echolocation to find objects and navigate spaces. A hungry bat emits a high-frequency sound (beyond the range of human perception) and hears it bounce off the doomed body of a mosquito. Some blind people use mobility canes to tap and listen for echoes, thus using echolocation to sense walls and doorways. A sonogram uses sound instead of light to see inside the body, creating pictures by bouncing sound waves against hidden structures.

Dutch designer Sanne Gelissen plays with the direction of sound in Sound Scene, a beautifully crafted speaker that directs sound waves to a precise location. Most sound systems are designed to fill a space with music, enveloping the whole room. Gelissen's system uses a concept similar to a flashlight, whose reflective bowl focuses light in a single direction. The speaker in Sound Scene points inward at a large parabolic bowl, which reflects the sound waves back toward the listener at a specific location. The bowl, reminiscent of the horn on a gramophone, is made of glass fiber laminate, a hard surface designed to reflect sound waves. The shape of the bowl targets common mid-tone frequencies. Sound Scene creates an intimate experience that isolates and personalizes sound.

Cities have sonic signatures. Shared_Studios, founded by Amar C. Bakshi in Washington, DC, creates two-way audio/video connections between dozens of cities around the globe, allowing a person in New York or New Haven to speak with someone in Iraq, Rwanda, Mexico, or Detroit. Curators living in these different areas have collected sounds that are unique to these locations.

Sound is synesthetic

Sound primes us to see. When a dog snarls or brakes screech, images rush to our minds. Filmmakers build suspense with ominous soundtracks. Musicians and audio engineers call a sound "bright" or "dull" depending on its overall frequency. The clash of a cymbal is considered wide and flat, while the voice of a flute is bright and sharp. Such terms assign visual and tactile qualities to sound.[4] People with synesthesia link certain sensations in a consistent or systematic manner—as do people with more ordinary sensory responses. Metaphors such as "piercing cry," "soft whisper," or "coarse language" assign tactile characteristics to sounds.[5]

Researchers in Spain wanted to learn if taste could be associated with qualities of music. They asked a group of jazz musicians to create short improvisations in response to the basic tastes—salty, sour, sweet, and bitter. They analyzed the resulting music and looked for patterns. In response to sourness, the musicians tended to create compositions with short notes that were high pitched and dissonant. In response to a bitter taste (such as coffee or dark chocolate), the musicians tended to create compositions whose notes were slower, lower, and more softly differentiated (*legato*). They found similar correlations for sweet (long, low, and soft) and salty (*staccato*, with quick, sharply separated notes). In a second experiment, the musical pieces were played for ordinary listeners, who then assigned taste labels to each composition. Participants affirmed the inclinations of the musicians to a degree substantially higher than chance.[6]

Sound is energy

Sound always results from an action—a string has been plucked, a rock has been thrown, or a door has been slammed. Many of the words used to describe sounds in English imitate the sounds of actions: *bang, bump, crunch, smash, tap, tinkle, whistle, whomp*. Objects and materials make sounds when they fall, break, or bend, or when they crash into other things. When these actions occur, energy is released as sound.

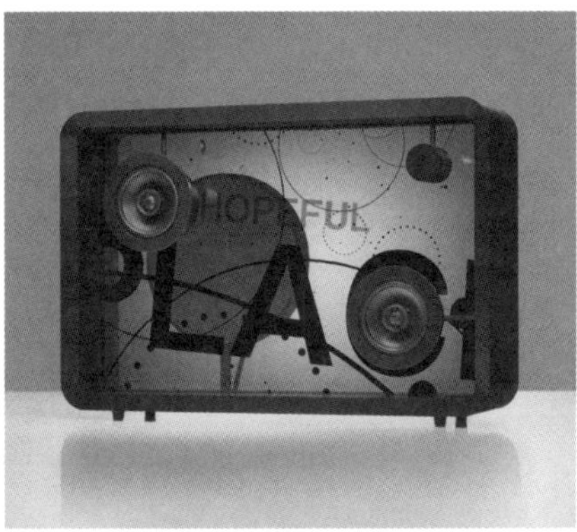

COTODAMA Lyric Speaker, 2016; Naoki Ono (monom) (Japan, b. 1981) and Lyric Speaker team (Tokyo, Japan, founded 2016); ABS, galvanized steel, acrylic plate; 52 × 14 × 35 cm (20 ½ × 5 ½ × 13 ¾ in.); Photo by Hisashi Ootsu

Sound is communication

Sound and gesture are the wellsprings of language. Humans construct intricate discourse when they speak, and they express emotion when they laugh, scream, or sing. Jin Saito's Lyric Speaker connects sound to words. Saito believes that to fully experience a song, you must grasp its words. He told us, "In Japan we believe that words have souls. People have souls. Dogs and cats have souls, and words have souls. This speaker shows the souls of lyrics. It makes music and lyrics into a whole." The Lyric Speaker downloads a song's lyrics from an online database and generates typographic animations in real time, based on the mood and structure of the music. (An algorithm analyzes the music for its soft/hard and positive/negative characteristics.) For songs with no lyrics, the software generates geometric compositions. The animations vary each time a song plays. Rendered in subtle shades of black and white, motion graphics pulse across the speaker's glass skin. The words and shapes appear on screen in sync with the music.

Sound signals danger

Sound alerts humans and other creatures to their environment in 360 degrees. Hearing keeps us tuned in to crying babies and bumps in the night. Paying attention to sound can be a matter of life or death. Alarm fatigue is a problem afflicting hospital wards, air traffic control rooms, and other environments that pelt workers with beeps, buzzes, and sirens. Repeated false alarms and confusing signals breed exhaustion and indifference. Some systems are so annoying, users shut them off completely—with potentially catastrophic effects. An auditory display is a set of sounds representing the state of a system. Sounds in an auditory display might range from a gentle background noise that signals normal functioning to alerts demanding attention and action. A shrill, blaring siren can cause a state of momentary shock, requiring operators to lose valuable response time before regaining their focus. Some sounds function best in the background. The rhythmic whir of a machine could indicate that a system is running normally; a sudden break in the pattern is cause for concern. Effective auditory displays, designed in conjunction with visual and tactile signals, reinforce multisensory information.[7]

Designers and engineers are studying the effects of sound on human behavior. Joel Beckerman and his colleagues at Man Made Music are researching a unified language of auditory alerts for use in hospitals. Although studies show it is difficult for humans to differentiate among more than six different alarm sounds, the average number of alarms in an ICU has increased from six in 1983 to more than forty different alarms in 2011. Beckerman says, "We envision creating a standardized, open-source sonic language that hospitals around the world can use." Instead of letting each device make its own special blips and beeps, the system will employ a limited and universal sonic vocabulary.[8]

Sound is material

Felt pads keep chair legs from screeching against a hard floor. An oak door clunks solemnly shut, while an aluminum screen door quivers and squeaks. The clatter of glass and tableware in a café spins a bright cloak of ambient sound. The density, elasticity, plasticity, and "squashiness" of a material affect the sounds it makes when it collides with other materials. Sound waves move quickly through matter that has densely packed molecules, such as steel or diamond. Waves are deadened and absorbed by materials like cotton, wool, or foam rubber. LABA, designed by Eason Chow and Pravar Jain, is a series of prototypes for audio speakers that alter sound based on the materials used and the shape of the speakers' earlike horns. Each horn amplifies and reflects sound in a different way, creating different auditory effects. A glazed ceramic horn maximizes the reflection of sound waves, while a horn lined with wool localizes sound to the zone of the listener. A horn laced with silicone at its periphery amplifies sound and gives it a warm tone.

Sound is experience

Designers create interfaces that shiver and ping to communicate actions. Architecture shapes sound—and sound shapes architecture. A tree falls in a forest. From the point of view of physics, it doesn't matter if the forest is empty when the proverbial tree hits the ground. Molecules bang back and forth against one another with or without a live audience. From the perspective of psychology, however, it matters very much if sensing creatures occupy the forest when those leaves shiver and those branches snap. Designers engage with the lived, bodily phenomenon of sound. Fabrics, rugs, and wallcoverings soften the echoes in a room. Trees, traffic, and fountains set the tone of a city. Beeps and buzzes mark our interactions with products. Whether heard with the ears or felt with the body, sound envelops us in the rich murmur of being.

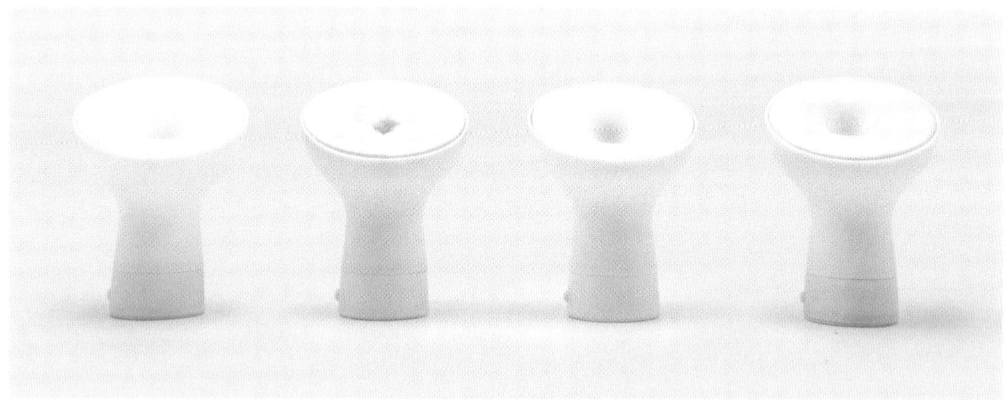

LABA Speakers, 2017; Eason Chow (Singaporean, b. 1989) and Pravar Jain (Indian, b. 1993); 3D-printed nylon, wool, ceramic, plastic, electronics; Each: 14 × 11 × 11 cm (5 ½ × 4 11⁄32 × 4 11⁄32 in.); Courtesy of Eason Chow

It is now estimated that humans can, in theory, smell at least one trillion distinct scents, but no one has made a definitive claim regarding the number of smells an individual can differentiate. Unlike hearing and sight, whose mechanics and molecular biology have been exhaustively mapped in the course of the twentieth century, there is little agreement on how smell works.

1. Our sense of smell is beyond doubt a tool of great precision. Strange, then, that in the history of Western philosophy it should be so little discussed, and so often dismissed as subjective. Smell has been held in low esteem since the height of the Enlightenment. When Condillac, in his *Treatise on the Sensations* (1754), imagined a statue that would be granted all the capacities of thinking and feeling one by one, smell was the first capability he bestowed upon it, because he held smell to be the most primitive of senses and the one that contributes least to the mind. Condillac maintained that, should his statue smell a rose, it would not thereby gain any concept of the rose as an entity distinct from itself. When it smells a rose, it simply exists within the sensation of the scent of a rose. Smell, this position implies, teaches us nothing about the outside world, but produces pleasant or unpleasant sensations that go on to determine what we desire, rather than what we know.

Essay first published as "Notes on Smell" in *Cabinet*, Issue 32: Fire (Winter 2008/09). Reprinted here with revisions. Figures redrawn by David Genco

1.1 This demotion of smell has continued more or less uninterrupted, as demonstrated by the manner in which Septimus Piesse attempted to defend the utility of perfumes in his 1857 book *The Art of Perfumery and Methods of Obtaining the Odors of Plants*: "Of the five senses, that of smelling is the least valued, and, as a consequence, is the least tutored; but we must not conclude from this, our own act, that it is of insignificant importance to our welfare and happiness. By neglecting to tutor the olfactory nerve, we are constantly led to breathe impure air, and thus poison the body by neglecting the warning given at the gate of the lungs. Persons who use perfumes are more sensitive to the presence of a vitiated atmosphere than those who consider the faculty of smelling as an almost useless gift."

A. Chlorine (Cl_2 at room temperature and pressure) is a pale green gas that was described by the soldiers that first encountered it in Ypres in 1915 as having a distinctive smell partway between pepper and pineapples. The characteristic acrid odor we associate with chlorinated swimming pools is not that of chlorine itself but of chloramine (NH_2Cl), the product of a reaction between chlorine and an organic molecule. When a pool smells intensely of chloramine, it's an indicator that the water is dirty, not clean, and the persistent smell that we carry for hours after a swim is the smell of free chlorine molecules reacting with our hair and skin. We become conscious of chlorine, in its peculiar chlorineness, at a concentration of three parts per million. At five parts per million it produces a choking sensation. At thirty it induces coughing and vomiting. At sixty it begins to corrode the lungs.

2. Kant makes almost no reference to smell in the *Critique of Judgment* or elsewhere in his writing on aesthetics. He does, however, discuss smell at length in his *Reflexionen zur Anthropologie*. There, he makes a curious distinction between the senses by which we as rational beings come to know things, and the senses that work on a more intuitive basis. Looking at things, hearing them, and even touching them require *Wahrnehmung*, or perception. But smelling things, like eating them, involves a sort of carnal knowledge, *Einnehmung*, or ingestion. By smelling things, we absorb them directly into our bodies, and consequently they provide what Kant otherwise attributes only to God: unmediated knowledge of the thing in itself. To prevent this from becoming a crisis for

his epistemology, Kant argues that experiences of smell or taste are things that we are interested in, personally, and compromised by in both senses of the word. This prevents us from the sort of disinterested contemplation that aesthetic experience requires. Kant's dogmatic exclusion of taste and smell from the aesthetic has been either reproduced without question or thrown out of court (see Frank Sibley's essay "Tastes, Smells, and Aesthetics"), but no one seems to have considered that maybe he was half-right. Smell is deeply connected with the unconscious, divorced from representation, and consequently in some respects more primal than the other senses. It indicates a royal road to our animal and emotional being, offering a way of thinking, or at least of drawing conclusions, that is not conceptual but intuitive.

2.1 Smells have two qualities that make them ill-suited to the Enlightenment project of establishing a firm foundation for our knowledge of the world. First, they do not persist. Most smells are fleeting—the smell of violets (methyl ionone) is famous among perfumers for persisting for only about half the duration of an inhalation before it becomes imperceptible. Other scents are more persistent, but even the most penetrating perfume becomes undetectable to the wearer after a short period of time.

2.2 Second, as Kant writes in *Reflexionen zur Anthropologie*, "all the senses have their own descriptive vocabularies, e.g. for sight, there is red, green, and yellow, and for taste there is sweet and sour, etc. But the sense of smell can have no descriptive vocabulary of its own. Rather, we borrow our adjectives from the other senses, so that it smells sour, or has a smell like roses or cloves or musk. They are all, however, terms drawn from other senses. Consequently, we cannot describe our sense of smell" (our translation).

2.2.1 Kant's observation does not seem to be a limitation of his Baltic Sea dialect. There are also no words in the English language that are exclusively devoted to describing a smell. All the other senses have a specific vocabulary that is part of everyday speech and in no way technical (*bright, loud, hard, soft, smooth, bitter*, etc). Smell proceeds entirely via euphemism. Typical words for describing citrus scents include fruity, refreshing, sweet, sharp. "Fruity" is derived from a noun. "Refreshing" is stolen from an affect. "Sweet" belongs to taste. "Sharp" to touch. The word citrus, in toto, is useless for anyone who has not smelt citrus already, and none of the descriptive words belong to the sense of smell except in a metaphorical sense.

B. A curious piece of trivia claims that all medical anesthetics are olfactants, that is, they have a peculiar and identifiable smell, even though smell is not part of their purpose. From chloroform on, synthetic molecules designed to knock you out (things you couldn't possibly have evolved to be able to experience) have distinct odors.

3. Freud said that "wishes are immortal." In this respect, smells and wishes are the same. The passage of time, which rots and corrodes the content of visual memory, has no measurable impact on the olfactory memory. On the condition that a smell is linked to an emotionally significant episode, the ability of specific smells to trigger episodic memories is immortal (the Proust Effect). Strangely, we are terrible at recalling the impression of smells—nearly as bad as we are at remembering physical pain. It's easy to recall the shape and color of a lemon, but almost impossible to conjure up its absent scent.

3.1 Speaking of Proust. Those oft-cited madeleines that are supposed to have triggered the reminiscences of *À la recherche du temps perdu* are traditionally flavored with almonds. Almonds have a sweet, penetrating, enduring odor that makes them particularly well suited to forming memories around. It is this quality that makes almonds such a common feature in recipes associated with annual rituals such as Christmas. It is questionable whether Proust would have been able to fill as many pages if his memory had been triggered by a highly anosmic scent, such as violet.

C. Is the sense of smell really subjective? Zookeepers have long noted that the smell of tiger urine resembles fragrant basmati rice. It was only in the course of the 1980s that Indian biologists realized that the same molecule is active in both—2 acetyl-1-pyrroline. Furthermore, it's been noted that we can detect certain pyrazines, such as 2-isobutyl-3-methoxypyrazine—which is found in peas and paprika—at a concentration of 1 part in 500,000 million, that is, virtually molecule by molecule.

4. The olfactory bulb in humans is relatively small compared to that in, say, a white-eared opossum, a West European hedgehog, a polar bear, or a domestic dog, especially when taken in proportion to the size of the brain. But the number of human genes that encode scent turns out to be unexpectedly large. According to Linda B. Buck and Richard Axel's research, about one thousand genes code for proteins that are expressed only in the olfactory epithelium. This means that roughly 3 percent of the human genome is devoted to the olfactory system. That's an enormous share.

4.1 The olfactory bulb feeds directly into the limbic system, the seat of both long-term memory and the emotions. The results of smelling are processed here, and loaded with associations, before they even reach the upper cortex, where language is composed. This is unlike the sense of sight, in which knowing and naming are intimately interconnected activities. In a peculiar way, smelling short-circuits conscious thoughts. It bonds to memory and emotion before it subjects itself to concepts, and emerges as already a part of the bodily unconscious.

4.2 Although there has been substantial research on the olfactory bulb, olfaction is dwarfed by the other senses in the amount of research committed to it, and ignored in undergraduate studies (a 2008 textbook on cognitive neuroscience offers a chapter on sight, another on touch, but exactly two sentences on smell). This might have something to do with the following: no one agrees on how smell works. Although the problems posed by hearing and sight on the cellular level were to a large degree cracked by the 1950s and 1960s, there is still no consensus on how a molecule of olfactant entering the nose brings a single neuron to fire.

4.3 In 1996, Luca Turin—a research biologist and well-known perfume reviewer—resurrected an exotic theory of the sense of smell that had first been mooted and dismissed in the 1950s. It suggests that the smell of a compound is not dependent on the shape of the molecule (although this is the standard hypothesis, as "lock and key" ligand-binding is the mechanism by which most chemical signaling within the brain takes place, as well as the way in which the immune system functions). Rather, Turin solves the combinatorial problem of smell by arguing that embedded in the cell membrane is a kind of electron-tunneling spectrograph, and so the smell of a molecule is dependent upon its chief vibrational resonance.

D. The port wine magnolia has small purple and white inflorescences that smell distinctly like nail polish remover (acetone) and wine jujubes. The scent is strong, sweet, and slightly nauseating. Other magnolias smell like citrus. Not exactly like citrus, but somewhat like citrus. Is acetone a pollutant that is actually found in cheap port wine?

5. The relationship between smell, long-term memory, and emotion is not a trivial one, and it's not meaningless to say that they're all one thing. Everyone knows that smell evokes strong memories, but the relationship works both ways. The olfactory bulb is the only part of the brain that continues to grow throughout our lives, and constantly generates new neurons (Buck and Axel won a Nobel prize for figuring this

out). The ability to recognize common smells is now used as a diagnostic tool in identifying neuro-degenerative diseases. People with memory loss—Alzheimer's patients—have massively reduced sensitivity to smell.

E. Real musk is obtained from the dried gland of a wild male deer, and fresh from the wild it has a repulsive smell. Harvesting musk involves hanging out in forests during mating season with a high-powered rifle, shooting a medium-large mammal, cutting out a small gland, and then taking and preparing that gland for a luxury product. Hunters can't tell whether the deer in their sights is a buck or a doe, and consequently half of the animals they shoot are the wrong sex. That's one reason for synthetic musks. Another is that real musk is a mélange of chemicals that will cause some wearers to break out in hives. The first synthetic variant—Musk Xylol—was produced in 1888, and as the industry bible by Steffen Arctander notes, it is a close relative of trinitrotoluene, or TNT. Attempts to synthesize Musk Xylol in commercial quantities have been responsible for serious explosions in fragrance laboratories, and the death of more than a few fragrancers.

6. It is as if, when chemistry evolved out of alchemy to become an Enlightenment science, smell was left behind. Appropriately, the perfumer behaves more as a member of a medieval guild than as part of a contemporary scientific discipline. Alchemists guarded their mysteries, whereas chemistry is based on peer review and the broadest possible dissemination of results. Perfumers are likewise notoriously secretive about their ingredients, even though the field involves the mass production of tons of refined chemical products. They are even loath to talk about how they arrange their fragrance libraries (this seemingly innocent question was in fact the impetus for this text). There is a legal reason for this: it's not possible to patent a scent. You can patent the individual synthetic molecules that might be used in a scent, but you can't patent what something smells like in the same way that you can patent the way in which a product looks and feels. Knockoff perfumes are prosecuted for copying the packaging of the original, not for smelling identical. As a result, perfumers are particularly clandestine about what's in their bottles. The other reason for their secretiveness is that, even if they want to talk about what they are doing, they seem to find it pretty difficult.

6.1 Systems of smell resemble medieval bestiaries that have swollen in population without gaining in order. Aristotle classified smells into five categories. Carl Linnaeus's system contained seven categories, but by the early twentieth century Hendrik Zwaardemaker's had risen to nine. René Gerbelaud's system from the 1950s encompassed forty-five categories, and a decade later Steffen Arctander's included eighty-eight separate groups. Even more striking than the increasing complexity of the proposed systems is the parallel proliferation in the taxonomies themselves. A comprehensive taxonomy of taxonomies is hardly possible, but we can enumerate a few.

6.2 Ernst Crocker and Lloyd Henderson's 1927 model derives many of its terms from Zwaardemaker's model of 1895, which itself draws from Carl Linnaeus's original taxonomy of 1756. According to Crocker and Henderson's ingenious scheme, each odor can be considered in terms of the extent to which it is fragrant, acid, burnt, or caprylic (goaty), each on a scale of 1 to 8. Thus, vanillin has an odor of 7122. Unfortunately, there is often disagreement as to the precise score to give a scent on each of its characteristics, although Crocker and Henderson do try to provide a structured language for comparing scents.

The Crocker-Henderson system ranks smells from 1 to 8 in four dimensions. Butter is somewhat acidic and goaty, but neither burnt nor fragrant, so its number is 1514. See Stephen W. D. Dowthwaite, "Odor Classification," → perfumersworld.com/article/odor-classification

CROCKER-HENDERSON SMELL SYSTEM (1927) APPLIED TO BUTTER

FRAGRANT	1							
ACID					5			
BURNT	1							
CAPRYLIC (GOATY)				4				

Drom Fragrance Wheel; Developed by Drom, a global scent company founded in Germany in 1911

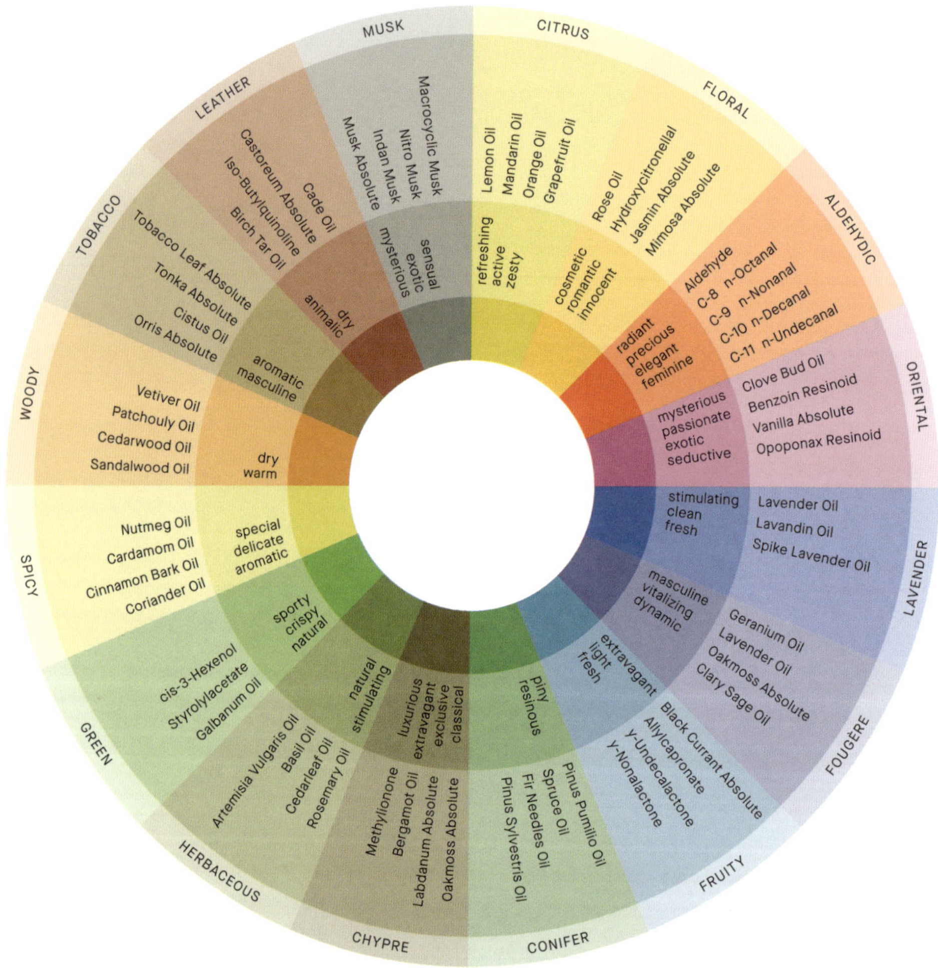

6.3 Some industrial scent manufacturers arrange smells into a sort of "color wheel" in order to describe them. But this is a weak analogy, as smells, unlike colors, do not naturally form a continuous spectrum. The Drom spectral wheel, for instance, implausibly places citrus directly next to musk, but spatially opposite "fruity" scents. Different wheels have been proposed, but their insufficiency is highlighted by their proliferation.

6.4 Even fragrance wheels specific to the perfume industry (such as Michael Edwards's 1983 version) are not designed as an objective tool for the fragrancers, but as a marketing guide for clients. To make matters worse, it seems that we are particularly susceptible to being suckered when we are told what we "ought" to be smelling. As Trygg Engen notes: "The associative strength of an odor-name pair is weak and asymmetric and is easily influenced by the verbal factor" (p. 502). In other words, if someone offers you a bad synthetic frambinone and tells you it's strawberry, you'll believe them, and if they ask you to sniff onion and tell you it's garlic, you'll notice nothing amiss.

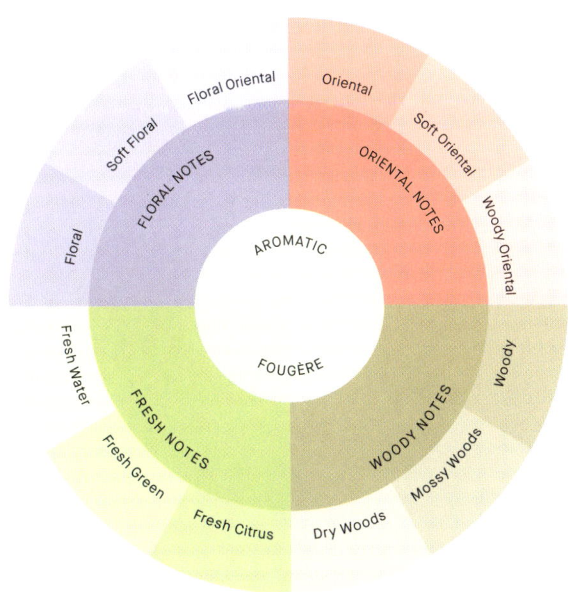

Fragrance Wheel, 1983;
Michael Edwards

6.5 There have been more inventive attempts to taxonomize odor. In the nineteenth century, Septimus Piesse arranged smell on a musical scale to show how harmonious perfumes could be composed, a better (more multidimensional) approach than a linear spectrum. He was the first to apply the term "note" to a distinctive odor, as well as introducing the terms "chord," "harmony," and "progression," all metaphors that are still current in the perfume industry. Piesse proposed that "sounds appear to influence the olfactory nerves in certain definite degrees," and that "there are octaves in odors like octaves in music." Piesse took his model quite literally. According to his theory, a harmonious fragrance can be composed by bringing together those odor notes that correspond to harmonious musical chords. Conversely, discord, a cacophony of smells, is the result of combining olfactory notes that would produce discordant sounds if played musically together. In his invention, Piesse resembles Des Esseintes in Joris-Karl Huysmans's *Against Nature*, the great novel of dandyism, who composes for himself a "taste symphony" by assigning a different note to each liqueur. Via this artifice, Huysmans's character could play himself his favorite refrains from classical music by sequentially tasting various spirits.

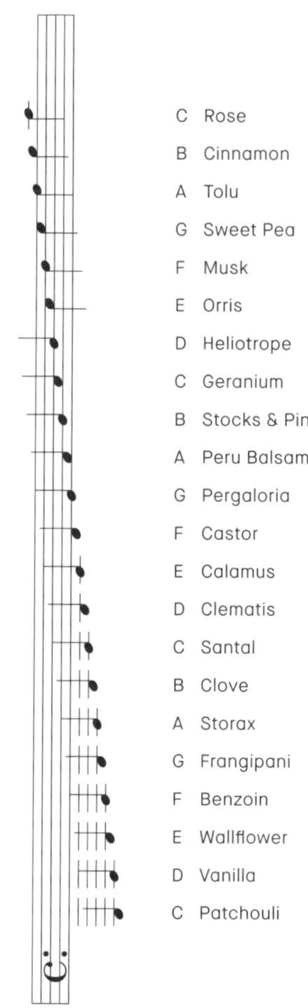

A music-inspired taxonomy of scent offered by English chemist and perfumer George William Septimus Piesse in his seminal book *The Art of Perfumery* (1857)

6.6 Perhaps one of the most interesting models is the Henning Odor Prism, or Henning Olfactory Prism (1915–16). The prism has six apexes and five faces, and allows for any smell to be described in terms of the six categories: flowery/fruity/putrid/spicy/burnt/resinous. This would not be a substantial addition to extant theories, except that Hans Henning goes on to argue that all smells can be described as being on the surface of the prism, but not within it. Therefore, a smell cannot be spicy, burnt, and resinous as well as being putrid, and likewise, a fruity, flowery, putrid, and spicy odor cannot exist. In making assertions of this kind, the Henning Prism is at least putatively falsifiable, unlike most other smell models. This is no small virtue.

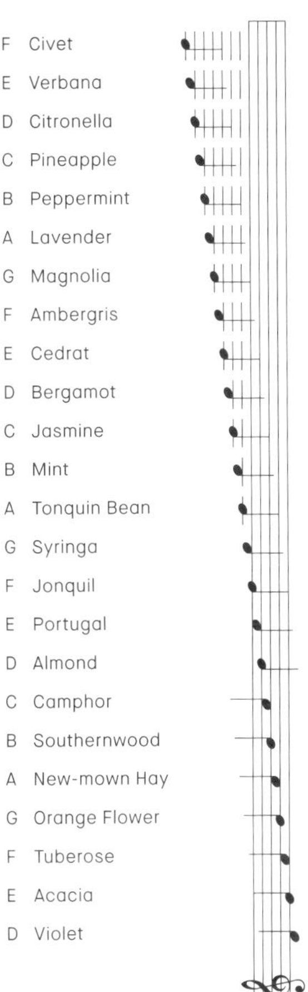

6.6.1 The Henning Prism becomes more interesting when one notes the subgroupings that the on-the-surface rule implies. Cover two of the terms at a time, and look again at the set of characteristics flowery / putrid / spicy / burnt versus the set fruity / putrid / burnt / resinous. It could be argued that both groups have enough terms to adequately describe any smell, and there is a risk of that, but that isn't what Henning intended. What is it about these two groups that make them mutually exclusive? Certainly the flowery / fruity / spicy / resinous—the general realm of attractive smells—can coexist, but not together with the putrid and burnt. The putrid and the burnt both mark out forms of decomposition. The putrid indicates metabolic decay carried out by simple life forms, whereas the burnt is the rather more chaotic decay caused by heat (both processes are marked by increasing variety but reducing complexity in the organic molecules present). Whereas flowery and fruity scents may, in their freshness, have much in common, according to the Henning Prism they differentiate themselves from each other in their odor profile during decomposition. Also, it is noteworthy that the flowery / fruity / putrid (less stable) and the spicy / burnt / resinous (less volatile) take opposite ends of the Henning Prism.

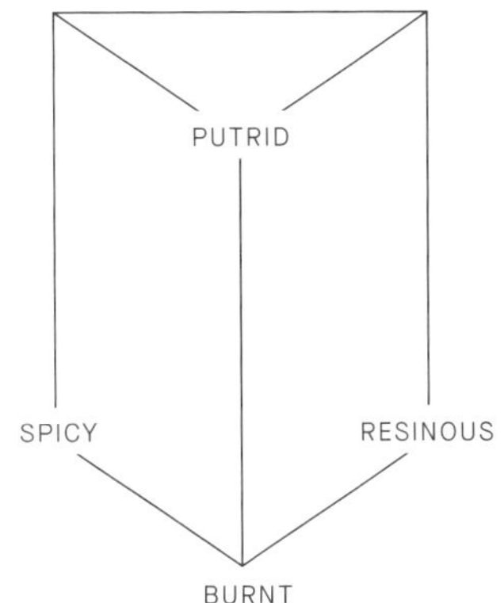

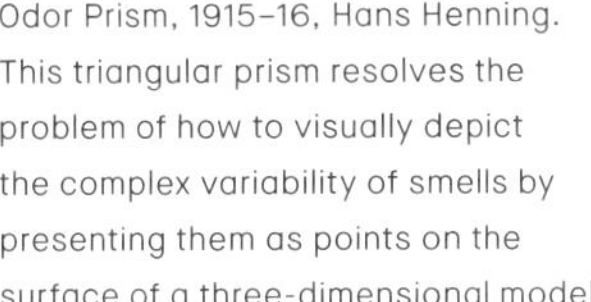
Odor Prism, 1915–16, Hans Henning. This triangular prism resolves the problem of how to visually depict the complex variability of smells by presenting them as points on the surface of a three-dimensional model.

6.6.2 Intriguingly, the Henning Prism also suggests the possibility of charting "smell trajectories," that is, the characteristic changes in smell as a perfume's volatile top note lifts to reveal its middle and base notes, as when a fruit ripens or when an organic product undergoes metabolic decomposition. By what habitual route does an unripe peach slowly lose its spicy, flowery characteristics to sweeten into an odor more fruity and perhaps more resinous? And via what path does this scent become putrid as the peach begins to rot? Is it curved, or straight?

6.6.3 Henning attempted to relate different chemical groups to the various sections of his prism, noting, for instance, that the category of the putrid is marked by volatile sulphides. Unfortunately, while some molecules might have predictable characteristics, as in a bad grammatical model, there are nearly as many exceptions to each category as well-behaved instances that fit the rules.

F. Ambergris is another highly valued ingredient in perfumes. It is made of a sort of fatty hairball, coughed up by a sperm whale, that then floats upon the surface of the ocean. Over time it darkens to black, and its scent mellows until it becomes what is described as a "soft, suave, dry-mossy, musty, and seaweed-like fragrance that is extremely difficult to duplicate with complete fidelity." The trade in ambergris is now banned, and a wholly synthetic version of the scent, Ambroxan, is sold in its place.

6.7 In 1951, Dr. Paul Jellinek proposed a new scheme for the classification of scents. Although a professional perfumer, his system (which was restated in *The Psychological Basis of Perfumery*, 4th Edition, 1997) has the virtue of attempting a degree of generality. The schema, however, is tendentious in the worst sense. As Jellinek held that the sense of smell is enthralled by sexuality, he arranges all odors on a scale based on their purported psychological effect. One axis connects the erogenic to the anti-erogenic; another axis runs from the narcotic to the stimulating. Following Jellinek, cheesy smells are both highly erogenic and slightly stimulating, whereas fruity

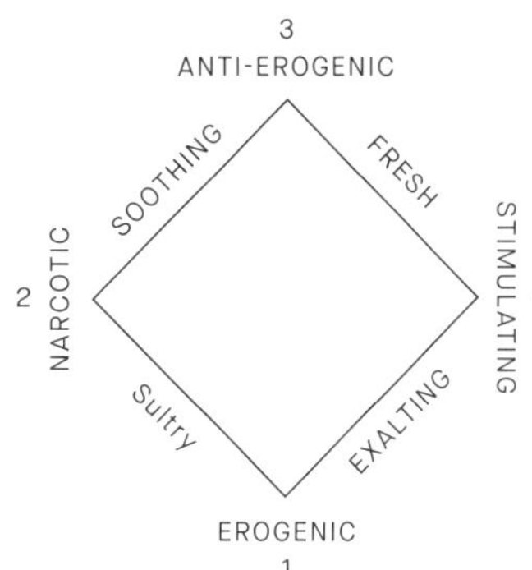

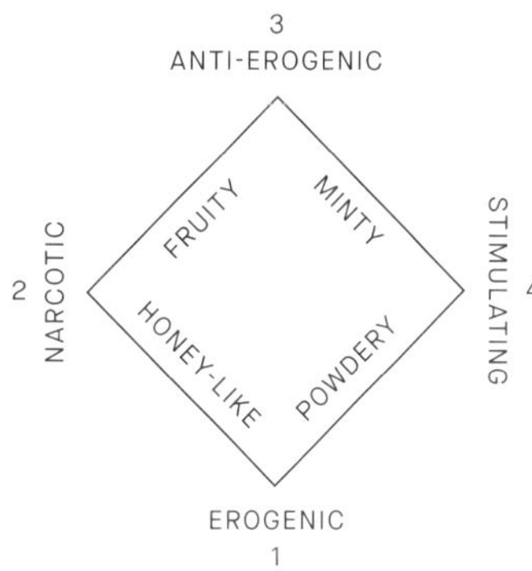

Dr. Paul Jellinek's classificatory system, 1951

smells are anti-erogenic and somewhat narcotic. The problem, of course, is that as soon as one questions the psychological model behind the classification, the schema collapses. And in spite of all the enthusiasm about pheromones, they remain more or less mysterious. It's also not advisable to buy synthetic pheromones from dispensing machines in toilets, as androstenones, the closest pheromones to humans that have been extensively synthesized, are from the porcine family (*Suidae*). The only mammals that you are likely to arouse irresistibly are pigs.

7. Luca Turin's thesis of the vibrational basis of smell has come up against entrenched opposition from the scientific establishment. Perhaps, here again, it is the enchantment of the diagram that is responsible, for should his argument prove to be correct, the wire-frame and space-filling molecular models that mesmerize fragrance designers worldwide would have precious little relevance in predicting how a chemical will actually smell. The thousands of line drawings of organic molecules that fill fragrance textbooks will turn out to be as much a fetish as Piesse's musical scale, because we have been studying the wrong characteristics.

7.1 In the 1980s, the chemist Roman Kaiser developed a procedure based around gas chromatography and mass spectrometry that promised the possibility of objectively capturing and recording the olfactory molecules in a sample of air. Artists and experimenters have seen in the invention the possibility of a new media format, something akin to a photography of smell. But according to Professor Kaiser, the enthusiasm is misplaced. Because the sense of smell is nonlinear in its sensitivity, a powerful scent at an undetectably low concentration—such as a pyrazine—can have a stronger impact on the senses than a pervasive gas. As a result, no currently imaginable technology can offer a reliable means to capture, store, and reproduce the scent of a place.

G. Oak moss has a particularly wonderful smell—neither vegetable nor animal, but richly aromatic. The moss grows only on oak trees, and only in the most established and ancient woods. For a very long time, the majority of it was harvested in Yugoslavia. However, it soaks up radioactive waste more effectively than just about any other life form, and ever since the Chernobyl disaster in the Ukraine, it has been exceedingly rare and expensive, because so much of it is too contaminated to use.

8. In conclusion, smell is not subjective; rather, it is simply very hard to communicate objectively, that is, to talk about and achieve any sort of consensus. One possibility would be to unwind the "color wheel" model, and ask how many dimensions it would have to incorporate in order that all its observable contradictions disappear. Much like experimental versions of Mendeleev's original periodic table, there are interesting possibilities for new spatial models for representing scents. Perhaps future models of smell will have to address similar orders of complexity, and the solution just hasn't been drawn up yet. Alternatively, there may simply be no way to represent visually the variability presented by scents.

9. In *Civilization and Its Discontents*, Freud tells an originary myth, in which Man goes from walking on all fours to standing erect. As he does so, the genitals are exposed, the sense of sight is privileged, and the sense of smell is denigrated. Whether or not the story refers to an actual historical event doesn't matter; Freud's point is that somewhere in our development, we learn shame for what has become the spectacle of shit and lose the capacity to smell it with any finesse. However, there's a simpler physical explanation for why walking on two legs might lead to a demotion for the sense of smell: olfactants are heavier than air, and consequently they fall to the ground. If you want to make a map of how your room smells, you need to get down on your hands and knees.

10. And finally, how do professional perfumers arrange their smells? *Alphabetically*, of course.

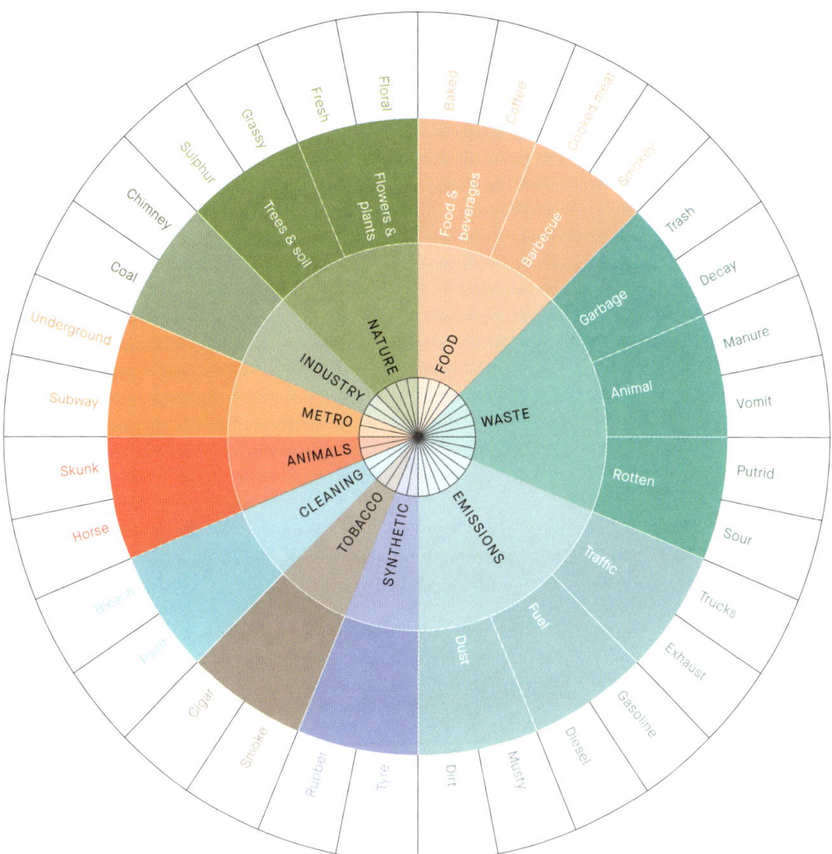

Urban Smellscape Aroma Wheel, revised 2017; Kate McLean (British, b. 1965), Daniele Guercia, Rossano Schifanella, Luca Maria Aiello; Courtesy of Kate McLean

To arrive at this taxonomy of urban smells, researchers collected hundreds of smell words during smellwalks with participants in cities in the UK, Europe, and USA. They matched this word list with descriptors appearing in or tagged to thousands of geo-referenced photographs and messages on social media. The wheel depicts a hierarchy of urban smells. The inner circle contains the top-level categories, such as nature, food, and waste. Second-level categories occupy the next ring, and words from the smell dictionary appear in the outer ring.

Flavor engages all the senses. As you bite into a ham sandwich and feel its layers mash together inside your mouth, the tongue seems to be the master of sensation, roused by grains of mustard, plumes of salt, strands of protein, and an earthy afterglow of rye. A simple bite of sandwich mobilizes more than the tongue, however. Texture, aroma, temperature, and appearance, as well as language and memory, all contribute to the complex experience of flavor.

Flavor is taste

Bundles of cells called taste buds populate the folds of the tongue and the back of the mouth. Responding to chemicals in food and drink, taste buds are tuned to differentiate just five channels: sweet, salty, sour, bitter, and umami. The tongue's five unique receptors transmit their signals separately to the brain, where the "taste cortex" creates a sensory map. "The beauty about taste is that it has limited chemical space. There are only five basic qualities and each of them has an innate and very well-defined meaning and valence," says Dr. Charles Zuker, scientist at Columbia University College of Physicians & Surgeons. "So the taste system provides a powerful platform to understand how the brain functions: how complex, hardwired circuits operate, how they are modulated, and how they are used to guide actions and behaviors."[1]

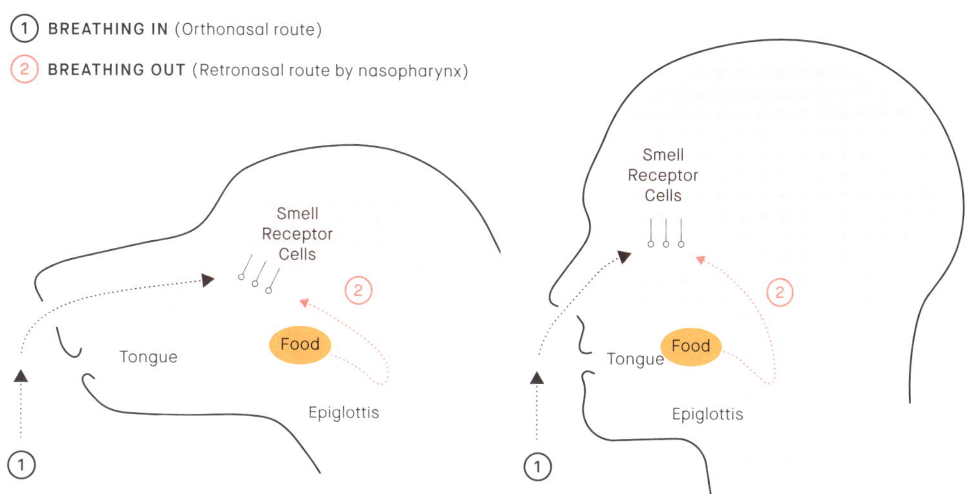

Dogs are talented sniffers. They distinguish odors with astonishing precision while inhaling air through their noses. Their long snouts enhance their sniffing skills. Humans outperform dogs when it comes to experiencing smells while breathing out. Humans can sense a vast number of different flavors, a process that relies on the retronasal route (air passing out, not in). Odor compounds travel on a direct route from the back of the mouth to the nasal cavity. Diagrams by David Genco, redrawn from Gordon M. Shepard, *Neurogastronomy: How the Brain Creates Flavor and Why It Matters* (2012). Used with permission © 2012 Columbia University Press

Flavor is smell

The olfactory bulb is a more sophisticated instrument than the human tongue, with its sharply limited sensory range. Smell receptors help the brain detect at least one trillion different aromas. Smell is thus the most discriminating of all the human senses. The eye can differentiate several million colors, while the ear makes sense of fewer than half a million tones.[2] Gordon M. Shepard's work on "neurogastronomy" upends the myth that humans have a poor sense of smell. Dogs, of course, are legendary sniffers, capable of tracking a fox through dense undergrowth or detecting a tiny bag of heroin deep inside a cargo hold. Sniffing, however, is not where humans excel. To sniff is to breathe in, drawing air into the nose to receive smell.

The triumph of the human nose occurs not when we breathe in, however, but when we breathe out. This process is called "retronasal olfaction." (Sniffing is "orthonasal olfaction.") The process of chewing food and mixing it with saliva releases volatile compounds, bathing the tongue and mouth with aromatic matter. Air passing out of the body carries smell molecules to receptors located at the top of the nasal cavity, and it is here where some of our most powerful messages about food are born.[3]

Flavor is primal

The taste buds that pepper the tongue and mouth transmit data to the brain stem, a primitive area in charge of involuntary actions such as breathing and digestion. In the brain stem, taste triggers preconscious responses such as attraction or revulsion. The brain stem sends along taste signals to higher-level areas of the brain, where they merge with aroma and other sensations to build a full perception of flavor.

Flavor is emotional

In contrast to the simple tongue, the madly sophisticated nose communicates with the olfactory cortex in the brain's limbic system. This higher-level brain structure is dedicated to memory and emotion. The olfactory cortex also connects to part of the brain controlling judgment and planning. Our ability to differentiate an enormous range of flavors reflects the highest human faculties of thought and consciousness—faculties that rely on our extraordinary sense of smell.

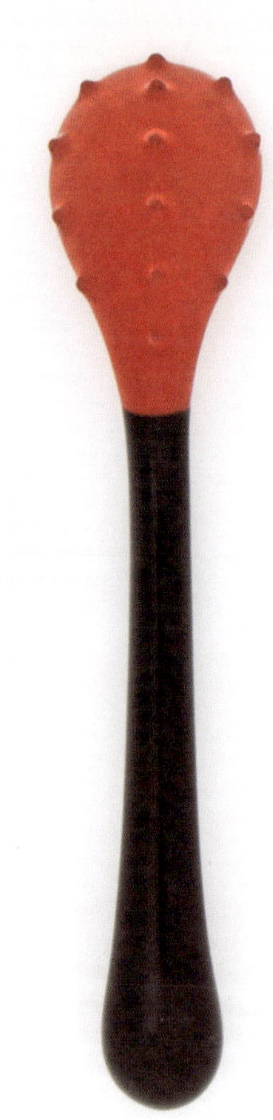

AEIOU VI Rear Bump Series, from the Sensory Dessert Spoon collection, 2016; Jinhyun Jeon (South Korean, b. 1981), Studio Jinhyun Jeon (Eindhoven, Netherlands, founded 2012); Ottchil-lacquered plastic; 2.8 × 2.2 × 13.3 cm (1 ⅛ × ⅞ × 5 ¼ in.); Courtesy of Jinhyun Jeon

Flavor is tactile

The sensation of eating doesn't stop with taste and smell. Touch receptors embedded in the skin of the mouth and tongue react to food's unique physical qualities. The movements of the tongue and jaw further shape our perception, as we experience the relative hardness, resistance, or granularity of the food we eat. Food can be smooth, slippery, gooey, gluey, glossy, stretchy, creamy, or fluffy. A slice of apple or a wedge of cheese changes as we chew, crush, swish, and swallow it. A spoonful of pudding slides down the throat, while a hunk of sirloin gives up a mighty fight. We also react to food's physical temperature and to the perceived heat of pepper or the coolness of mint. This diverse group of responses constitutes the mouthfeel or mouth-sense of food. Mouthfeel is a somatosensory phenomenon: *soma* (body) plus sensory. These embodied responses loom large in our perception of food and drink. Texture and temperature contribute to our instinctual belief that flavor resides in the mouth rather than the nose.

Flavor is visual

Visual cues—especially color—influence our perception of flavor. Color perception may have helped early humans know when fruit was ripe on the tree and find the yellow bananas in a sea of green. A human's ability to see color thus conferred an evolutionary advantage.[4] Vegetables pulped into a gray mass repel the appetite. Such mush suggests rot and decay—as compared to a fresh, bright salad. Designers use color to influence flavor experiences when they create packages, patterns, and surfaces that evoke or amplify sensations of taste and smell. A deep, warm brown evokes the buttery bitterness of chocolate. A greenish hue of yellow evokes the woodsy balm of citrus. A purple jellybean tastes something like a grape.

Flavor is aural

People munching popcorn in a movie theater hear it from inside their own heads. They can also hear the munching sounds of moviegoers in surrounding seats, as well as the clatter of ice cubes and the crinkle of candy wrappers. Eating makes noise. In Japan, slurping soup is an acceptable sign of gustatory pleasure; not so at a traditional Western dinner table. Sound and texture merge in words like "crispy," "crunchy," "crackly," and "fizzy." The English word "snack" sounds as crisp as a bag of pretzels or chips. Experimental psychologist Charles Spence studies the effects of sound on flavor. In a 2004 experiment, participants were asked to eat and evaluate Pringles potato chips. A Pringle is produced from a smooth potato slurry, yielding a perfectly blond, uniform wafer. As the subjects ate these identical salted snacks, Spence's team piped crunching sounds into headphones worn by each subject. Unbeknownst to the subjects, Spence's team was altering the loudness and frequency of the sounds. Participants tended to believe that the chips consumed with a louder, higher-frequency sound track were fresher than those with a quieter, lower sound.[5]

Schematic Illustrations of Ingredient Pairs, 2011; Yong-Yeol Ahn, Sebastian E. Ahnert, James P. Bagrow, and Albert-Laszló Barabási. The flavor of food is determined in part by chemical compounds that exist in many different ingredients. Coffee and beef have 102 flavor compounds in common; shrimp and lemon have only nine.

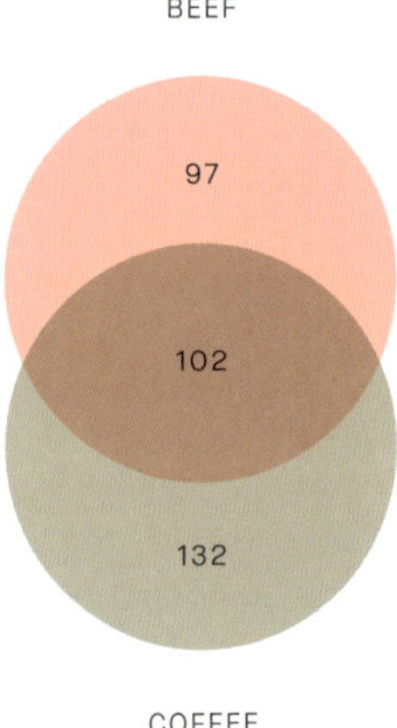

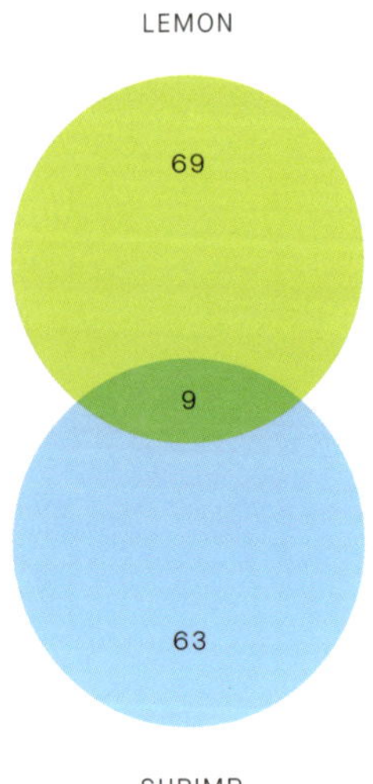

Flavor is contextual

Environmental factors change our flavor experiences as well. Designs for menus or packages prime our judgment of an item's freshness, cost, nutrition, and flavor. According to Brian Wansink, who has devoted his career to improving public health with behavioral psychology, "Most of us don't overeat because we are hungry. We overeat because of family and friends, packages and plates, names and numbers, labels and lights, colors and candles, shapes and smells, distractions and distances, cupboards and containers."[6] Wansink encouraged the US food industry to introduce 100-calorie snack packs, an antidote to king-size portions.

Flavor is a Gestalt

The brain fuses together scent, taste, texture, and other qualities. Flavor is a unified sensory object—a Gestalt—that unfurls in time and space. The flavor of strawberries is not merely sweet and tart; it derives its flowery, fruity aroma from a cocktail of chemicals, including acids combined with alcohol (called ethel esters) and furaneol, a chemical also found in pineapple, which has a nutty, caramel aroma.[7] The juicy meat of a strawberry is not the fruit itself, but is in fact auxiliary tissue beaded with hundreds of achenes, each one a tiny fruit enclosing a tiny seed. Those seeds give the strawberry its pocked and pebbly skin. A strawberry is a complex organism with a layered anatomy. Strawberry is also a myth, a cultural idea. It is the pink stripe that follows chocolate and vanilla. It is a symbol of sensory delight, a crucial node in a dictionary of iconic flavors.

Foodpairing® is a digital platform for developing new flavor combinations by matching ingredients that have common flavor components. Some chefs believe that foods with overlapping tastes harmonize, even when the combinations are surprising or nontraditional. Paired here: asparagus and cherry. The Foodpairing® tool includes a database of ingredients and methods for making and analyzing matches. Courtesy of Foodpairing® Inc.

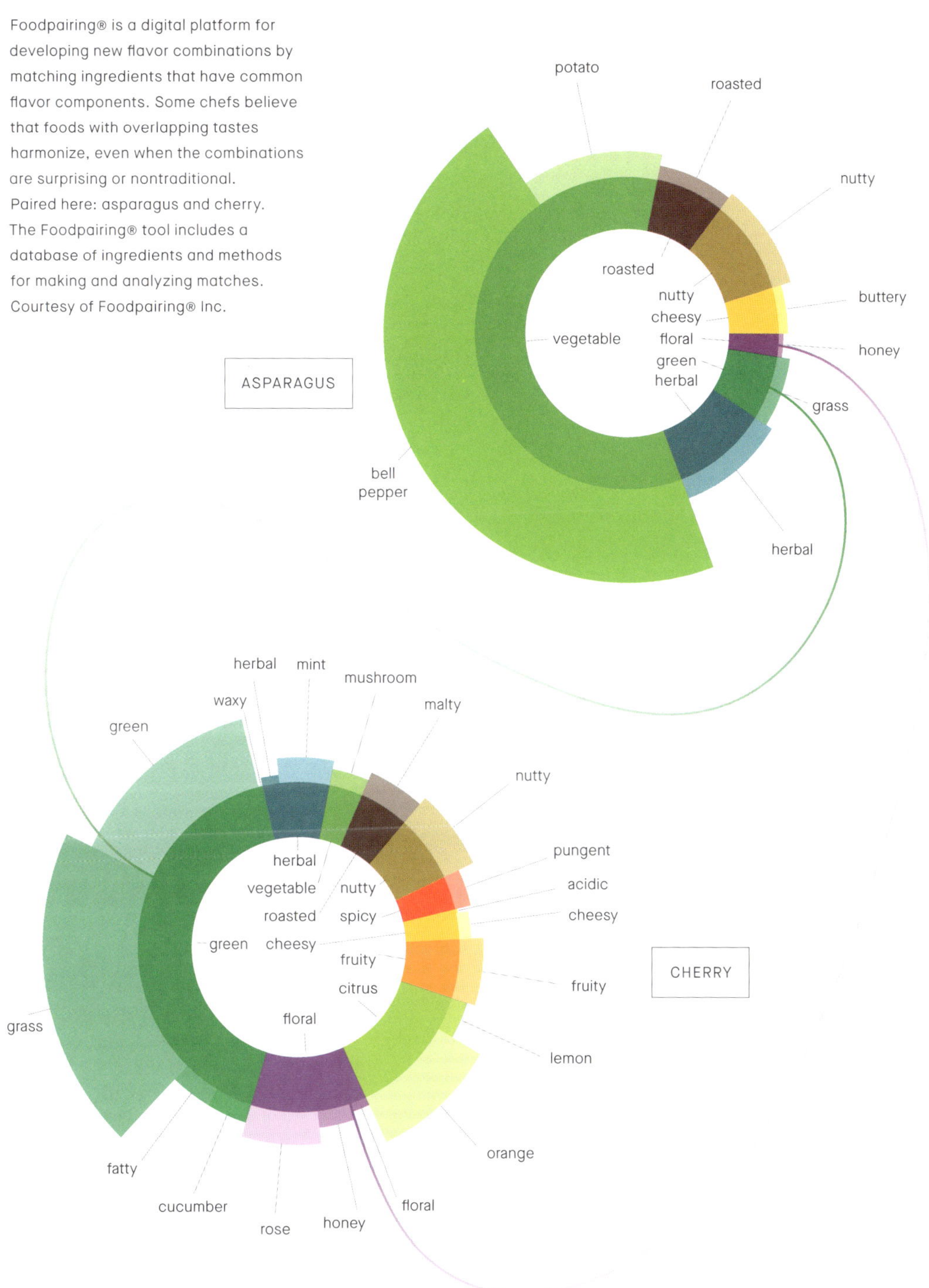

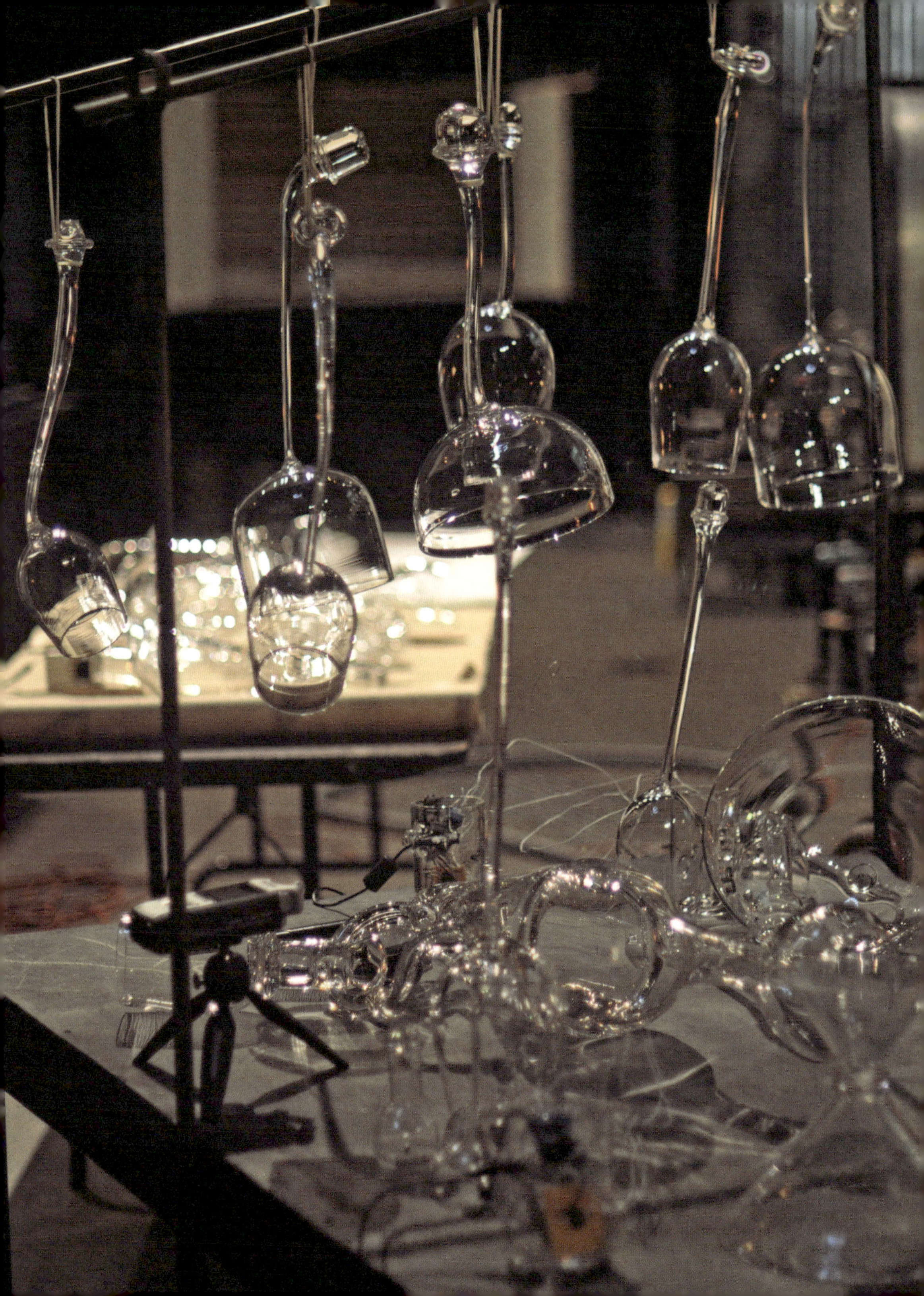

Sensory Materials

Paper or plastic, silk or wool, rubber or resin? Materials define the character of places and things. A surface could be hot or cold, hairy or slick. It could absorb waves of light or sound, or send echoes bouncing around a room. The tangible qualities of things include shape, smell, texture, rigidity, buoyancy, and weight. Light and air have presence, too. A humid day weighs us down with wetness and warmth. Fluorescent lights make a super-chilled supermarket feel even colder. Sensory design considers the many ways that materials impress the human mind and body.

Tympanum Temperament, 2014; Lili Maya (American, b. 1965) and James Rouvelle (American, b. 1967), Maya + Rouvelle (New York, New York, USA, founded 2009); Glass, magnets, electronics; Sizes vary; Courtesy of Maya + Rouvelle

In 1930, a young critic and historian of design named Beatrice Warde compared good typography to a crystal goblet. A properly designed page of text, she said, is a transparent vessel for content. Likewise, a glass of fine wine is best served in a clear glass vessel—not in a chalice crusted with gems. Among graphic designers, Warde's metaphor of the crystal goblet triggered decades of debate about form and content. She loved glass because it disappears. She exhorted designers to stay in the background, letting content take center stage.

Consider for a moment the materiality of glass. What do you see, touch, and hear? Not quite invisible, a glass of water shows itself in gleams of light. Glass pings to life as it jostles with the stuff around it. Shimmering with potential menace, glass speaks when a rock sails through a picture window or when cubes of ice drown their sorrows in a tumbler of scotch. Glass finds danger in its own fragility.

Artists Lili Maya and James Rouvelle play with the sonic qualities of glass in Pulse, Drift, Ping, Echo, assembled for Cooper Hewitt's exhibition *The Senses*. Scattered across a tabletop are a dozen or so overturned cones, domes, and droopy tubes of glass. Tiny spheres of metal roll around unbidden inside each upturned vessel. The spheres tap against the glass, making a gentle, irregular pattern of sound.

This piece is the latest in a series of installations begun by Maya + Rouvelle in 2014. Earlier pieces in the series include Tympanum Temperament, shown here. The glass artifacts were handmade by glassblowers during artist residencies at the Tacoma Museum of Glass and Pilchuk Glass School. Maya told us, "The glass pieces stem from goblets and vessels, while playfully hinting at shapes derived from the inner workings of the ear and from engine parts and plumbing fixtures." Maya and Rouvelle designed the pieces to ring and resonate, not to hold water. A glass element resembling a melting champagne flute is a delicate horn designed to conduct sound.

The little spheres rolling around inside the vessels are neodymium magnets. These powerful, rare-earth magnets appear in many commercial products, including cordless

Tympanum Temperament (detail), 2014; Lili Maya (American, b. 1965) and James Rouvelle (American, b. 1967), Maya + Rouvelle (New York, New York, USA, founded 2009); Glass, magnets, electronics; Sizes vary; Courtesy of Maya + Rouvelle

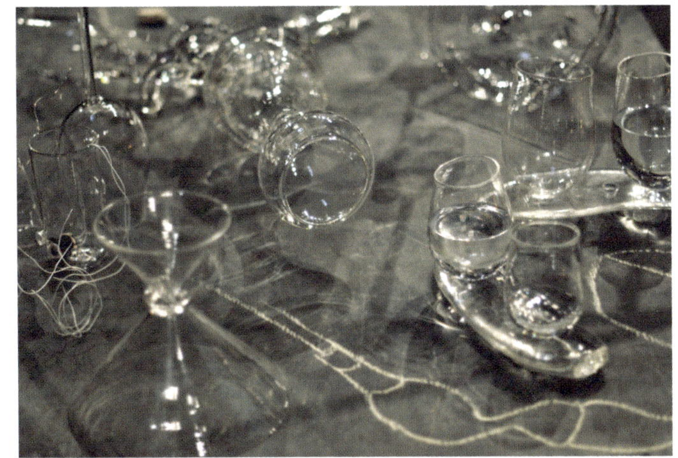

power tools and computer hard drives. Electromagnets installed beneath the tabletop produce magnetic fields. Sensors detecting changes in the electromagnetic field surrounding the piece instruct the electromagnets to switch their polarity from north/south to south/north. This causes the tiny spheres to change direction. The spheres assert their own dynamics as well, influencing one another and the larger magnetic field, in turn affecting the sensor that controls the electromagnets. Rouvelle explains, "What you see and hear on this tabletop is an example of chaos: a system of dynamic, individual elements influencing each other through complex feedback loops." Intricate relationships yield a rhythm that is random yet textured, like the sound of falling rain.

Cooper Hewitt asked Maya + Rouvelle to add a new sensory dimension to their piece: touch. Typically, the duo's glass installations are too dangerous for direct interaction. If a visitor were wearing a metal ring, one of the tiny super magnets could leap against the surface of the glass and shatter it to bits. To create a tactile experience, Maya + Rouvelle assembled a landscape of low, reclining sculptural objects tethered to the table. Inside are mechanisms that tap against the glass or gently vibrate in response to visitors. The pulsations vary in response to the same sensors that control the electromagnets, producing a tactile variant of this series of fascinating works.

A wineglass feels smooth to the touch. It seems to have its own temperature as well. A glass vessel feels warmer in our hands than a metal fork or a chunk of marble. A tin cup filled with hot coffee will burn your hands faster than a cup made of Styrofoam. Corian countertops feel warmer than granite or stainless steel. (Each surface also absorbs sound differently.)

Why do materials have different perceived temperatures? Glass, oak, and velvet are poor conductors of heat. When you walk across a concrete floor in bare feet, heat quickly flows into the slab from your body. A wool carpet will have the opposite effect; energy stays with you longer, because wool is a weak heat conductor. The pockets of air in the carpet heighten the impression of warmth. The piled surface prevents air from flowing across it and carrying away heat, and air itself is a poor conductor. Likewise, smooth bedsheets feel cool against your body because air flows freely against their surface, while fuzzy flannel sheets trap air and feel cozy. Fiberglass (made from tiny filaments of glass) is a great insulator because glass doesn't conduct heat well, and the space between the filaments slows down the flow of air and the transfer of heat.[1]

Air is thus a crucial component of materials. It hides among the fibers of a felt curtain, and it fills the cells of a foam-rubber mat. Air is also an active, dynamic medium unto itself. Daniel Wurtzel is a sculptor who works with air. He creates clouds of fabric, glitter, or mist that rise and fall, ripple and swirl, driven by currents of air. For a production of Shakespeare's *Tempest*, he sent panels of silk soaring out into the audience to conjure a ravenous storm. For the Winter Olympics in Sochi, 2014, he made sheets of paper rise out of giant books to form a turning, twirling, diaphanous tower—a metaphor for snow and for the tradition of Russian literature. Wurtzel's Feather Fountain brings viewers closer. Vents circling the round base shoot streams of air inward across the fountain floor. The air currents meet in the center, making hundreds of feathers levitate toward the ceiling. At a certain height, gravity takes over and the feathers float back down, only to be picked up again by the ceaseless draft. The feathers

Feather Fountain, 2008; Daniel Wurtzel (American, b. 1962); Feathers, mirrors, fiberglass ring; 35.6 × 236.2 cm diam. (14 in. × 7 ft. 9 in.); Courtesy of Daniel Wurtzel

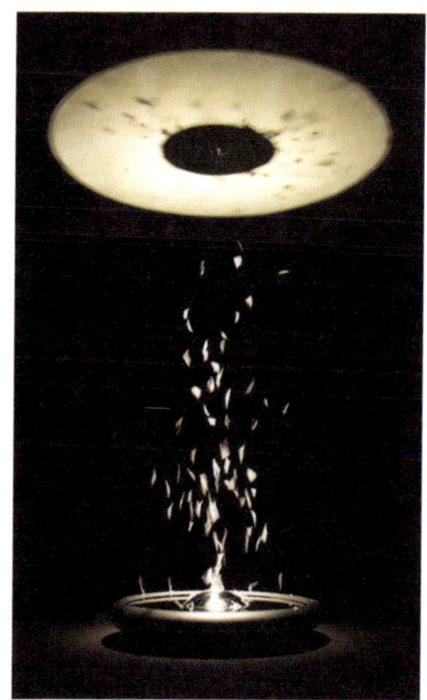

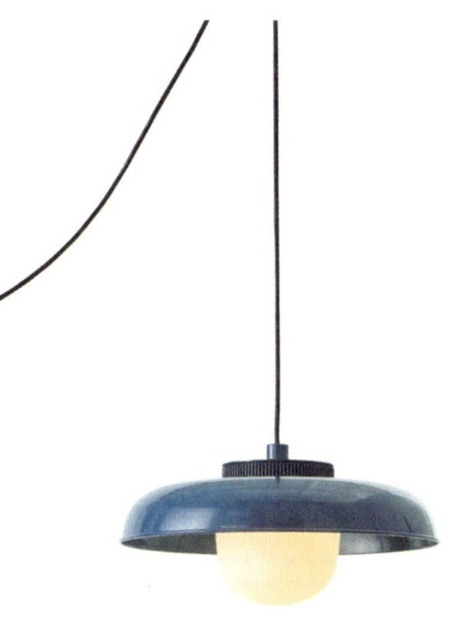

Lighting Fixture, Meyer Davis Hoist Pendant; Rich Brilliant Willing (New York, New York, USA, founded 2009); Cast glass diffuser, steel shade, aluminum module; 36 × 18 cm diam. (14 × 7 in.); Courtesy of Rich Brilliant Willing

plink like raindrops when they make landfall. Each feather is itself a brilliant piece of aerodynamic design. A curious thing happens when a wayward feather drifts outside the bowl of the fountain, says Wurtzel: "People tend to pick up the lost feathers and put them back into the air column. Visitors are naturally curious to see what happens."

Light is a material, too. Light models form with shadow and contrast, and it confuses the eye with reflections and glare. Light is a symbol of truth, but it's also a trickster. Changing with time, it makes everything it touches change, too. It strikes us as warm or cool, hard or soft, depending on its intensity and color temperature. Industrial designer Theo Richardson, talking to us about how light shapes the character of a space, said, "Light surrounds us like a fragrance."[2] His company Rich Brilliant Willing (RBW) designs and manufactures light fixtures in Brooklyn, New York. From the cool white of daylight to the warm honey of a candle, light bathes people and things in a tactile glow. Richardson told us, "A room consists of layers of sensory experience—from cut glass to shaggy carpet to raw wood to the light falling from a fixture."

Studio Banana, a multidisciplinary design studio with outposts in Spain, Switzerland, and the UK, generates playful objects with lifelike personalities. Their Kangaroo light is a sheet of quilted silicone with twenty-four LEDs hiding inside. Different settings allow the bendable, portable Kangaroo to blink, pulse, or emit a steady glow. Sensory deprivation is

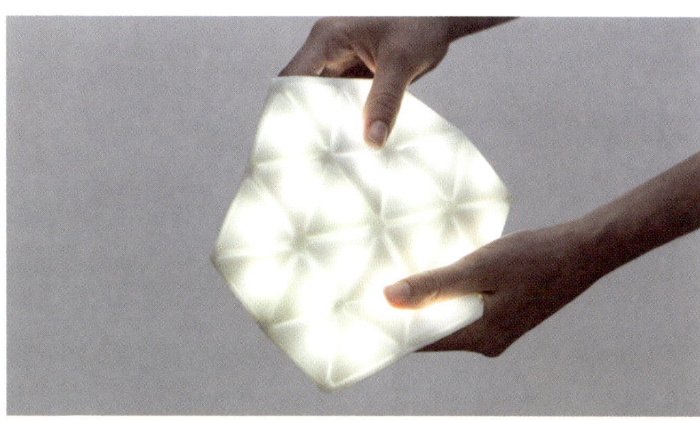

Kangaroo Light, 2014; Studio Banana (Madrid, Spain; London, United Kingdom; Lausanne, Switzerland, founded 2007); Silicone, LEDs, lithium-ion battery; 19 × 19 cm (7 15⁄32 × 7 15⁄32 in.); Courtesy of Studio Banana

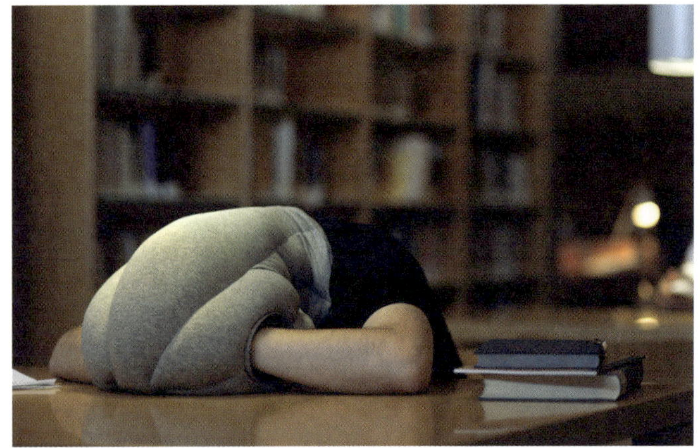

OSTRICHPILLOW Original, 2012; Studio Banana (Madrid, Spain; London, United Kingdom; Lausanne, Switzerland, founded 2007); Viscose, elastomer, polystyrene microbeads; 45 × 28 × 15 cm (17 11⁄16 × 11 × 5 7⁄8 in.); Courtesy of Studio Banana

another delight for Studio Banana. Their OSTRICHPILLOW is a napping tool for overworked millennials. This padded object shuts out light and sound, offering a modicum of privacy to persons compelled to sleep in public places, from office cubicles to airline seats. The masklike OSTRICH is a portable sleeping chamber—part pillow and part portable architecture. Accounting for a full upper-body experience, it includes holes for tucking the arms into a resting place beneath the head.

Materials change the sound of a room. Hard materials reflect sound, creating echoes that make a space noisy and blur the sounds of speech. Soft materials absorb sound, clarifying the sonic experience of a space. Furniture is an acoustic instrument. Wakufuru, designed by Johan Kauppi, is a family of tables and benches designed to be quiet both visually and acoustically. According to Kauppi, "Wood as a material always contributes a natural warmth to interiors. I wanted to find out if solid wood furniture could also reflect some of the sound atmosphere that is experienced in forests."[3] Produced by the

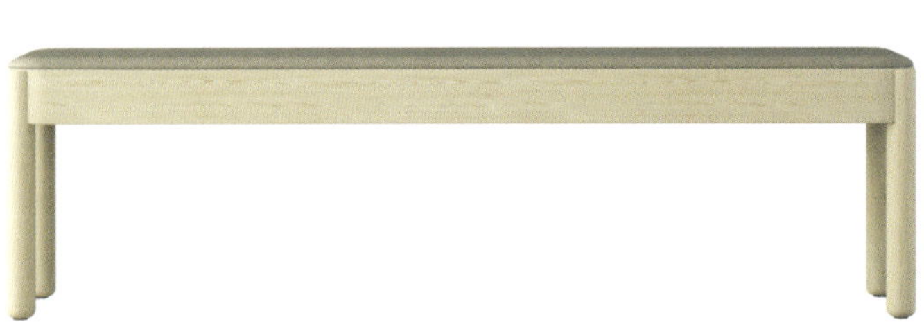

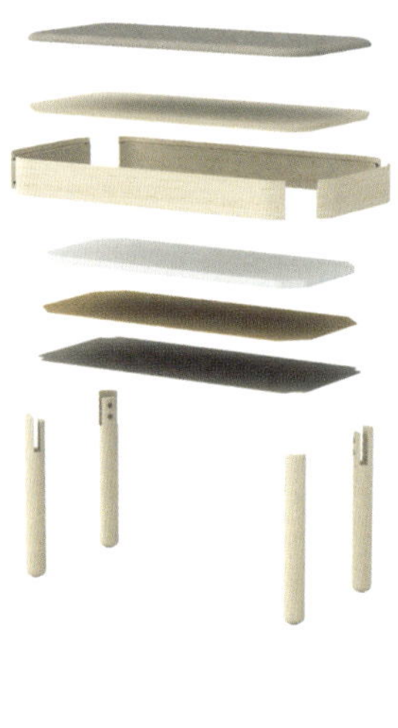

Wakufuru Bench and exploded view, 2017; Johan Kauppi (Swedish, b. 1975), manufactured by Glimakra of Sweden (Glimakra, Sweden, founded 1948); Wood, top in veneered MDF; Acoustic filling: formfelt, perforated board, and polyether; Sizes vary, up to 160 × 80 × 45 cm (5 ft. 3 in. × 31 1⁄2 in. × 17 11⁄16 in.); Courtesy of Johan Kauppi

THIS PAGE: Virginia San Fratello (American, b. 1971) and Ronald Rael (American, b. 1971), Studio Rael Fratello (Oakland, California, USA, founded 1995) and Emerging Objects (Oakland, California, USA, founded 2012); Courtesy of Emerging Objects

Swedish company Glimakra for cafes and public places, each piece has three layers of sound-absorbing material beneath the top surface. An air gap further dampens the sound.

Ronald Rael and Virginia San Fratello, founders of Emerging Objects and Studio Rael San Fratello, are avid explorers of the material landscape. By devising their own 3D-printing processes, they are creating forms and substances with unique structural and tactile qualities. Trained as architects, they view themselves as material scientists and cooks, "inventing recipes that would allow us to ask questions about the future of architecture through the lens of 3D printing." Objects and structures printed from salt, cement, ceramics, and plant-based plastic binders are prototypes for new sustainable construction methods that could employ materials on hand at a site. Sensuality matters, too. Exploring materials that could be eaten or consumed, they have printed vessels from coffee, tea, sugar, curry, and the skins of Chardonnay grapes.[4]

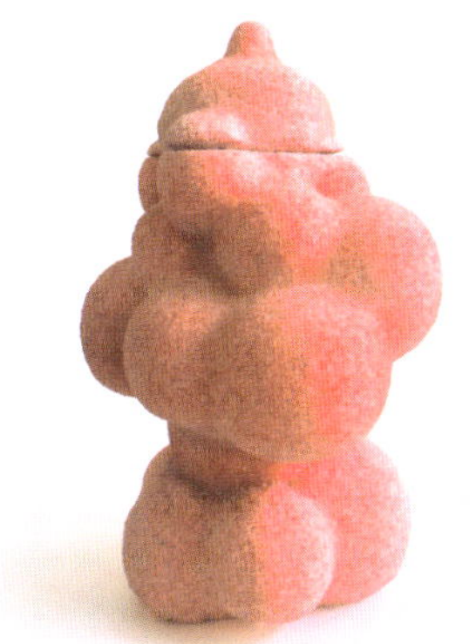

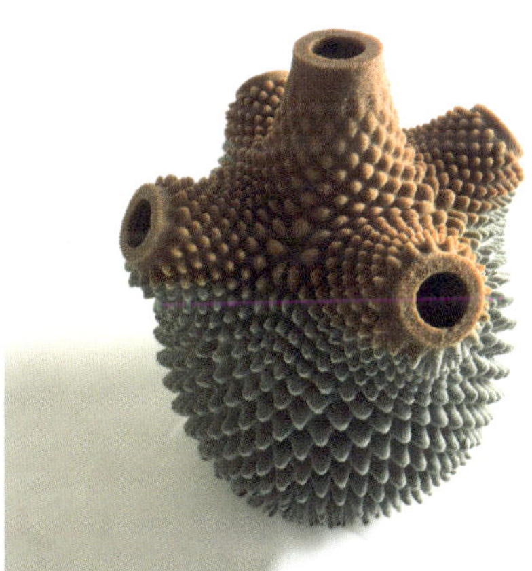

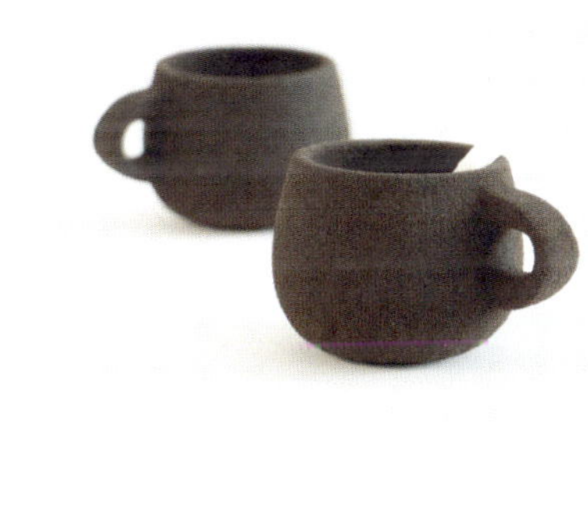

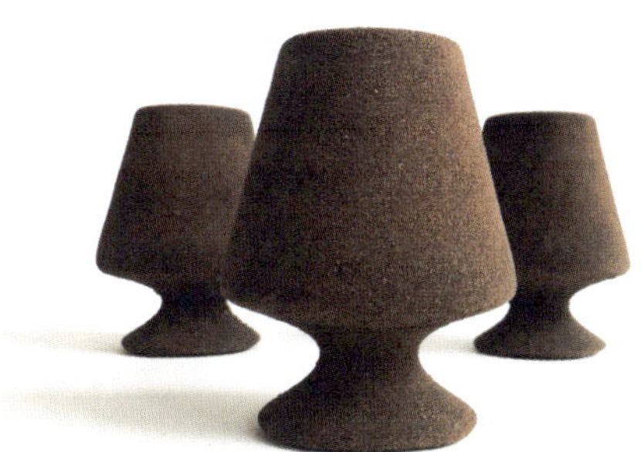

TOP LEFT: Cotton Candy Dish, 2017; 3D-printed sugar, aromatics; 30.5 × 15.2 × 15.2 cm (12 × 6 × 6 in.).
MIDDLE: Furry Curry, 2017; 3D-printed cement, curry; 15.2 × 15.2 × 17.8 cm (5 31⁄32 × 5 31⁄32 × 7 in.).
TOP RIGHT: Coffee Cups, 2015; 3D-printed coffee; Each: 7.6 × 8.9 × 5.7 cm (3 × 3 ½ × 2 ¼ in.).
BOTTOM RIGHT: Chardonnay Wine Goblets, 2017; 3D-printed chardonnay skins and seeds; Each: 11.4 × 11.4 × 9.1 cm (4 ½ × 4 ½ × 3 19⁄32 in.); Courtesy of Emerging Objects

Textured surfaces feel warm because they slow down the flow of air. Visible textures can add warmth to any work of design—even when the texture isn't physically touched. A rough concrete wall seen from a distance or a grainy scrim applied to a digital photograph changes our mental response to what we are looking at. We touch with our eyes. The mere illusion of texture evokes past interactions with real materials. A craggy surface simulated on a screen or printed on a wallcovering stirs expectations of touch, adding depth to our encounters with flat surfaces and virtual objects.

Layers of hand-torn paper give dimension and texture to Snarkitecture's non-repeat wallpaper, Topographies. Created with Calico, the wallcovering is a two-dimensional exploration of excavation as architectural process—Snarkitecture's signature aesthetic. To create the design, founders Alex Mustonen and Daniel Arsham stacked reams of oversize cotton rag paper and tore each sheet by hand, exposing the fibers. The contours of the torn sheets resemble the curved lines used in maps to show the topography of a landscape. The texture is reproduced in such high fidelity we can imagine touching the paper's pulp and enter an otherwise unseen landscape. The paper is treated as a three-dimensional structure with interiority, revealing and concealing a process.

Wallcovering, Topographies, 2017; Snarkitecture (New York, New York, USA, founded 2008), manufactured by Calico Wallpaper (Brooklyn, New York, USA, founded 2013); Vinyl; Non-repeating custom print; Photo by Lauren Coleman, Courtesy of Calico Wallpaper

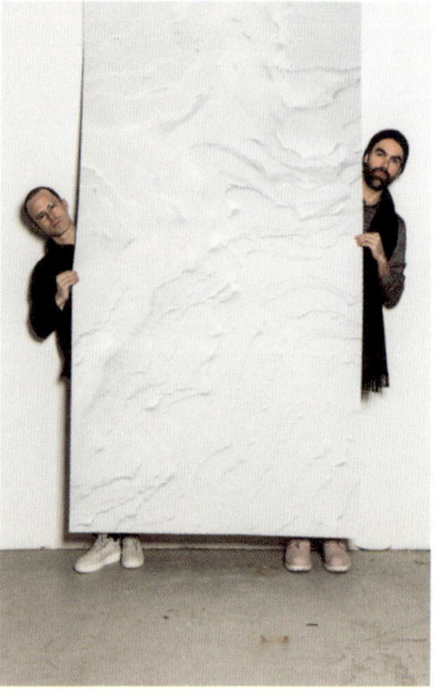

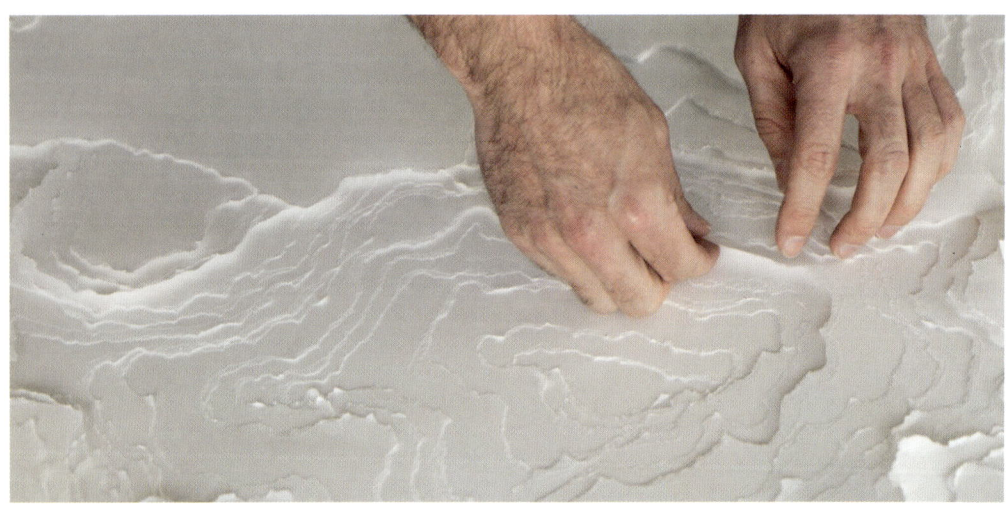

Treasures 1, 2016; Anny Wang (Swedish, b. 1990) and Tim Söderström (Swedish, b. 1988), Wang & Söderström (Copenhagen, Denmark, founded 2016); 3D software: 3Ds Max, Vray, Modo; Courtesy of Wang & Söderström

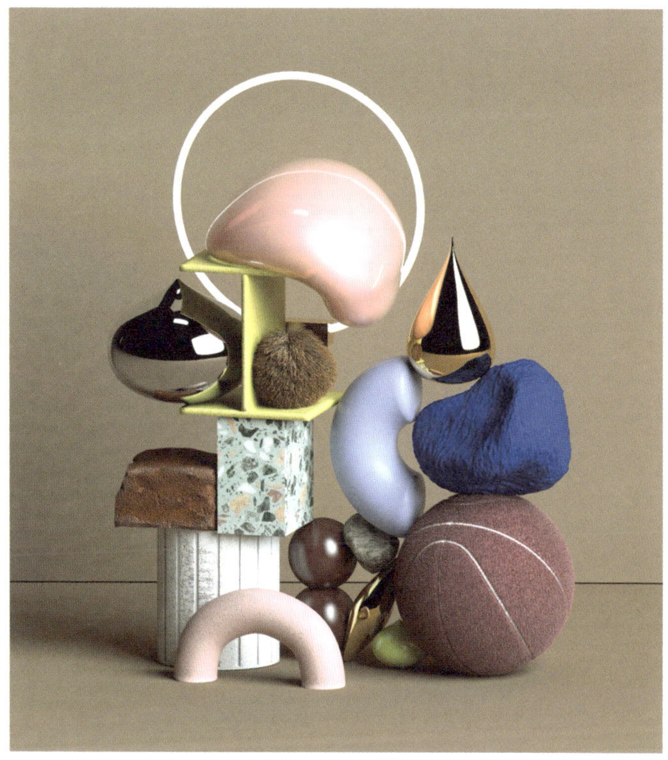

The hyperreal illustrations and animations of Wang & Söderström are populated with imaginary objects, constructed entirely with 3D software. Candy-colored objects stacked in a compact still life beg to be touched and tasted. Blobs of metallic gel shimmer in a sugary pink void. Vases manufactured from paper-thin porcelain shatter along a slow-motion path of destruction. The surfaces coating this eerie artificial world are pebbly, furry, shiny, squashy, viscous, or reflective. This work pumps up the illusory effects of today's digital rendering tools. The 3D software used by architects, product designers, and game designers is stocked with dictionaries of simulated materials. A cube or a sphere can become wood, marble, or glass with little thought about the properties of physical things. Wang & Söderström amplify the fakery of product renderings and futuristic fly-throughs to create places and things glistening with toxic allure.

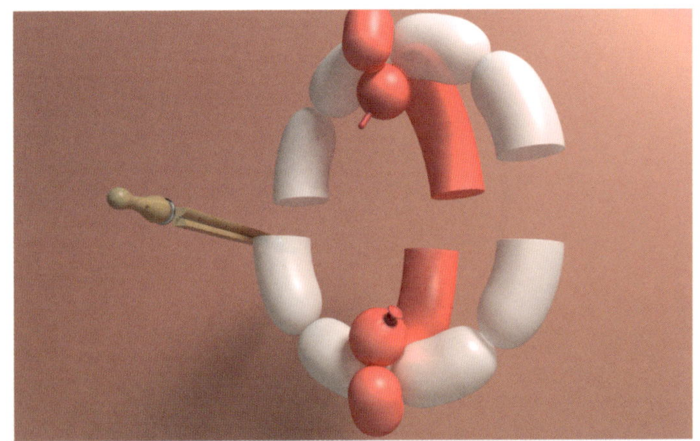

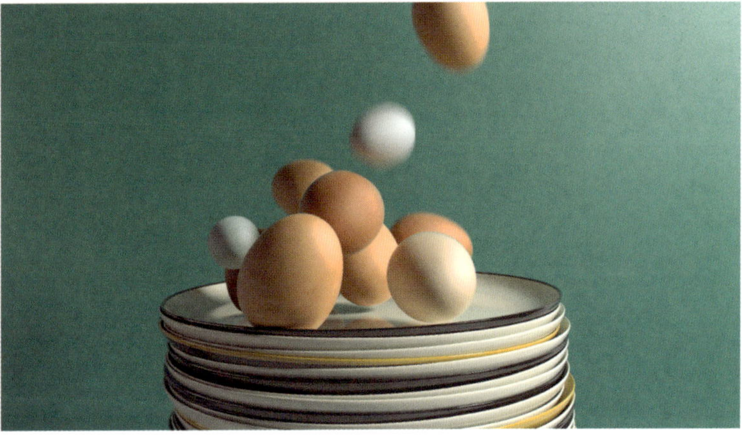

Artificial objects come to life in the 3D animation *For Approval*, produced by Mainframe and directed by Chris Hardcastle. We predict how an object will behave based on sight. *For Approval* subverts those expectations. Eggs dropped on a ceramic plate bounce instead of breaking, their shells deforming like soft rubber. Balloons should burst when pierced with a knife, but these are as dense as sausages. A glass of milk should spill when knocked over, but this glass melts away like water, leaving behind a solid white core of milk. The texture, weight, density, and brittleness of these simulated objects can be judged and understood through visual means—and then altered for narrative effect.

For Approval (stills), 2017; Chris Hardcastle (British, b. 1975), Ben Black (British, b. 1985), and Jack Brown (British, b. 1986), Mainframe (Manchester, UK, founded 2008); Autodesk Maya, V-Ray; Courtesy of Mainframe

Active Textiles, 2017–18; Self Assembly Lab, MIT (Cambridge, Massachusetts, USA, founded 2013); Steelcase (Grand Rapids, Michigan, USA, founded 1912); Designtex (New York, New York, USA, founded 1961); Textile combined with active polymers; approx. 101.6 × 50.8 × 35.6 cm (40 × 20 × 14 in.); Photo Courtesy of Self Assembly Lab, MIT

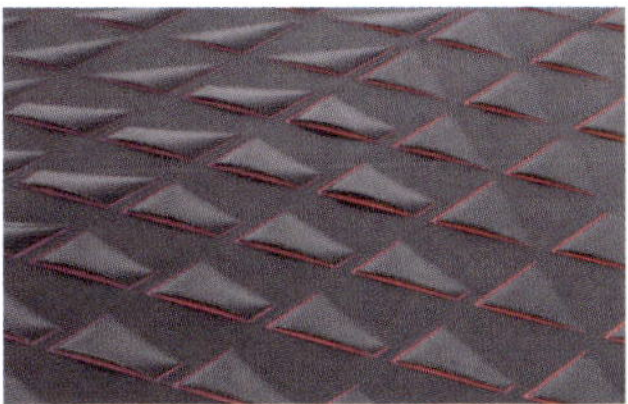

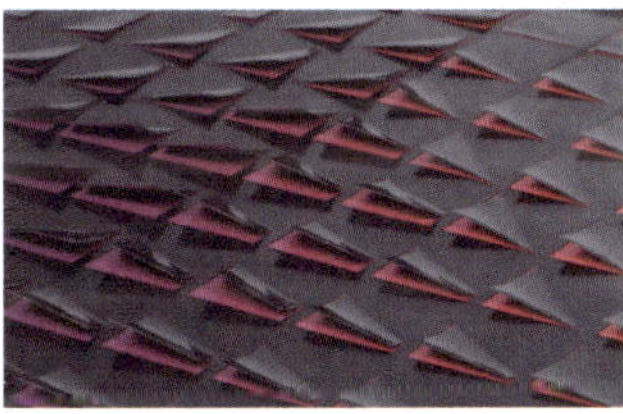

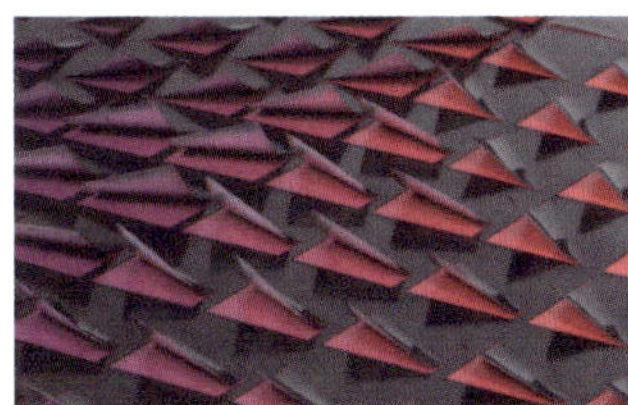

Designers consider warmth and texture (real or illusory) when choosing materials for products or rooms. When describing a classroom filled with hard furniture and fluorescent lights as "cold," we mix and match the qualities of materials—tactile, emotional, acoustic, and kinetic. Weight and sound are important, too. How heavy is a book or a bar stool? Is a table or chair designed to be moved around or left in place? A plastic chair is easier to pick up than a metal one, and it clatters less when stacked. Is a curtain designed to drift in the breeze or cloak a room in stillness? Conservator and fashion curator Sarah Scaturro spoke to us about sound in the history of fashion. When Christian Dior launched his "New Look" in 1947, with its narrow waists and wide skirts, he was not only celebrating the end of wartime austerity but also reviving the rustle of Edwardian silk from his childhood. Beads, straw, and high-heeled shoes all make distinctive sounds. Velvet offers the opposite. Its deep pile absorbs sound as well as light.[5] Black-box theaters and hotel ballrooms are hushed by floor-to-ceiling velvet curtains.

Materials respond to their environment. Skylar Tibbits, codirector and founder of the Self-Assembly Lab at MIT's International Design Center, conducts research into methods of "programming" synthetic or natural materials through means of self-folding, tension, or curling. All materials react to something—temperature, moisture, or friction. Laser-cut wood veneer bends, folds, and curls in on itself based on the striation of the cut. Textile structures can be designed to expand and contract in response to temperature changes. Imagine jackets, sneakers, or car seats that adapt and respond to their user's body temperature. As Tibbits tells us, "by printing or otherwise assembling materials to optimize their response to other conditions, they can be programmed to fold, curl, and respond."[6]

For Cooper Hewitt's *Senses* exhibition, Tibbits collaborated with Designtex and Steelcase to demonstrate how programmable materials can enter our living spaces. Perforations in a composite textile are programmed to open and close in response to light and heat. In front of a light fixture, the textile's perforations open to reveal patterned shadows cast on the wall around it. Turn the light off and the textile contracts and closes to reveal another texture. As a curtain in a window, the textile's perforations could be programmed to close in response to bright sun, providing necessary shading, and to open when a cloud passes. The textiles seem to breathe, like gills in the water, with textures and patterns that are both functional and poetic.

Materiality invites an embodied response, influencing how we interact with something. We bristle away from a porcupine's quills. We stroke a cat's long fur and pat a dog's matte hair. We sit erect in hard plastic chairs and slump and curl ourselves in the cushioned support of couches. Touch provides a universal interface, guiding our gestures and interactions. For Roos Meerman, tactility humanizes our interaction with technology. She designs tactile interfaces whose materiality invites desired gestures, rather than instructing users to wave or flap their arms in front of a screen. The Tactile Orchestra is an installation she created with KunstLAB Arnhem. In it, users stroke a wall covered in a furry material to control the intensity and instruments of a musical composition. The "furriness" directs the interaction. As Meerman tells us, "almost everyone approaches something furry with the same response. They want to stroke it."[7]

For the *Senses* exhibition, Cooper Hewitt invited Meerman to create a new version of her Tactile Orchestra installation. Synthetic fur covers a wall that is curved to undulate like a wave. Users stroke and sweep the fur with their hands, arms, and bodies, activating a piece of a musical composition that plays from binaural speakers overhead. The music is composed of string instruments. As Meerman explains, the string instruments more closely align with the act of stroking than would, say, percussion instruments. The composition is divided into six sections, tuned to different parts of the wall. When a user strokes one section of the wall, the strings programmed to that section play. When another participant touches the wall, strings in their section are added to the

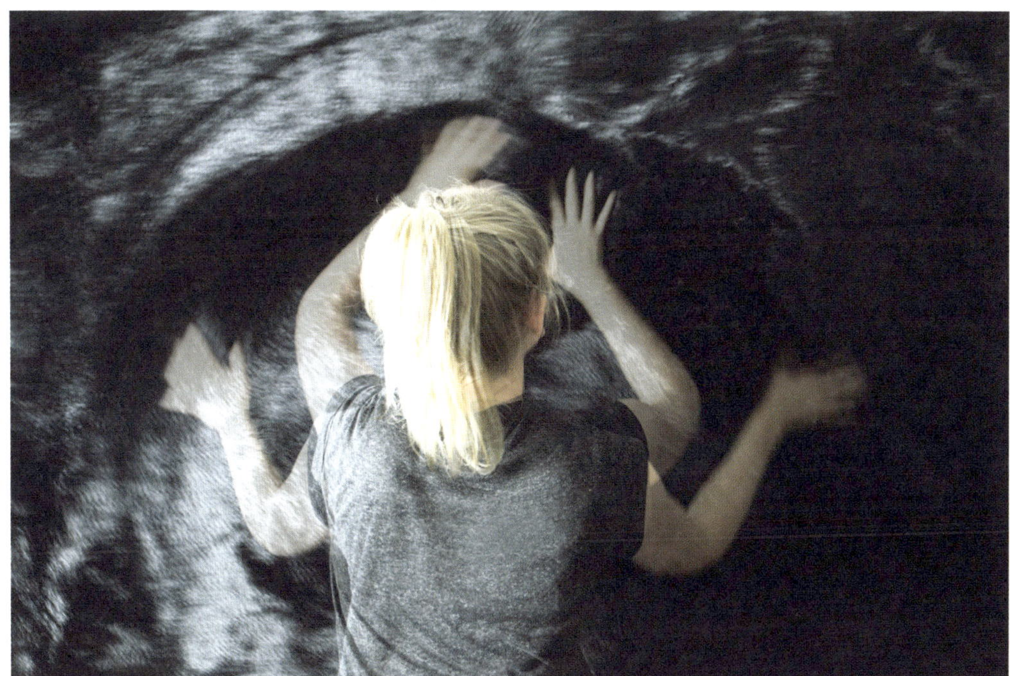

Tactile Orchestra, 2015; Roos Meerman (Dutch, b. 1991), Studio Roos Meerman (Arnhem, Netherlands, founded 2014) with Stefanie Hesseling (Dutch, b. 1985), Tom Kortbeek (Dutch, b. 1987) and Tim Rouschop (Dutch, b. 1988), KunstLAB Arnhem (Arnhem, Netherlands, founded 2014); Textiles, wood, electronics; 460 × 230 cm (15 ft. × 7 ft. 6 in.); © Xandravander Eijk

composition, which both participants hear. Multiple users are needed to "play" the full composition, suggestive of the orchestra itself. Meerman leverages our embodied response to material.

Materials are the flesh and bones of objects and buildings. Glass, wood, and silicone breathe, shift, and sigh. A curtain or bench absorbs sound. Light bounces, reflects, and floods the periphery—light is not a thing, but it changes everything. Textures speak to the eye as well as to the hand, incising flat surfaces with real or imaginary depth where the restless gaze can wander. Sensory design considers materiality across multiple dimensions, from the visible to beyond.

Renderings and prototype, exhibition design for *The Senses: Design Beyond Vision*, Cooper Hewitt, Smithsonian Design Museum, New York, 2017; Studio Joseph; Curtain made from Bolon fibers

Studio Joseph's exhibition design for Cooper Hewitt's exhibtion *The Senses* features curving transparent partitions woven from colored strands of nylon fiber. The fiber is manufactured by Bolon for use in floor and wallcoverings. Throughout the exhibition, rich textures form the interface between people and objects.

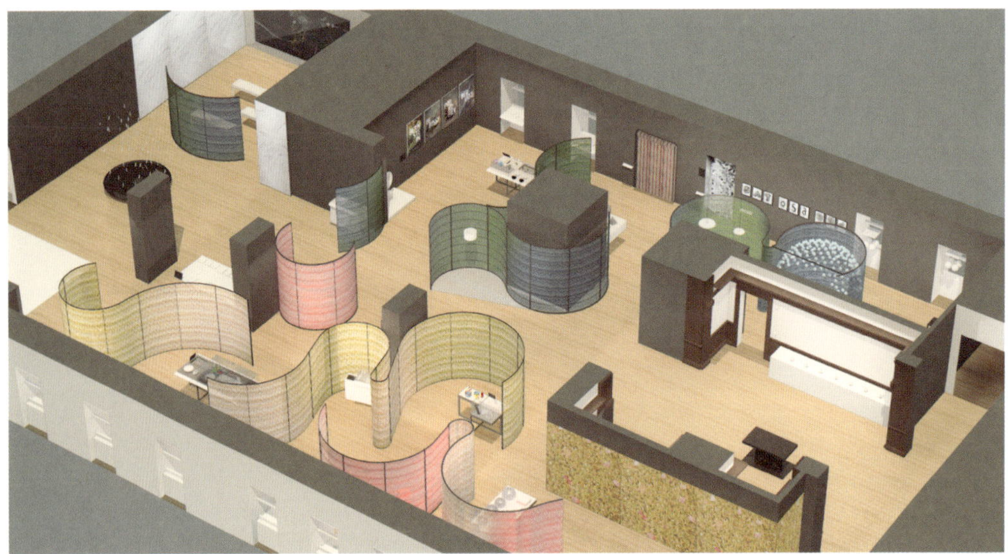

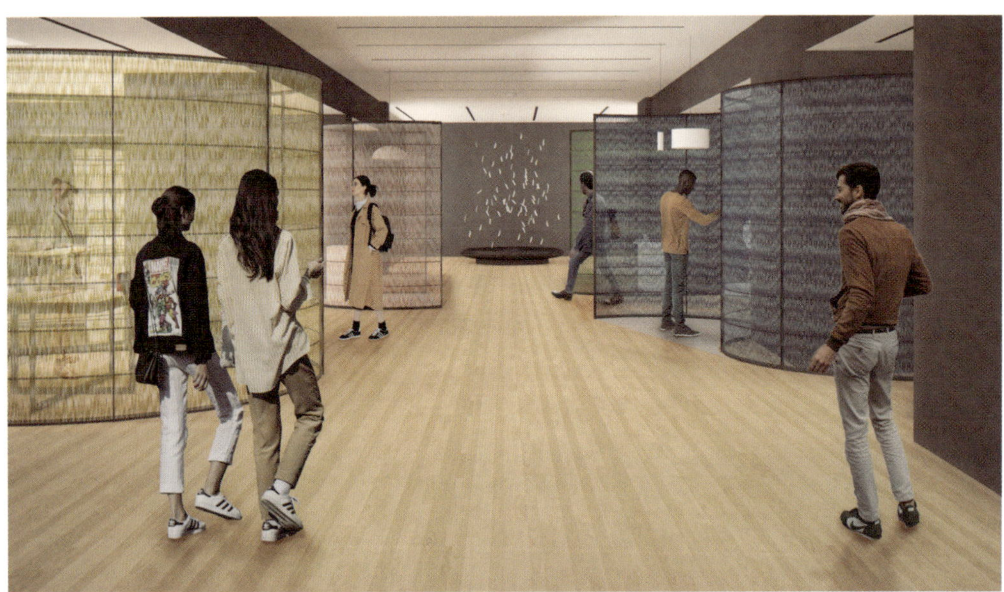

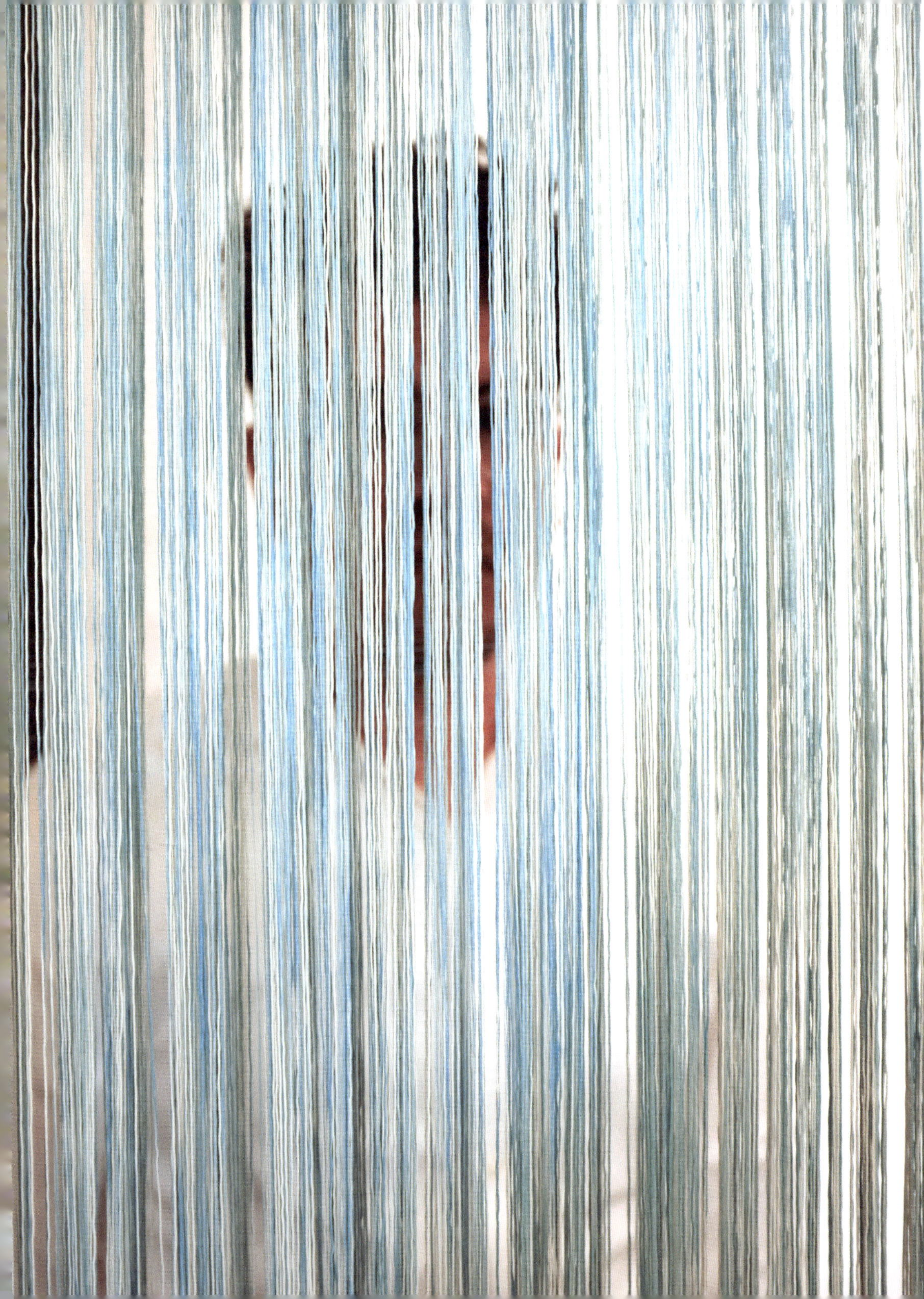

Rich Brilliant Willing

Designing with Light

No aspect of an interior more powerfully shapes our sense of well-being than quality of light. In a restaurant or hotel lobby, a warm, welcoming light puts us at ease. In the workplace, light sets the tone of our day, lifting the mood and inspiring productivity. At home, light enlivens mealtimes, morning routines, and the moments we spend with friends.

Despite its constant presence, light is notoriously difficult to describe. Our perception of light is relative, rather than absolute, and so while we can easily measure the universal qualities of light itself, our individual physiological functions challenge our understanding and ability to articulate our experiences. A number of factors influence what we see, including the contrast of light against its environment. The amount of light emitted by a small lamp, for example, appears much brighter at night than in the light of day. Additionally, the adaptive physiology that allows our to eyes adjust quickly to the dark also complicates our perceptions. Designing an environment with a desired sense of atmosphere, therefore, requires the consideration of light's quantifiable and perceptual qualities.

RICH BRILLIANT WILLING was founded in 2009 by Theo Richardson, Charles Brill, and Alexander Williams. RBW is a Brooklyn-based studio that designs and manufactures innovative LED fixtures. Cooper Hewitt invited RBW to create a lighting installation for *The Senses* exhibition, and to author the following guide to designing understanding light's qualities.

Light: How Much Is Enough?

Light is measured in several ways, including the amount of light at the source and the amount of light arriving on a given surface. In the International System of Units (the modern form of the metric system), the amount of light at the source is the lumen. The lumen is often incorrectly confused with the watt, a measurement traditionally stamped on incandescent lightbulbs indicating the amount of energy consumed. More efficient contemporary light sources, including the LED, consume fewer watts yet yield more lumens.

Looking beyond measurements alone, an effective designer takes into account the human experience. These myriad considerations include intended application, desired ambiance, and the materiality of surfaces as well as age of users. In the realm of architecture and interior design, our innate inability to describe light poses an extra obstacle.

THINKING ABOUT LIGHT

- Envision your space with light before considering fixtures. Which surfaces should draw attention? Which should recede? Where is the visual focus?
- Apply layers of light: an overall or ambient layer for comfort, focal lighting on important objects, and decorative elements that add sparkle and depth. Avoid bland, uniformly lit spaces.
- Light selectively, placing light where it's needed and minimizing it elsewhere.
- We see by contrast. In a softly lit environment, a little light can do a lot of good.
- Distribute light around the space; avoid concentrating all the lumens in one place. It is more comfortable—and more effective—to have multiple "points of light" than a few very bright fixtures.
- Adjust the quantity light with dimming controls. This will help in balancing brightness around the space and adapting the lighting for different activities and users.

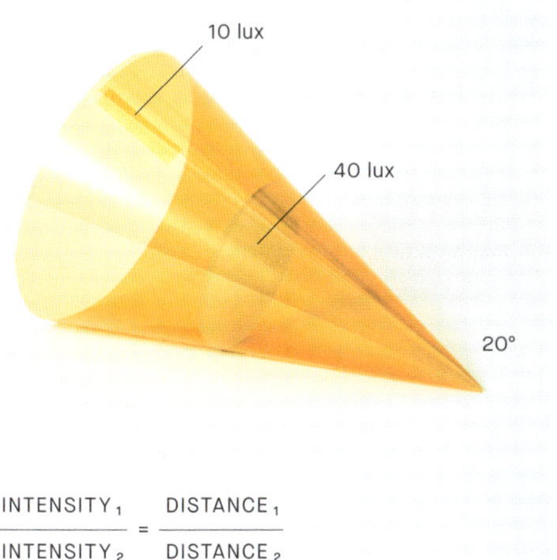

INVERSE SQUARE LAW

In the illustration, a 20° beam of light is represented by a cone. If the source were 100 lumens, then at a 5-meter distance, the amount light arriving at the surface would be 40 lux. (The lux is the unit of measure for the amount of light on a given surface in lumens per square meter.) According to the Inverse Square Law, to find the lux at E1, $E1=(d1/d2)^2*E2$. Doubling the distance between source to surface reduces the lux by $(2)^2$, or 4 times. Practically speaking, a larger room therefore requires more light.

A Whiter Shade of Pale

There are typically two reasons why someone would proclaim to dislike a certain type of light. Both reasons relate to colorimetry, the science of color perception. Sometimes light seems too cold in appearance, with a blueish cast. Other times, it appears too warm and yellow. The apparent color of light is described with Correlated Color Temperature (CCT). The standard CCT unit of measure is the Kelvin. The warm yellows of a match flame measure around 2000K, and the clear daylight of a bright blue sky measures upwards of 10,000K. Counterintuitively, warm colors have lower temperatures than cool ones. Ideal color temperatures match the intended purpose of a space. Cooler colors function well to promote a sense of alertness, and we tend to expect these environments to be brighter. The inviting, tactile quality of warmer colors fits more intimate settings, which tend toward lower light levels.

THINKING ABOUT LIGHT

- Color consistency among fixtures is important. Similar fixtures should look the same.
- Color temperature varies over the course of the day, influencing the activities and mood of a space.
- Dynamic color temperature is a feature of some LED products. Look for user friendly features such as Warm Dim or Dim to Warm. These LEDs get warmer as they dim, unlike standard LEDs, which get cooler when dimmed. Professional products such as Tunable White or Natural Light have more expansive and complex variables.
- Color temperature influences the appearance of interiors, finishes, and fabrics: cool light favors blues, greens, silver and gray; warm light favors reds, yellows, wood, leather, gold, and bronze.

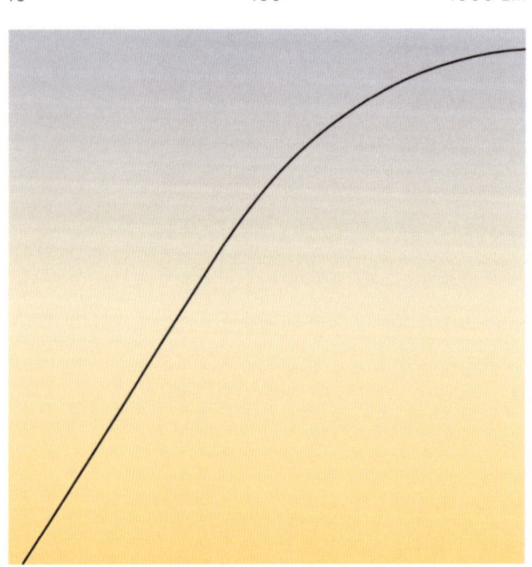

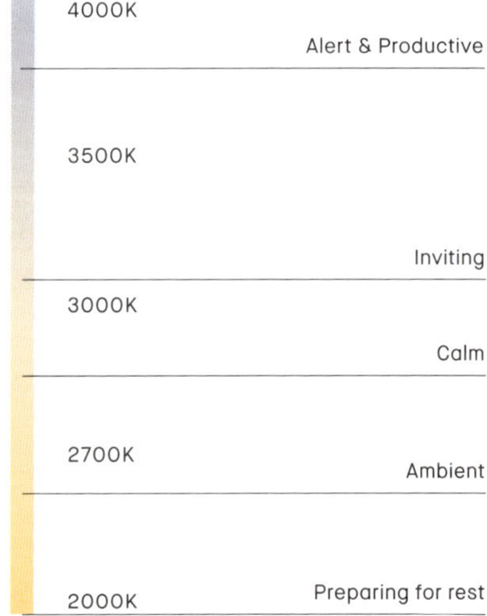

The Art of Fidelity

We count on the ability of light to produce expected and natural colors, such as skin tones or the appearance of fruits and vegetables. Deviation from naturalness, or a lack of fidelity, is a measurable characteristic of light.

The invention of the fluorescent bulb, infamous for casting skin tones in greenish, sickly hues, also gave rise to a testing method to address the hue shift and saturation of color caused by these new lamps. The CRI, or Color Rendering Index, was established in the 1960s to measure a light source's accuracy when illuminating an object against a specific benchmark: the incandescent bulb. The range of values was arbitrarily set so that the maximum CRI would produce a score of 100, and a warm white fluorescent would produce a score of 50.

Today's technologies (including LED and incandescent enhanced with neodymium) offer a wider, more saturated range of color. The aisles of many grocery stores likely offer greener bell peppers and redder steaks because the lighting has been designed to produce higher saturation of these specific colors. The resulting CRI scores of such highly saturated light sources are inherently lower than 100. CRI values above 85 are generally acceptable, and it is important to point out that higher scores do not necessarily correspond with greater preference in the general population. CRI testing today is achieved by comparing fourteen color chips (R1 to R14) to a reference source of the same color temperature. A score of 100 indicates a perfect match to the original benchmark, the colors as produced by an incandescent bulb.

There are two faults in the score. One lies in the benchmark itself—who is to say a limited set of fourteen swatches and the incandescent bulb represent colors optimally? The second fault is that a single metric score oversimplifies, combining saturation and hue shift.

TM-30-15, launched in 2015, is a more nuanced system of measuring and communicating color rendition. It measures fidelity against an expanded rubric of 99 color samples and presents results in a graphical form to describe hue shift and saturation that the CRI system fails to address.

THINKING ABOUT LIGHT

- Not all spaces will necessitate high color fidelity.
- Small differences in CRI values are generally unimportant, and values above 85 are typically acceptable.
- When choosing a source or fixture, select the appropriate color temperature first, then consider color rendering.
- For pleasing facial tones, choose light sources rich in red and evaluate the source on your hands or face.
- For specialized applications where color is critical, use the TM-30 metric to evaluate options.

QUALITY & FIDELITY

The Color Rendering Index, established in the 1960s after the introduction of fluorescent bulbs, uses 14 chips to measure fidelity (RIGHT). The new TM-30-15 system (LEFT) employs 99 color samples.

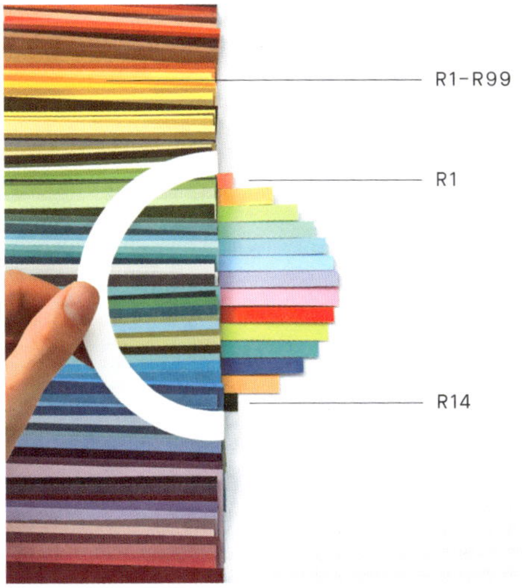

R1–R99

R1

R14

In Living Color

Rich Brilliant Willing is a studio founded on the idea that light is an experience and an essential component of effective architecture and interior design. Light's many variables—its intensity, color, and fidelity—can subtly or dramatically alter the atmospheric qualities of a space. In turn, light affects our sense of well-being, productivity, and mood. For many people, however, these nuances go unnoticed.

In order to recast light from the background of our perceptions to the foreground, RBW created the installation In Living Color for Cooper Hewitt's exhibition *The Senses*. This interactive installation emphasizes light's effects on our environment.

As visitors move below a series of light fixtures suspended from the ceiling, the fixtures respond to people's motion by changing in temperature and intensity, triggering a change in the atmosphere of the surrounding environment. Like the hiss of a background white noise that disappears with time, light is an ambient sensory detail that we rarely notice in our environment after we adapt to its baseline. When the white noise abruptly changes, however, the background in our environment becomes acutely apparent.

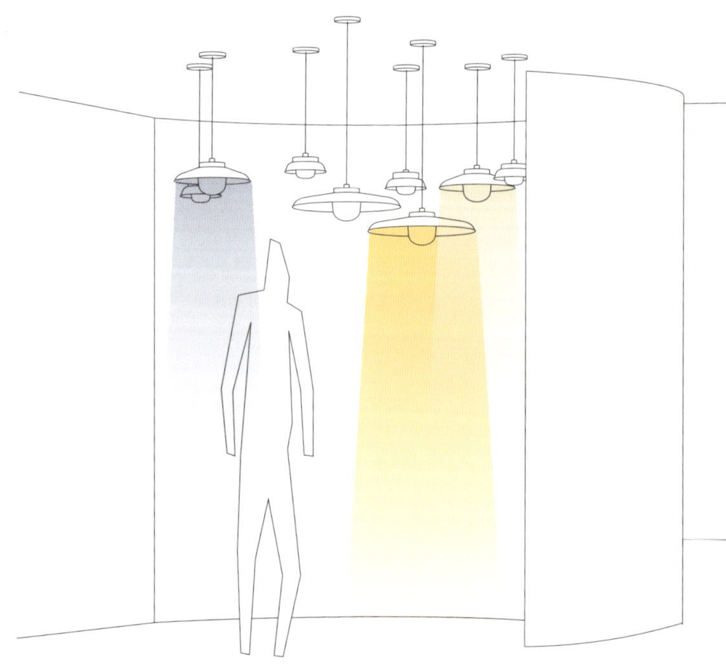

ADAPTIVE LIGHTING

Sensors embedded in the installation react to visitors. Meanwhile, the visitor's visual perception adapts to the changing lighting conditions.

Lighting Fixtures, In Living Color, 2018; Rich Brilliant Willing (New York, New York, USA, founded 2009); Light-emitting diodes, aluminum, glass; 15.2 × 182.9 × 15.2 cm (6 × 72 × 6 in.); Courtesy of Rich Brilliant Willing

UNOCCUPIED

2700K

A pulsating, neutral light at 2700K expresses warmth and attraction, beckoning people to enter. Lights at this temperature are standard in hospitality and dining atmospheres.

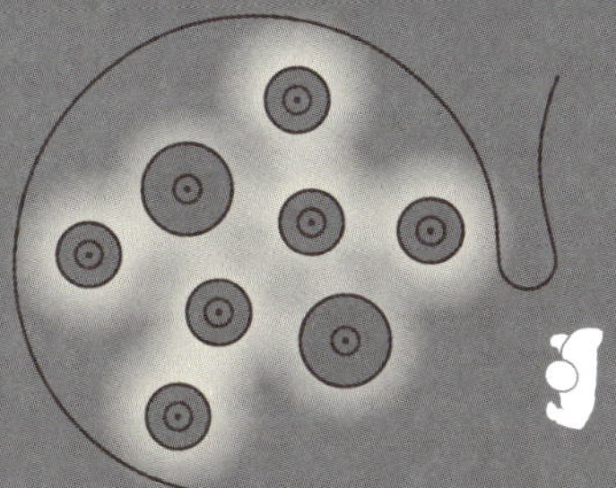

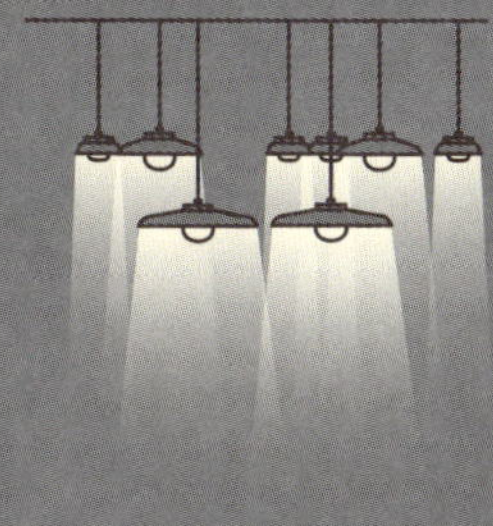

INHABITED

4000K

Fixtures respond to a visitor by slowly shifting to an energetic 5000K from the softer, warmer 2700K. This perceptible shift changes the ambiance of the space.

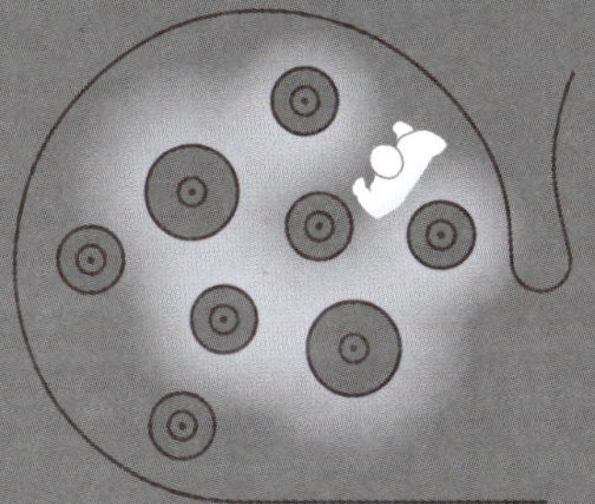

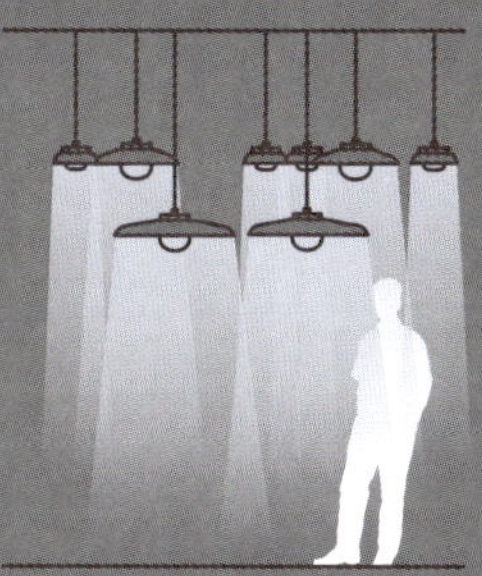

SOCIAL DYNAMICS

2200K

Sensing additional visitors, the fixtures change to create an atmosphere more conducive to social interactions.

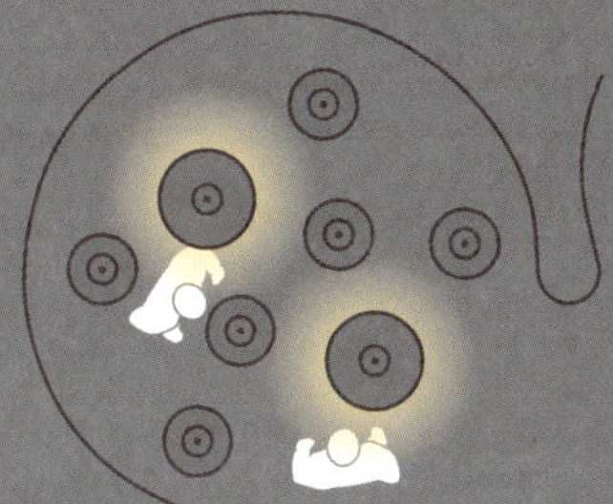

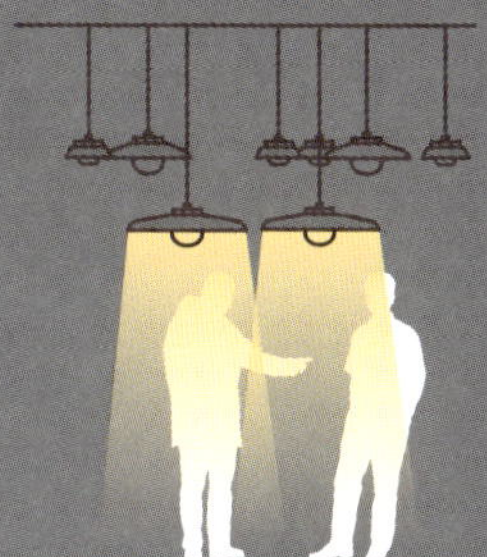

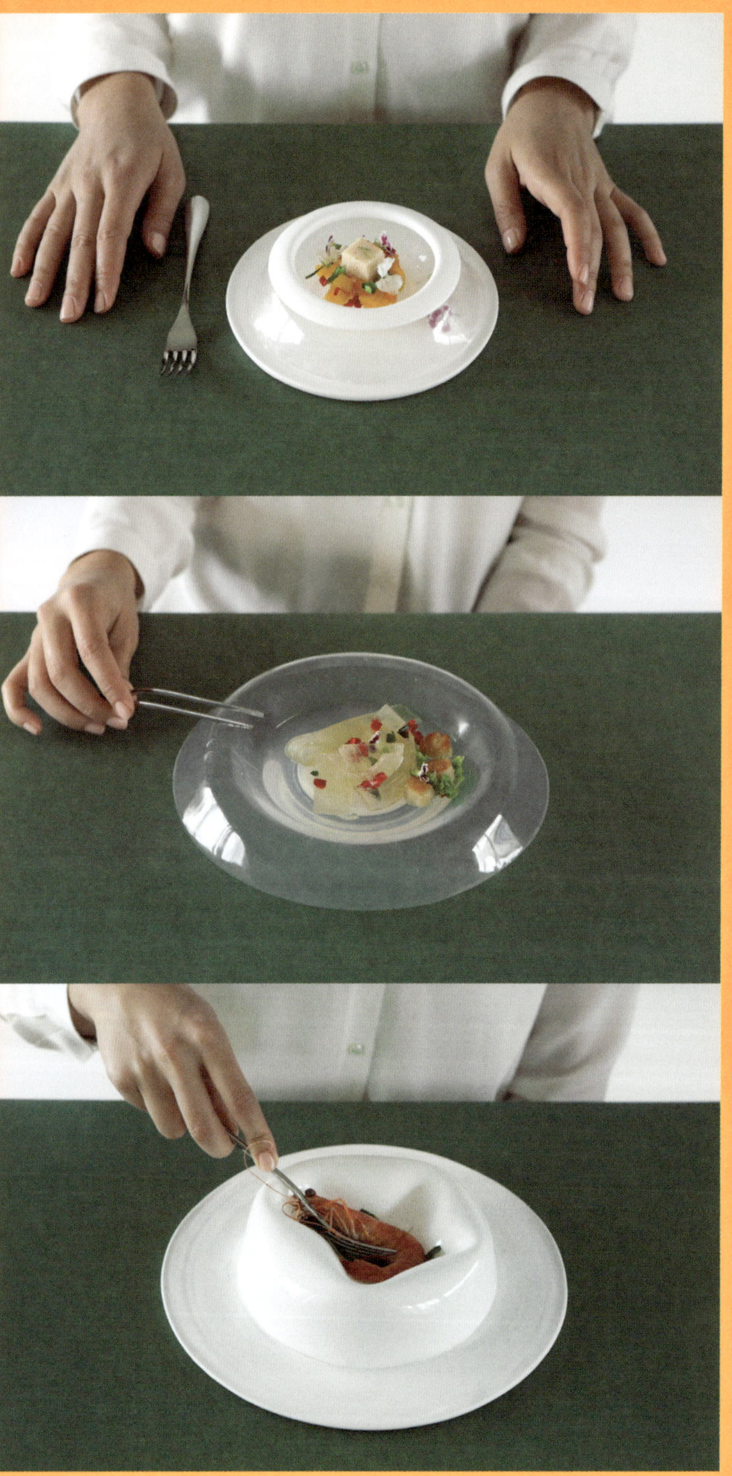

Folding Plate, from the Living Plates collection, 2017; Lina Saleh (Saudi Arabian and Italian, b. 1991); Silicone, porcelain; 6 × 18.2 cm diam. (2 3⁄8 × 7 3⁄16 in.)

Large Folding Plate, from the Living Plates collection, 2017; Lina Saleh (Saudi Arabian and Italian, b. 1991); Silicone, porcelain; 8 × 30 cm diam. (3 1⁄8 in. × 11 13⁄16 in.)

Breathing Plate, from the Living Plates collection, 2017; Lina Saleh (Saudi Arabian and Italian, b. 1991); Silicone, porcelain; 7 × 23 cm diam. (2 3⁄4 × 9 1⁄16 in.)

Photos by Nicola Tree, Courtesy of Lina Saleh

The Sensory Table

The table is theatrical. It is rooted in rituals, embellished by tableware, and activated by our behaviors and our interactions with one another, objects, and food. Designer Lina Saleh's Living Plates are central to the experience at any table on which they're set. The plates quiver in response to touch. They bend and conform to the weight of food. Saleh made the plates from silicone. One bowl flutters. Another dish pops into position. We might jiggle the table to set the plates in motion or caress their sides. The objects change our expectations of plateware from inanimate, static vessels for food to responsive objects to enhance eating.

Taste is social. We reunite with friends over a meal, negotiate a deal during a power breakfast, reconnect with a family dinner at day's end, welcome a guest with food and drink. We mark important events with food: weddings end in a lavish meal; birthdays are feted with cake; holidays are organized around feasts, whether breaking a fast or commemorating a harvest. As naturalist Diane Ackerman says, "If an event is meant to matter emotionally, symbolically, or mystically, food will be close at hand to sanctify and bind it."[1]

We create rituals around food that often underscore the company of others. Tea ceremonies are codified and choreographed rituals emphasizing the interaction between host and guests, vessels and utensils. Designer Bilge Nur Saltik created a collection of tableware, called Share.Food, which highlights our meal's companion. Users seated across from one another tip the vessels toward their companion in a ritualized offering of food and drink. The objects balance on an angled bottom. The undersides are neon pink, casting a soft glow on a table. Roxanne Brennen has created a series of dishes called Dining Toys, whose warm colors and delicate folds invite erotic foreplay with food. If taste is social, the table is our playground, awash in a play of color and objects that amplify eating.

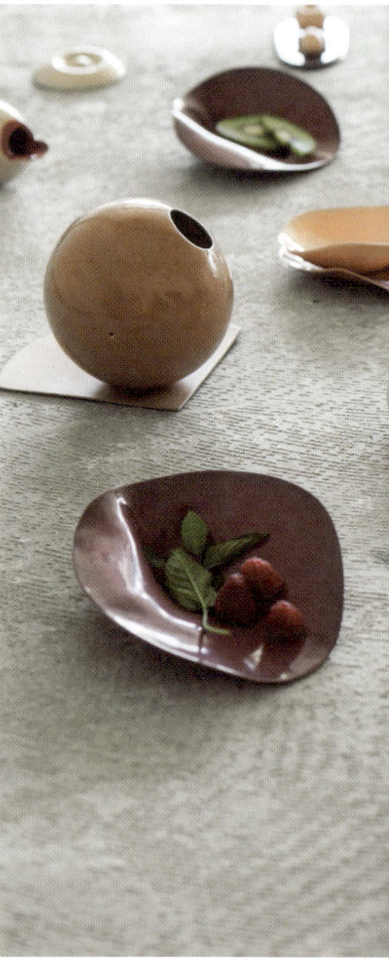

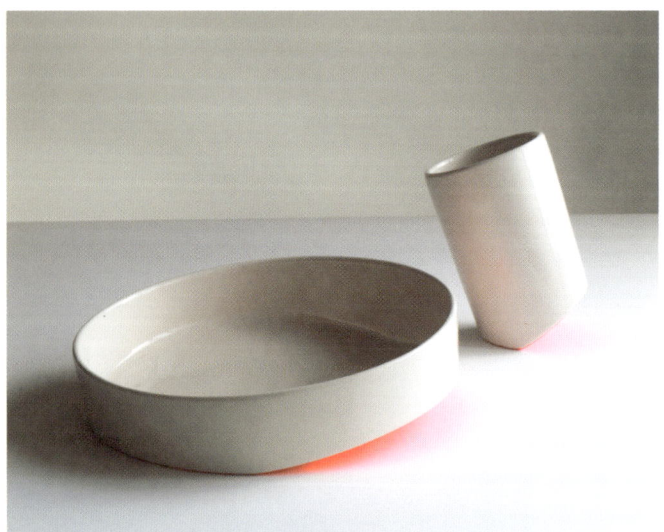

Plate and Cup, from the Share.Food Tableware collection, 2013; Bilge Nur Saltik (Turkish, b. 1988), Studio Bilge Nur Saltik (London, UK, founded 2013); Ceramic; Plate: 5 × 25 cm diam. (1 15⁄16 × 9 13⁄16 in.), Cup: 10 × 8 cm diam. (3 15⁄16 × 3 1⁄8 in.); © Studio Bilge Nur Saltik

Dining Toys, 2017; Roxanne Brennen (American, b. 1999); Glazed stoneware; Sizes vary, up to 7 × 20 cm (2 ¾ × 7 ⅞ in.); Copyright: Design Academy Eindhoven. Photograph: Iris Rijskamp

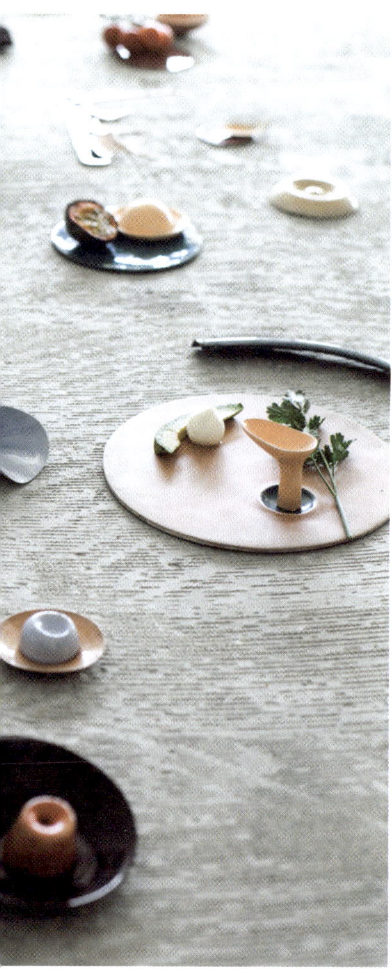

At its most elemental, taste is limited to the attributes detected by receptors on our tongues—sweet, sour, salty, bitter, and umami. Physiologically, these taste attributes help us infer the nutritional value of food. Sweet indicates calories. Sour cues us to ripeness. Salty signals electrolytes and mineral content. Bitter alerts us to poison. Umami is linked to protein.[2] These are useful roles for our survival. But with taste alone, we cannot distinguish chocolate cake from vanilla, just as coffee is nothing more than hot water with a bitter aftertaste. Flavor is what enables us to decipher the nuances of food and drink, to appreciate the complexity of Coke or differentiate a cherry lollipop from a grape one.

We experience flavor through olfaction—our sense of smell—not when we breathe in, but when we breathe out as we swallow food. This process is called retronasal olfaction. (See more on page 67.) Neuroscientist Gordon M. Shepard explains that smell and taste are so intertwined, we call the combined sense "flavor."[3] Even gastronome Jean Anthelme Brillat-Savarin, in his 1825 classic, *The Physiology of Taste*, recognized the entanglement of smell and taste: "I am tempted to believe that smell and taste form a single sense, of which the mouth is the laboratory and the nose is the chimney."[4]

Flavor is a cross-sensory experience, savored best when our other senses are piqued. A piece of chocolate cake is a rich, velvety brown. It is springy yet compliant against a fork, and its dense, creamy layers exude a cocoa aroma. And that's before taking a bite. Flavor combines smell and the oral sense of touch. It integrates tactility, vision, and sound in what experimental psychologist Charles Spence refers to as "flavor senses." Texture, appearance, temperature, weight, color, shape, and language impact our experience of taste.[5]

The table is the site of flavor, where we eat with not just our tongues, mouths, and noses, but with our eyes, fingers, lips, and ears. The table is where eating, an activity rooted in survival, is transformed into one of our most enjoyable pastimes. Brillat-Savarin gushes over the "pleasures of the table," the location of our multisensory experiences of taste.[6]

Like foreplay, the table teases our eyes and entices our fingers for the tastes to come. Design heightens our experience of eating. Design can trigger us to be more alert—a crisp white tablecloth and formal place setting signal a lavish meal. Or design can seduce us into gluttony—we eat more off a bigger plate. Consumer psychologist Brian Wansink has studied how visual perception of food quantity makes us overeat. The fullness of our "platescape" (a term Wansink uses for plates, bowls, and other food containers) influences how much we consume.[7] Marije Vogelzang, a pioneer in eating design, created a series called Volumes inspired by Wansink's research on visual cues and portion control. Her Volume objects are like prosthetics for our platescapes, to be nestled among food to give the illusion of a fuller meal. When we visually perceive more food, we are more satiated when done.

Vogelzang's Volumes modify eating by changing environmental cues. In place of smaller plates and bowls, these objects offer an entirely new typology to discourage overeating. Bulbous and odd, they resemble tubers and organs. One is nippled like the underbelly of a pig. Some cradle food among their protrusions. These unusual objects are made of stones covered in silicone in tantalizing colors. While intended to hinder overeating, they make us more aware of our food, inviting playfulness and experimentation with food's presentation. Evocative of body parts, they impede mindless consumption.

Volumes, 2017; Marije Vogelzang (Dutch, b. 1978), Studio Marije Vogelzang (Dordrecht, Netherlands, founded 1999); Rocks, silicone; Sizes vary, up to 8 × 8 × 10 cm (3 ⅛ × 3 ⅛ × 3 15⁄16 in.); © Studio Marije Vogelzang

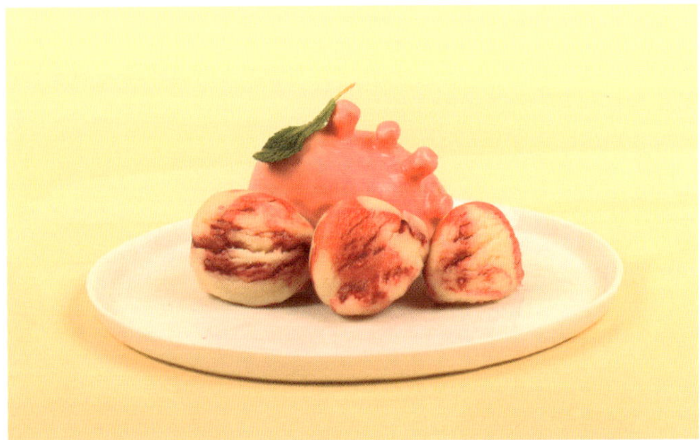

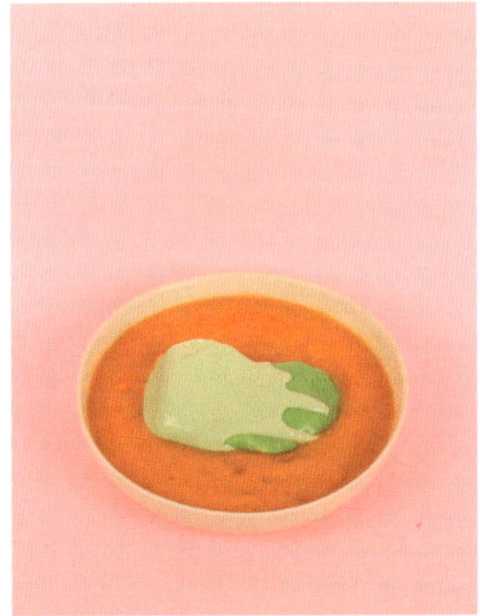

Double crenelated
bone structure
leaf shaped on twig
plant meat growing on
bone structure. Twig shaped.

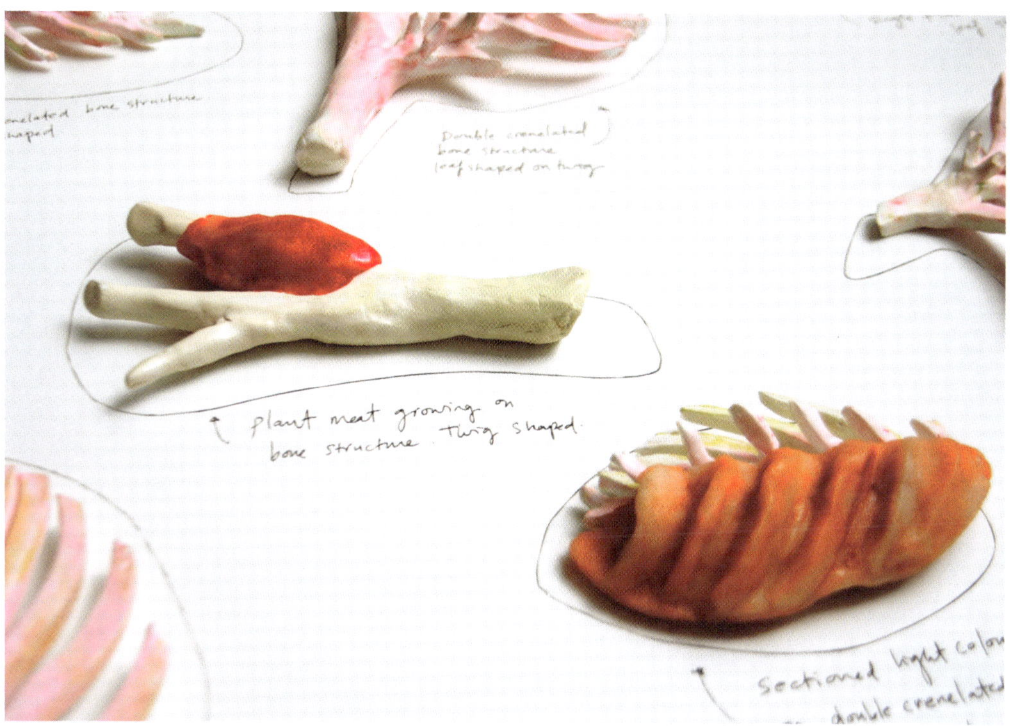

Plant Bones, 2016; Marije Vogelzang (Dutch, b. 1978), Studio Marije Vogelzang (Dordrecht, Netherlands, founded 1999); Paper-based clay, marzipan; Sizes vary, up to 5.1 × 12.7 × 20.3 cm (2 × 5 × 8 in.); © Studio Marije Vogelzang

Throughout her work, Vogelzang reimagines not just how we eat and the tableware that accompanies it, but what we eat. Plant Bones is a speculative project that proposes a future of plant-based meat grown by mutant plant species. Botanical specimens with ribbed, bone-like structures are made of cellulose and shaped like leaves—capable of growing a meat-like tissue onto their bony scaffolds. Imagine spare ribs, sans the pig. This scenario raises questions about the future of food, and it challenges our assumptions about the art of eating. Rather than using traditional utensils, could there be a future in which we apply or grow food to bone-like structures to finger and nibble, our tongues wrestling the food out from between the ribs?

Taste, like touch, is intimate. It requires physical contact. Saliva is key—food must dissolve in order to be tasted, much like molecules must evaporate in order to be smelled. Put a hard candy in your mouth and, for a fleeting moment, you don't taste it, until it begins to dissolve and assaults your tongue with the tang of tart cherry. Tongues are dexterous sensors. Packed with nerve endings, the tongue is sensitive to scalding tea and cooling menthol. It navigates the rough edges of a potato chip, the creaminess of an avocado, and the seediness of a grape. Our initial impression of a food is, in part, based on its texture. We profile foods as we put them into our mouths, scouting for freshness and quality. A rubbery pickle or a mealy apple signals that these foods may not be fresh, ripe, or even edible. Known as "mouthfeel," our physical interaction with food scans for all sorts of mouth textures when it touches our palate and we initially bite down—chewiness, cohesion, coarseness, bounce, graininess, and more.

As humans, we start out exploring the world with our tongues and mouths. New parents will alarmingly attest to a baby who puts anything in their mouth—balls and stuffed animals, dirty socks and cell phones. By "mouthing," babies learn about shapes and textures, hard and soft, smooth and rough, warm and cool, using among the most keenly tuned sense organs available to us out of the womb. The tongue and mouth are lined with sensory nerves that provide input to the brain about temperature, piquancy, roughness, shape, and so on. But how much of this input impacts taste?

AEIOU I Rear Bump series, from the Sensory Dessert Spoon collection, 2016–17; Jinhyun Jeon (South Korean, b. 1981), Studio Jinhyun Jeon (Eindhoven, Netherlands, founded 2012); Ottchil-lacquered and gold-plated SUS metal; Each: 2.2 × 2.7 × 13.3 cm (7/8 × 1 1/16 × 5 1/4 in.); Courtesy of Jinhyun Jeon

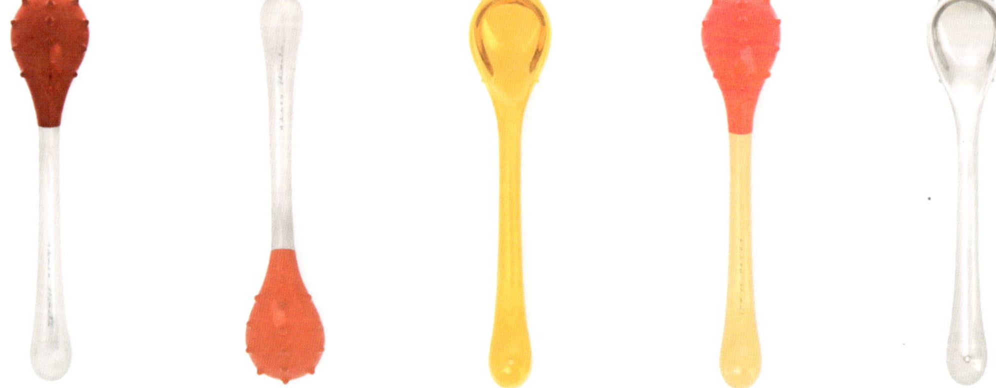

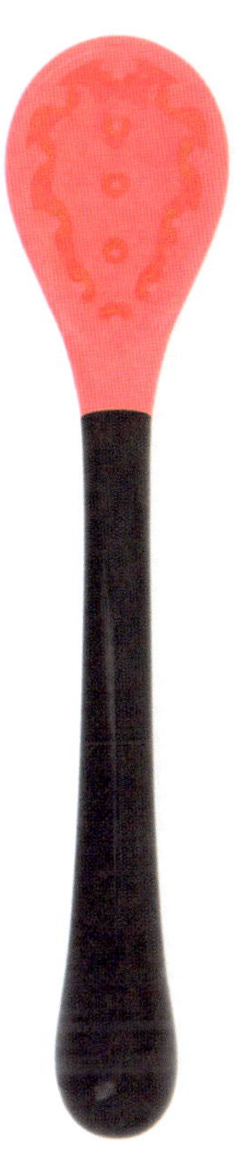

AEIOU VII Inner Bump series, from the Sensory Dessert Spoon collection, 2016; Jinhyun Jeon (South Korean, b. 1981), Studio Jinhyun Jeon (Eindhoven, Netherlands, founded 2012); Ottchil-lacquered plastic; 2.8 × 2.2 × 13.3 cm (1 ⅛ × ⅞ × 5 ¼ in.); Courtesy of Jinhyun Jeon

Texture and shape change what we taste. Spence has demonstrated that we associate sweetness with round shapes and bitterness with angular shapes.[8] The bulbous form of a lollipop, for instance, is designed to enhance our experience of its sweetness. Designer Jinhyun Jeon designs utensils with this in mind, discarding ideas of cutlery as a mere vehicle to get food into our mouths. Her Sensory Dessert Spoon series features instruments whose rough interiors and handles are designed to stimulate the fingers holding them as much as the tongue. Spoons are edged with bumps or rippled like waves to catch and pool food. Bulbous utensils are akin to lollipops and sex toys. More than just activating form, Jeon uses lacquered glass, plastic, aluminum, wood, or gold; each material is chosen for its temperature as well as for sonic properties that lull the tongue or clink against the teeth. The utensil tips are bathed in bubblegum pink and strawberry red. This is tableware that looks good enough to eat.

A table set with these utensils invites guests to dip and indulge, cradle, lick, and explore food. The implements heighten the experience of eating by calling attention to it, altering our rote behaviors—insert food, chew, swallow. They invite us to pause and consider how sensory cues impact taste. Are we more alert to the tang of yogurt eaten from a cool rough spoon? Does chocolate mousse eaten from a bulbous red utensil taste more decadent? These dessert spoons stimulate and deepen our flavor senses, asserting that the implements with which we eat change how we experience food.

Visual cues inform our perceptions and expectations of taste. Designer Verena Schreppel's Singlet tableware set consists of metal utensils cast with knit textiles that cover the handles—the part of cutlery we cradle with our hands and fingers, not with our mouths and tongues. From the neck up, the utensils resemble a spoon, knife, or fork; from the neck down, they appear soft and protected by a cozy knit. The visual cue of a perceived textile softens our tactile expectation of what is typically a flat metal handle. The utensils evoke *hygge*, that Danish quality of "coziness and comfortable conviviality."[9] Think of a crackling fire and wool socks, mulled wine and flannel blankets. This is tableware that changes the sensations in our mouths by beckoning the eye and hand.

Today we eat food directly from the package as often as off a plate, where visual cues change what we taste. We anticipate taste based on the way a package looks. The packaging of a Hershey's chocolate bar, for instance, is simple and iconic. A glossy dark brown with silver lettering, the wrapper is a simple and familiar indulgence, like the chocolate inside.

The packaging of Compartés Chocolatier, however, under the design and creative direction of its owner Jonathan Grahm in Los Angeles, is unbound from convention, suggesting the bars inside are, too. The cardboard packages are covered with Grahm's hand-drawn avocado halves or with palm trees on a pink-to-orange gradient background, inspired by an historic Beverly Hills wallpaper. The designs brim with collages of magical worlds—tiered cakes, gilt statues, and roses, or distant mountains, white-water rafters, and orange poppy fields. The packaging is rich in pattern, color, and symbolic imagery, designed to inform and inspire our taste perceptions.

Grahm carries the visual opulence to the design of the bars themselves. He covers his chocolate in colored sugar crystals or edible gold leaf, and mixes it with marshmallow cereal

Dessert spoon, Soup spoon, Fork, and Knife, from the Singlet collection, 2003; Verena Schreppel (German, b. 1977); Cast metal; Sizes vary, up to 0.7 × 4.3 × 20 cm (1⁄4 × 1 11⁄16 × 7 7⁄8 in.); © Verena Schreppel

Cup, from the Singlet collection, 2003; Verena Schreppel (German, b. 1977); Cast porcelain; 12.9 × 6.4 cm diam. (5 1⁄16 × 2 1⁄2 in.); © Verena Schreppel

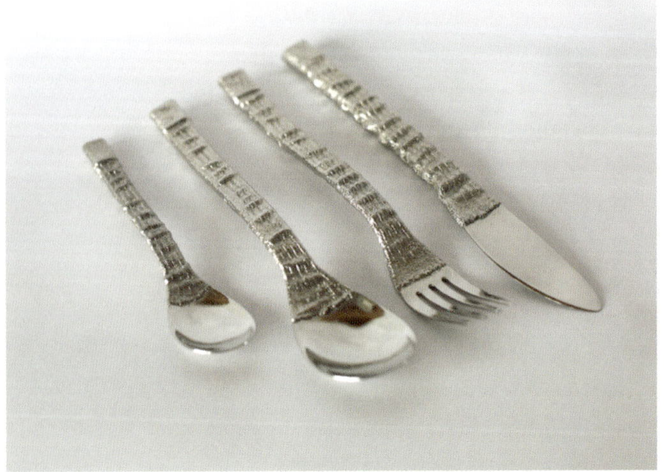

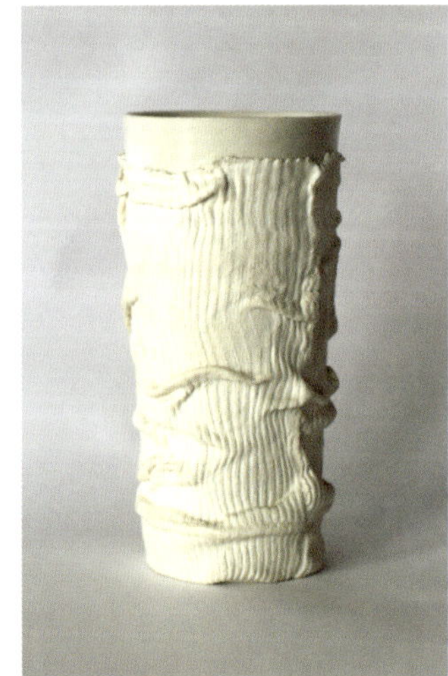

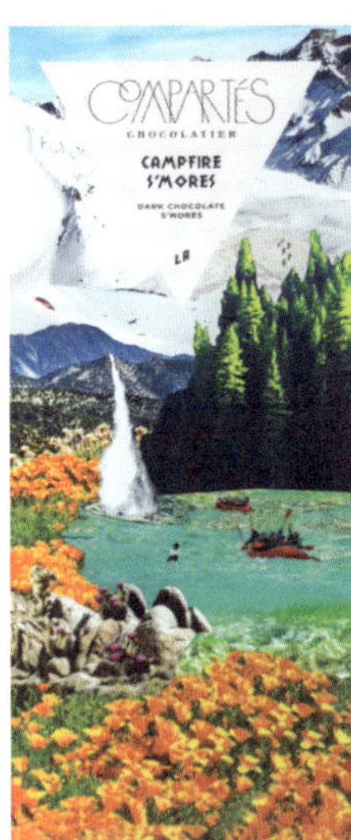

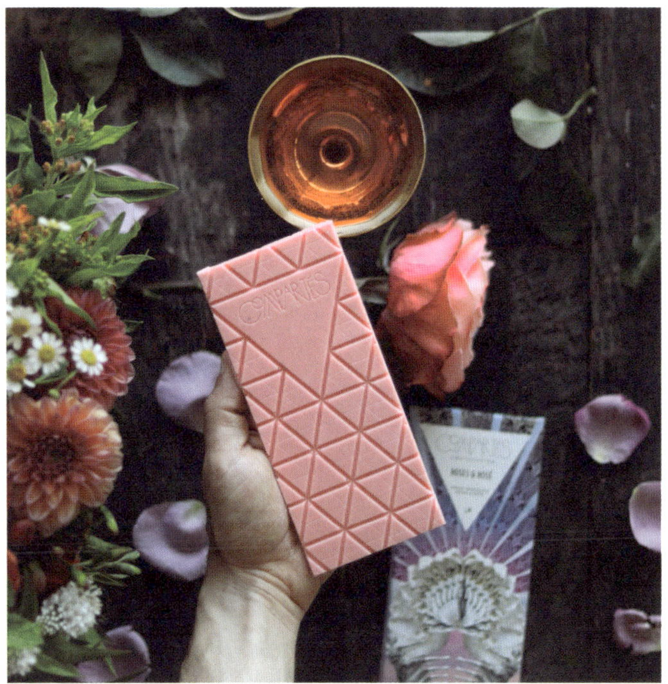

S'mores Dark Chocolate Bar Packaging and Roses and Rosé Chocolate Bar; Jonathan Grahm (American, b. 1984), Compartés Chocolatier (Los Angeles, California, USA, founded 1950); Paper, chocolate; Each: 19.7 × 8.3 × 0.95 cm (7 ¾ × 3 ¼ × ⅜ in.); © Compartés Chocolatier

or rainbow sprinkles. The designs are saturated and bold, luxurious and memorable. Perhaps the taste of the chocolate will be, too.

Color amplifies the sensation of taste and flavor. When we see a red jellybean, our brain may associate red with something sweet, like a strawberry or cherry, or with a hot flavor, like cinnamon. These color cues signal how we see flavor perceptively before we actually taste anything. We rely on color to determine ripeness and freshness of natural foods. A red strawberry will be sweet and tart. A green strawberry is not ready to be picked. Gray meat is troubling. Sugary candy comes in bright poppy colors, associating it with the intense shots of sweetness of natural fruits—orange (orange), pink (watermelon), green (apple), red (raspberry), and yellow (lemon). Taste attributes of color don't impact food alone. Spence and his colleagues have shown that the color of plateware affects the perceived saltiness or sweetness of the food eaten off it. Colorful plates make food taste both sweeter and saltier.[10]

Humans have embellished eating with colorful plates and glasses since ancient times, signifying the importance and joy of the table. Cooper Hewitt's collection has over one thousand tableware objects. The earliest example—an iridescent green bowl with lotus petal ornamentation—dates to the first century. Today we continue to decorate our tables with lush, colorful tableware. Bitossi's Spot glassware is a series of tumblers and pitchers whose bottoms are bathed in a creamy wash of color, creating a playful evocation of taste. The design suggests that a milky, colorful concoction has been swirled inside each glass to create the irregularly colored base.

Designer Matali Crasset and chef Pierre Hermé created a cake platter for Alessi consisting of orange and cream concentric circles nested around a chocolate brown center plate. Each layer or ring is a movable part, recalling the nested round cutters and baking pans used in pastry making. Made of melamine, the rings come together with a satisfying "clack."

Design duo Kollectiv Plus Zwei's series of benches and stools, Importance of the Obvious, evoke the sensory table. The designers layered wood, plastic, foam, and resin, and cut them like cakes and nougat. A stool's strata of colored resin resembles hard sugar candy. A bench made of layered foam and polystyrene conjures an ice-cream finger, seemingly topped with nonpareils.

Drinkware, from the Spot collection, 2014; Bitossi (Montelupo Fiorentino, Tuscany, Italy, founded 2007); Glass; Sizes vary, up to 24.5 × 8.5 cm diam. (9 5/8 × 3 3/8 in.); Photo © Bitossi Home

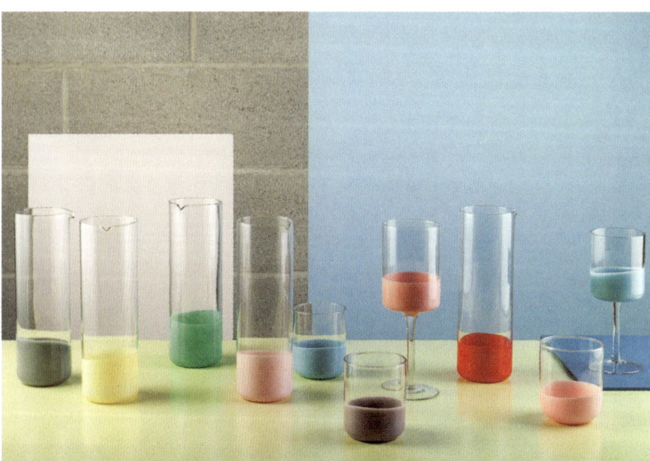

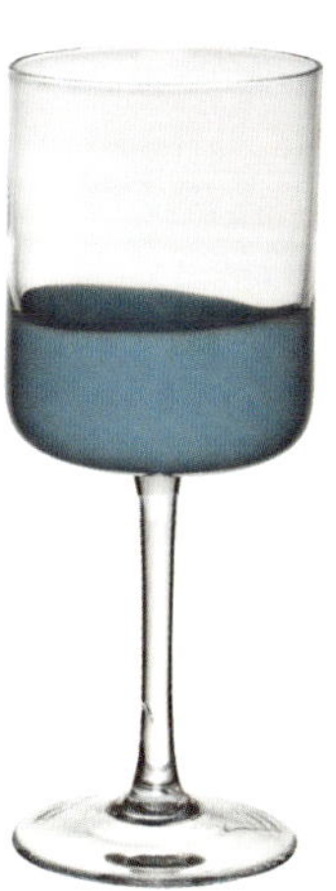

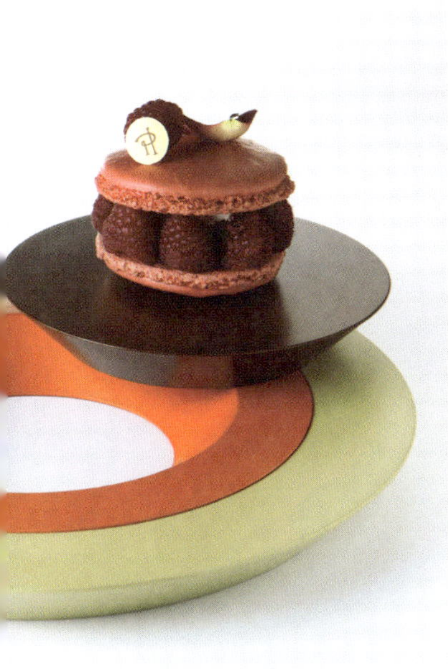

Essentiel de Pâtisserie Pastry Plate, 2010; Matali Crasset (French, b. 1965) and Pierre Hermé (French, b. 1961) for Alessi (Italy, founded 1921); Melamine; 2.5 × 29.85 cm diam. (1 × 11 3/4 in.); © Matali Crasset / ARTISTS RIGHTS SOCIETY (ARS), NEW YORK / ADAGP, PARIS, photo by Bernhard Winkelmann

Yellow-Rosa Pie Cut with Crumbs, from the Importance of the Obvious collection, 2013; Matthias Borowski (German, b. 1983), Kollectiv Plus Zwei (Vienna, Austria, founded 2014); Foam, polystyrene; 25 × 30 × 110 cm (9 13/16 × 11 13/16 × 43 5/16 in.); © Matthias Borowski, Kollectiv Plus Zwei, 2014

In the end, could taste be an illusion? Designers, marketers, scientists, and chefs certainly tease and tickle our senses to amplify taste. Cooper Hewitt invited designer Emilie Baltz to create an installation around color and taste that helps us understand how sensory illusions can enhance or alter our eating experience. For our exhibition, Baltz created Flavor-Factory, a space that manufactures new sensory perceptions about taste, arousing ideas about what we see as "sweet." Over-scale ice-cream cones, donuts, candy, and popsicles cover the walls of an all-white space, onto which provocative imagery is presented. The visuals ooze, mold, gurgle, and crawl. They are fuzzy or fizzy, saturated pink or worrisome gray. They are gross or lusciously inviting, toying with our perceptions and expectations of taste.

Have you ever drooled at the sight of something delicious? It's a gustatory response, stimulated simply by sight. We eat with our eyes before we even take a bite, translating cues about color, texture, temperature, and ripeness that change what we taste. A white jellybean tastes less like strawberry than a red one. A drippy ice-cream cone is savored less in our haste to finish it. The next time we sit at the table, perhaps we will stop to consider how the sensory cues hitting us will impact our next bite. It may not taste the same.

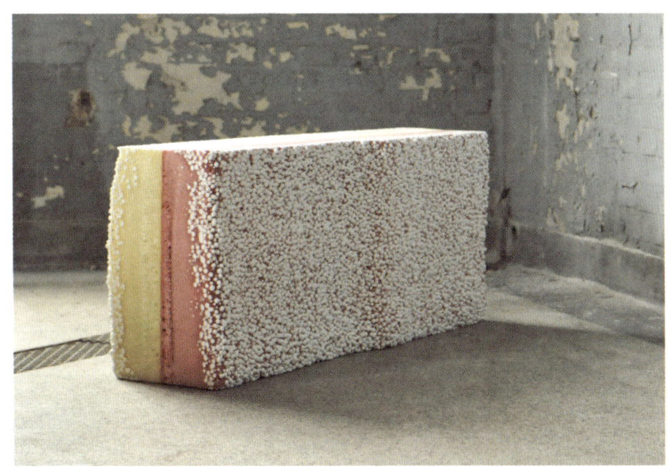

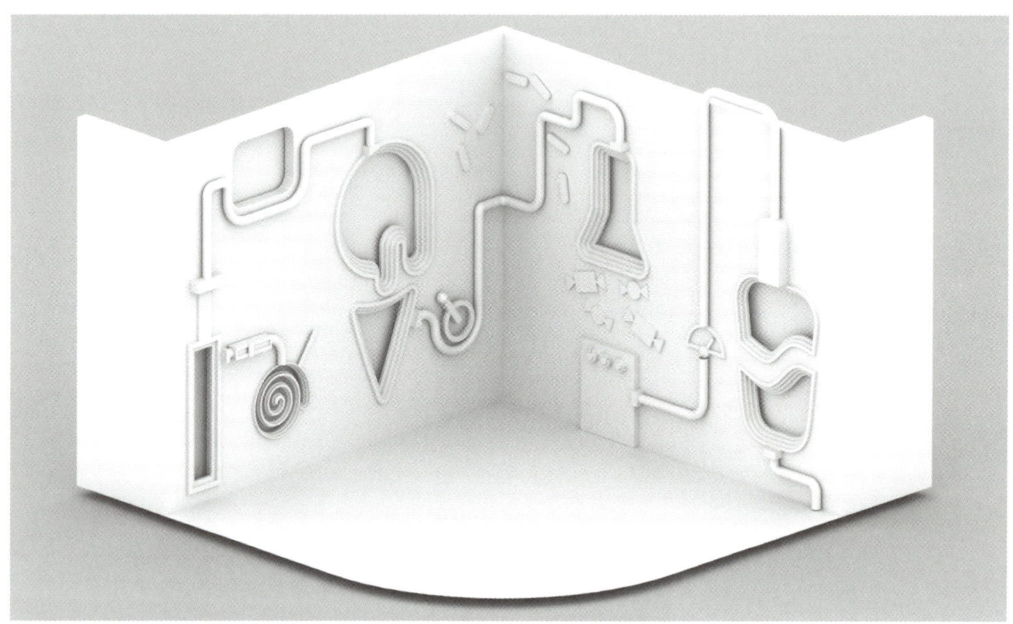

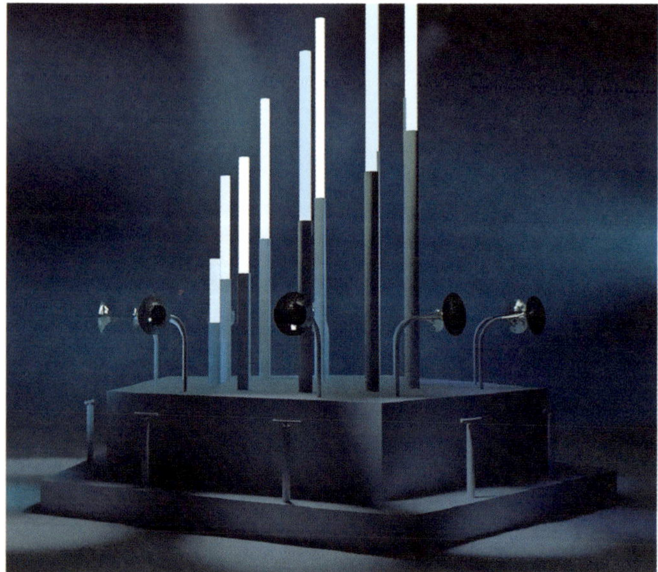

FlavorFactory (New York, 2018); Emilie Baltz (French-American, b. 1979); Digital renderings; Commissioned by Cooper Hewitt, Smithsonian Design Museum; Courtesy of Berke Ilhan

Dream Machine (New York, 2017); Emilie Baltz (French-American, b. 1979); Interactive installation; Sound design by Antfood Studios; Technology by Smooth Technology; Fabrication by No.4 Studios; Scent by Givaudan. Ten horns dispense light, sound, and scent. Each sensory chord is keyed to a human emotion, from happiness to fear. Multiple players create a sensory symphony.

Importance of the Obvious collection, 2013; Matthias Borowski (German, b. 1983), Kollectiv Plus Zwei (Vienna, Austria, founded 2014); Foam, polystyrene, resin, wood; Sizes vary, up to 25 × 30 × 110 cm (9 13/16 x 11 13/16 × 43 5/16 in.); © Matthias Borowski, Kollectiv Plus Zwei, 2014

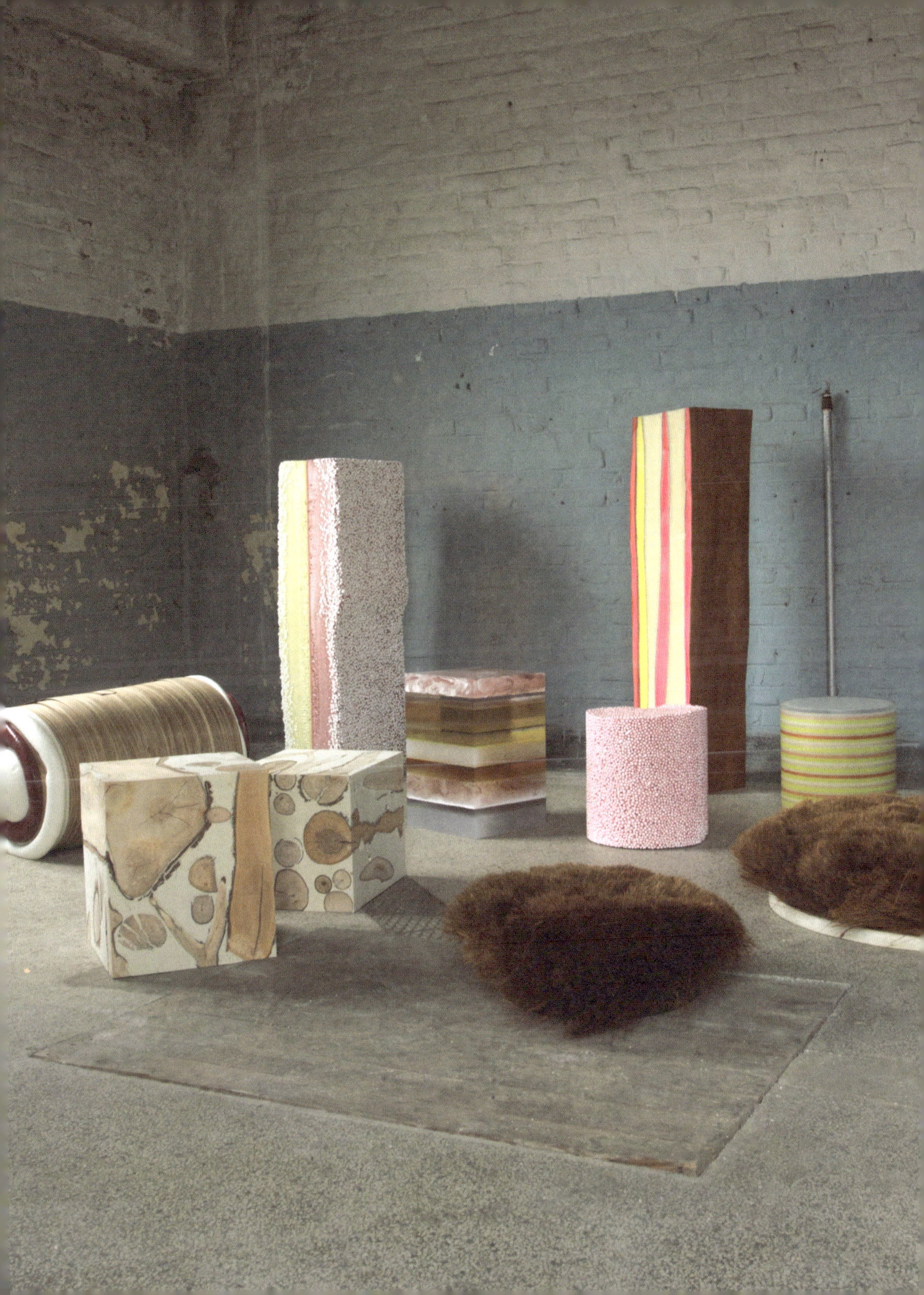

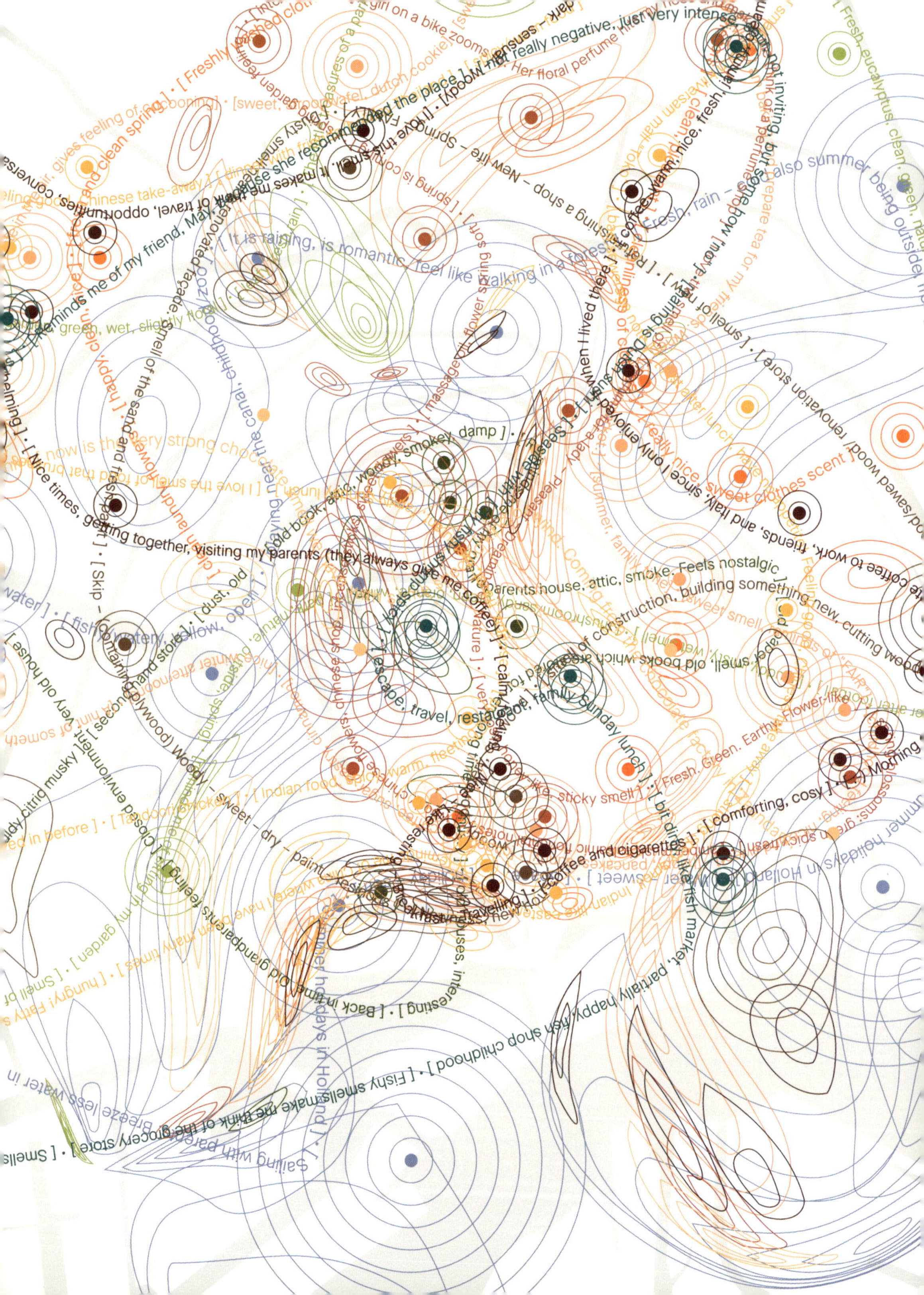

Freshly washed clothes
girl on a bike zooms
sweet, stroopwafel, dutch cookie
Her floral perfume
not really negative, just very intense
Fresh, eucalyptus, clean, green, nature
also summer being outside
Fresh, rain
Chinese take-away
Fresh and clean spring
I love this smell, it makes me think of travel, opportunities
Reminds me of my friend, May, because she recommended the place
renovated facade
New life – Spring is coming
Refreshing a shop
warm, nice, fresh, jammy
It is raining, is romantic, feel like walking in a forest
green, wet, slightly foggy
happy, clean
smell of the sand and the sea
when I lived there
since I only enjoyed
and Italy
coffee to work, friends
sawed wood/renovation store
really nice, sweet clothes scent
old book, attic, woody, smokey, damp]
now is the very strong chocolate
Nice times, getting together, visiting my parents (they always give me coffee)
Parents house, attic, smoke. Feels nostalgic
building something new, cutting wood
smell of old books which are
Skip – containing plywood) second hand store
dust, old
fishy, watery
Closed environment, very old house
escape, travel, restaurant, family Sunday lunch
calm feeling
sticky smell
Fresh. Green. Earthy. Flower-like
comforting, cosy] • [Morning
Indian food
Woody – sweet – dry – paint
coffee and cigarettes
bit dirty, like fish market, partially happy, fish shop childhood
Back in time, Old grandparents feeling
Summer holidays in Holland
Fishy smells make me think of the grocery store
Sailing with parents
Breeze less water in
Smells

Scentscapes Smell is perhaps our most primal sense. It is interwoven with life and tied to breath. It is one sense we cannot tune out or turn off. Hold your nose to prevent smelling and you die. More than perception of external stimuli, smell is our ingestion of it. Smell happens when odor molecules enter the nasal cavity and are absorbed by our mucous membranes. These membranes contain receptor cells bearing olfactory cilia, or microscopic hairs, that sweep in odor molecules, swaying in the current of our mucosa's watery solution like sea anemone on a coral reef. The signals head directly to our olfactory bulb—the bud of our limbic system—where they are processed as our sense of smell. Breathing is a sensory act.

Smellmap: Amsterdam (detail), 2013-14; Kate McLean (British, b. 1965); Courtesy of Kate McLean

Olfaction has long been key to survival. When we were organisms in the ocean, smell guided us to food and away from danger. When we flopped onto land, smell was so important that the olfactory tissue at the base of our nerve cord grew into a brain. The olfactory bulb remains rooted to our limbic system, the center of emotion and memory, where processes to guarantee our survival are triggered, like hunger, sexuality, and aggression.[1] The limbic system is home to the amygdala, hippocampus, and thalamus, where our brain modulates emotions and creates, consolidates, and accesses memories. The signals of smell are just a few synapses away from these structures. Emotion and memory are wired to our nose.

Smell can be vividly precise and move us profoundly: a beloved grandmother's perfume; deteriorating leaves as fall begins to turn; orange and cinnamon at the holidays. Marcel Proust famously describes the involuntary memory that arises from smell when a madeleine soaked in tea unexpectedly awakens a cascade of memories. We react with powerful emotions when exposed to a smell from our past, which maintains its memorable peculiarity over time. As Russian author Vladimir Nabokov wrote, "Nothing revives the past so completely as a smell that was once associated with it."[2]

Yet smell is evasive. It lacks a vocabulary. To describe a smell is to dance around it. We reference its source (cut grass) or a physical property (effervescent). We borrow words from other sensations like taste (sweet), tactility (sharp), or vision (bright). Scent designer, artist, and researcher Sissel Tolaas, featured in Cooper Hewitt's 2016 *Design Triennial*, has developed a dictionary of dedicated descriptive smell words, called the Nasalo Lexicon. These fantasy words are untethered to any existing dictionary. "Daadoo" is the smell of dead leaves. "Ihkonka" is a urine smell. "Giish," the smell of money. Smell doesn't have a quantifiable spectrum, like color or musical tones. No neat and tidy chart captures its essence. Smell furls and plumes and spins and winds and curls and disperses in the air, uncontained by our efforts to describe and quantify it.

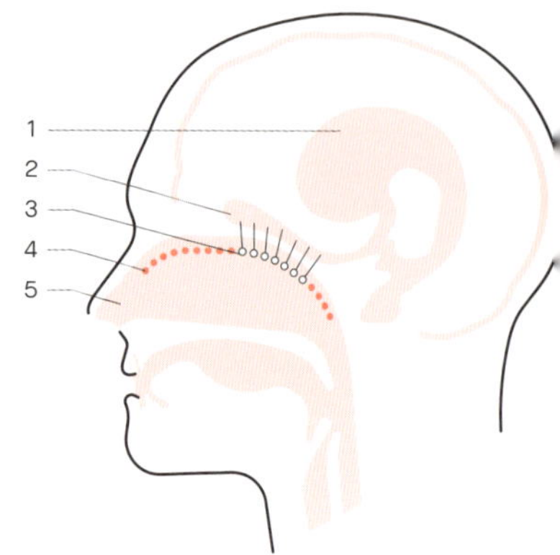

THE ORGANS OF OLFACTION

1 Limbic System
2 Olfactory Bulb
3 Sensory Cells
4 Mucous Membrane
5 Nasal Cavity

AFIISH	**African shops**
BEETEE	**concrete**
BIISH	**rubbish**
BEESH	**mixed barbeque**
CAA	**traffic**
CAMECC	**vehicle repair**
CHIISH	**Chinese shops**
CLESH	**clean sea**
CLII	**nature**
DAADOO	**dead leaves & compost**
DUSBI	**dusty brick**
EER	**ferrite**
ENGEA	**sport**
FAATS	**bad food oils**
FAFEES	**fast food**
FIIWAA	**dirty water, channel**
FIIPAA	**paint fixative, printing**

Nasalo Lexicon (selection); Sissel Tolaas (Norwegian, active in Germany, b. 1962); Courtesy of Sissel Tolaas

How do we navigate contemporary smellscapes? Kate McLean is a graphic designer and researcher who maps urban scentscapes. To create a smellmap, McLean conducts smellwalks to gather data. Participants identify and record aromas, called "smellnotes," indicating an odor's location, intensity, description, and associations. For Smellmap: Amsterdam, McLean led smellwalks with forty-four local residents over four days. The participants identified 650 smell impressions, of which eleven scents were selected for the map to represent Amsterdam. McLean organized the smells into one distinctive background odor ("canal"), seven episodic smells (like "herring carts," "leafy fresh rain," and "warm, spicy"), and three curiosity aromas (like "laundry"), and ascribed them colors based on the visual landscape. Smells emanate from sources indicated by dots, which McLean speculatively plotted; smell sources are often transient. Concentric rings around each source suggest the smell's intensity and range, distorted by the wind, drifting and mingling with other smells. The maps

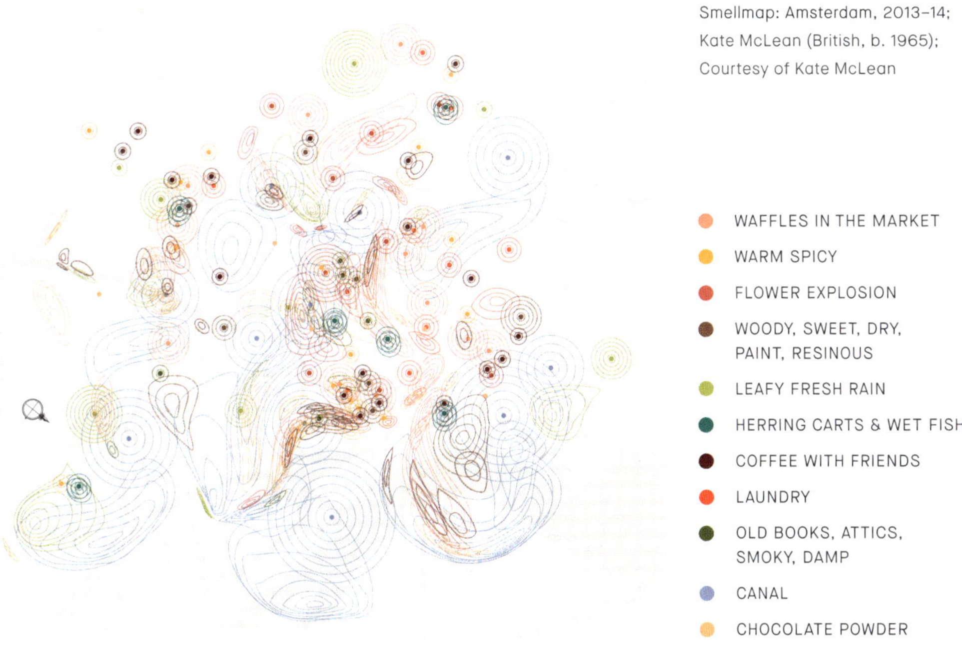

Smellmap: Amsterdam, 2013–14; Kate McLean (British, b. 1965); Courtesy of Kate McLean

visualize the lived experience of a place. They intimate a sensory heritage that is temporal yet ancient, suggesting a time of olfactory navigation in which smells guided us to food, mates, and safety.

Celebrated perfumer Christopher Brosius creates a series of scents called Secret History. These perfumes reference memories of specific points in time for their creator, underscoring the subjective nature of smell. The series includes At the Beach 1966, a scent that smells like original Coppertone suntan lotion and the cold sting of the North Atlantic, with notes of wet sand, driftwood, and the boardwalk. Greenbriar 1968 is Brosius's memory of his grandfather, a blend of sawdust, worn leather work gloves, pipe tobacco, and dirt smells. Winter 1972 recalls fresh snow, wool mittens, and a frozen earth and forest. Brosius believes that the ultimate user of a perfume is not other people but the wearer. Smell is deeply personal.

Winter 1972 is the scent that inspired Snow Storm, the installation that Brosius created for Cooper Hewitt's *Senses* exhibition. In it, dozens of pale blue snowballs hang from the ceiling, each one made of hand-felted wool infused with the Winter 1972 scent. A wool carpet underfoot contains faint glimmers of the scent that are released with each step. The smell inhabits and shapes the space. Wool, Brosius says, holds aromas for a long time.

His approach to scent has evolved since founding his first fragrance company, the Demeter Fragrance Library, in 1993. Demeter (featured in Cooper Hewitt's 2003 *Design Triennial*) creates single-note scents based on such unusual sources as baby powder, turpentine, and Play-Doh, like a dictionary of smells. It designs "linear" smells to be perceived quickly, all at once, rather than as changing over time. With that vocabulary, Brosius founded I Hate Perfume in 2004. The company's contrarian name reflects his wary view of the scent industry and his disdain for assumptions about how a perfume should smell or function. Moving scent off the body, Brosius designs home sprays with names like Burning Leaves and In the Library for

Snowball, from Snow Storm installation, 2017–18; Christopher Brosius (American, b. 1962); Wool; 10.2 cm diam. (4 in.); Photo by Matt Flynn © Smithsonian Institution

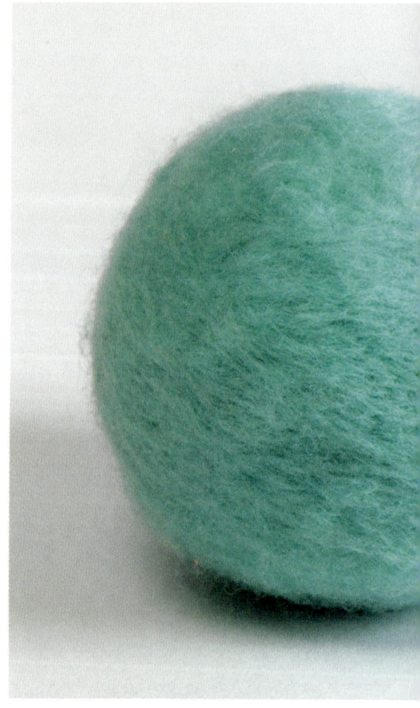

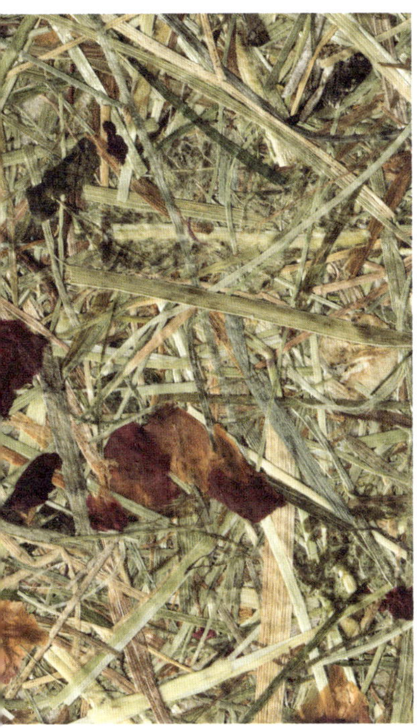

Organoid Rose, 2016; Martin Jehart (Austria, b. 1973), Organoid Technologies Gmbh (Fließ, Austria, founded 2012); Alpine hay, rose petals and buds, HPL carrier board; 305 x 130 × 0.11 cm (10 ft. 1⁄16 in. × 51 3⁄16 in. × 1⁄16 in.), Photo by Matt Flynn © Smithsonian Institution

use on soft fabric, curtains, or couches. For an exhibition in Philadelphia, he created ten fluffy blankets, each infused with a different interpretation of vanilla, from synthetic vanillan to expensive Tahitian vanilla to a scent derived from cut wood. An installation in Brosius's Bushwick-based gallery and laboratory features a curtain, a flask, and a closed book. "The scented curtains were a gateway that people walked through," he told us. "Olfactory experience affects space."[3]

Smell shapes our interior landscapes. The Japanese have long used cedar in bathrooms not only for its antiseptic properties but for its clean, citrus-like scent. Arab builders mixed rosewater and musk in the mortar of mosques, so the spaces exuded the fragrance when heated in the noonday sun. Modern Western architecture has largely removed olfactory experiences in the built environment. Seeking more control over interiors, architects rationalized spaces and neutralized the air, removing smell, humidity, and temperature fluctuations. In urban environments, we sometimes close our windows in retreat from the exhaust and fumes of the air outside. Encased in our buildings, we are anesthetized to smell in its absence from our spaces. The air is sterile. Organoid is a line of surface materials made from Alpine hay mixed with herbs and flowers. Manufactured into flooring, wallcoverings, and acoustic panels, Organoid introduces gentle scents into a room.

How do we reintroduce environmental scent? Christophe Laudamiel is a master perfumer and "scent composer," a chemist and creator who founded DreamAir, a New York–based company that develops scent for spaces, products, and bodies. Laudamiel is French and an advocate for the art of perfumery—both on the body and in the environment. He makes air an aesthetic experience, designing ambient environmental scents that evoke the dead of night or a field of wildflowers. For the 2013 Istanbul Biennial, Laudamiel developed a scent based on the Bosphorous waterway. He paired wood notes—to evoke the brown rocks and trees lining the landscape—with rose, a smell considered masculine in Muslim countries, like what you might find in a menswear shop.[4]

For a 2017 show at Dillon + Lee gallery in New York, Laudamiel developed avant-garde smells like Cocaine, The Whip, and The Orchid No9, olfactory compositions exploring spirituality, addiction, and sex. Green Fairy in Chelsea is the scent of absinthe embedded with wormwood, anis, fennel, and coriander, suggesting the delirium and exaltation of 1920s Paris. These smells evoke stories and places, moods and landscapes. Laudamiel says, "Your mind makes a movie from what you smell."[5]

Designing perfume is as much about chemistry as it is about art. Laudamiel has a master's degree in chemistry from the European Higher Institute of Chemistry in Strasbourg, France, studied for his PhD at MIT in Cambridge, and taught chemistry at Harvard University before receiving a creative perfumery degree from the Proctor & Gamble European Center in Brussels. He deeply understands reactions and interactions between chemicals, how their volatilities and diffusion enhance or disrupt an olfactory experience. One difference in the molecular structure of a smell, Laudamiel says, "could mean the difference between a vanilla scent and the odor in a dentist's office."[6]

Smell is three-dimensional. Laudamiel and other perfumers describe smell as an architectural form. It envelops us. Base or foundational notes ground a scent; middle notes act like an internal structure holding a smell together, sometimes imperceptible in a scent's final impression; top notes, the exteriority of a scent, grab our attention. Material sensations are often used as metaphors to describe smells—sharp or round, warm or cool. "Scent designers build volume and textures," says Laudamiel. "A scent can be cold, fuzzy, or fluffy."[7] For Cooper Hewitt's exhibition, he selected two "scent sculptures" inspired by contrasting tactile experiences. The first, called Fear, is cold and electric, like touching a knife. Laudamiel started working on this scent when the chef Hector Blumenthal asked him to make a fear smell to accompany a dinner. They visited a bomb shelter in London—a dark, underground place with chalky rock walls. Laudamiel says that the scent

How To Smell

1. **Close your eyes.**
2. **Breathe naturally. Do not sniff or change your breathing.**
3. **Give your nose time to get accustomed to the scent.**
4. **To refresh, breathe your own skin (no coffee beans, please).**
5. **Your brain is learning a new language. It will not explode.**

—Christophe Laudamiel

smells like "wet stones, a rusty fence, and electricity in the air." The second smell, Volatile Marilyn, recalls Marilyn Monroe's white dress, soft skin, and airy freshness. This scent is more than innocent, however: "It is tormented in the middle."

How does smell move and disperse? The air around us is turbulent, flowing like a river. Odor molecules, invisible to the naked eye, are light enough to be swept around in the current, plumes of fragrance furling around us. Scientists have visualized smells by pointing a laser at fluorescent odor molecules. They discovered that odors creep, moving less like a puff of cumulus cloud and more like the rolling coils of thick cigar smoke. Filaments of smells are like tentacles that stretch and extend before they buckle and fold on top of one another.[8] When we sniff, we may tug a tendril from a nearby odor plume into our nasal passage. "Roses," our brain glistens momentarily before the plume passes, trailed by a blank pocket of air devoid of odor molecules.

In a hotel lobby or living room, plumes of fragrance designed for an interior environment can be delivered through a variety of scent players. These devices contain canisters loaded with scents, often in liquid form. The fragrances are heated, diffused into a space with a fan, and cooled before cycling again. Laudamiel's custom fragrances are often diffused into an environment using scent players, programmed to emit aroma throughout the day.

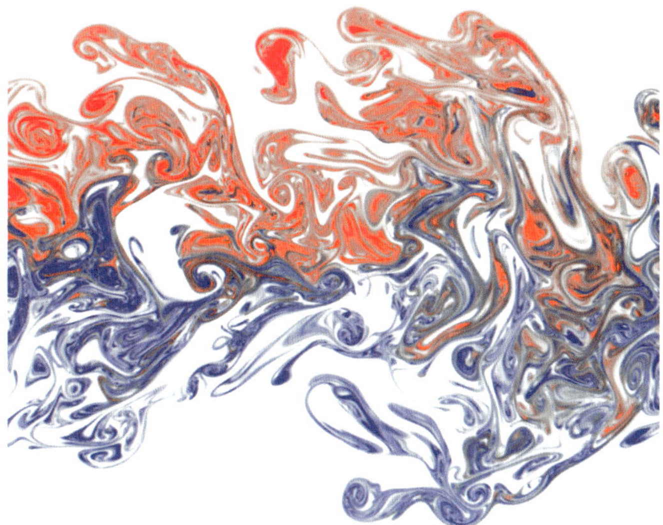

Visualization of two odor fields (one red, one blue) using 2-color laser-induced fluorescence; John Crimaldi and Mike Soltys, University of Colorado, Boulder; Courtesy of John Crimaldi and Mike Soltys, University of Colorado, Boulder

Smell can also be delivered into our spaces more passively. Walls can be studded with smell. Brooklyn-based wallpaper company Flavor Paper produced the first scratch-n-sniff wall-covering in 2007 with Michael Angelo, a celebrated hairstylist whose Wonderland Beauty Parlor in New York City features mirrored walls, a fuchsia settee, and a Mylar waterfall dotted with Barbie mermaids. Among their scratch-n-sniff wallpapers is Cherry Forever, a pop art homage of glossy red cherries on a yellow chrome background. The wallpaper is hand-printed and seeded with microcapsules of fragrant oil. When a user rubs the cherries on the wallpaper, the capsules break open to release the scent—a celebration of the effervescent fifties, a full-fruity embrace of the synthetic cherry fragrance.

By contrast, Cyrano is a portable, digital scent speaker, effectively the first software platform for scent. Users insert scent disks into the device and control it with a smartphone app called oNotes. Loaded with scent disks, Cyrano can be programmed to diffuse a sequence of different scents based on mood or time of day. The scents are designed to stimulate or relax users, to trigger memories or boost productivity. "Surfside" elicits escapism; "Einstein" is reenergizing; "Central Park" induces relaxation. Research shows that smell can make us more alert, stirring us to attention as much as it can seduce us to linger.[9] Beyond boosting our mood though, Cyrano's

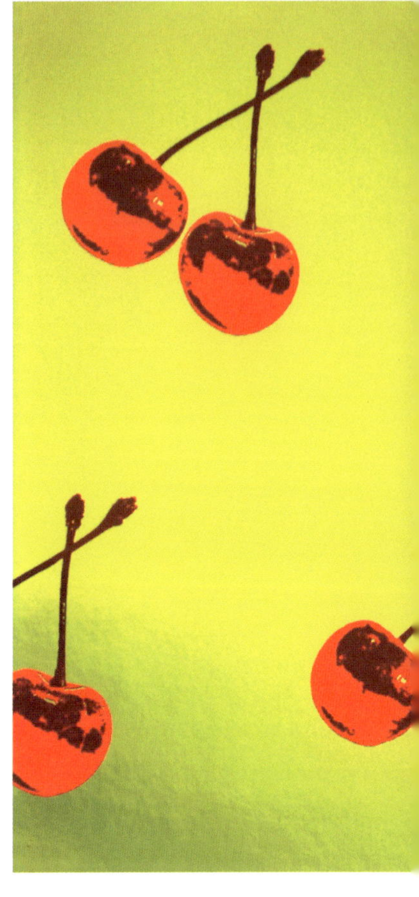

Sidewall, Cherry Forever, 2007; Michael Angelo (American, b. 1970) for Flavor Paper (New York, New York, USA, founded 2003); Screenprinted, microencapsulated scented oils; 457.2 x 75 cm (15 ft. × 2 ft. 5 17⁄32 in.); Gift of Flavor Paper and Michael Angelo, 2007-36-1; Photo courtesy of Flavor Paper

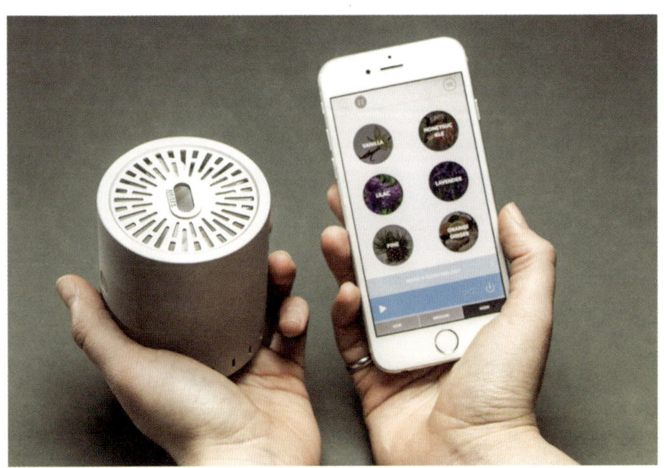

Scent Player, Cyrano, 2017; oNotes (Cambridge, Massachusetts, USA, founded 2013); Aluminum, plastic, electronic components, scent cartridge; 7.6 × 7.6 × 7.6 cm (3 × 3 × 3 in.); Photo by Wayne Earl Chinnock

founders envision a day when the device can be tuned to other content—a movie or song, perhaps—heightening our experience. Hans Laube's dream of Smell-O-Vision is closer than we thought.

For now, Cyrano's changing scents are dubbed "mood medleys." By playing a sequence of different scents, Cyrano combats olfactory fatigue, the phenomenon of losing awareness of a smell over time. When entering a new space, we stop noticing the odor of flowers, pets, or disinfectants after twenty minutes or so. In evolutionary terms, this phenomenon lightens the brain's sensory burden, reserving attention for new signals of danger or opportunity.[10]

Smell can promote well-being for stressed-out urban millennials and aging populations alike. The Ode Dementia Player is a personal scent player that serves dementia patients, for whom weight loss and malnutrition are common conditions. The device is designed to diffuse food smells into a room to stimulate appetites, like a mealtime prompt. Patients in nursing homes and care facilities are often removed from sites of food preparation and their associated smells. Designed by UK-based Rodd Design, Ode's ovular housing is humble and elegant, intended to sit on a table in a living room or bedroom. A user can program three canisters of fragrance to be diffused for two hours at a time around breakfast, lunch, and dinner.

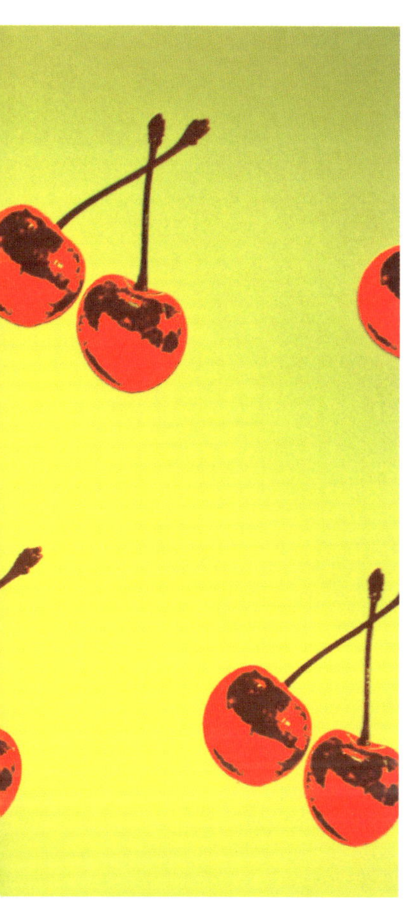

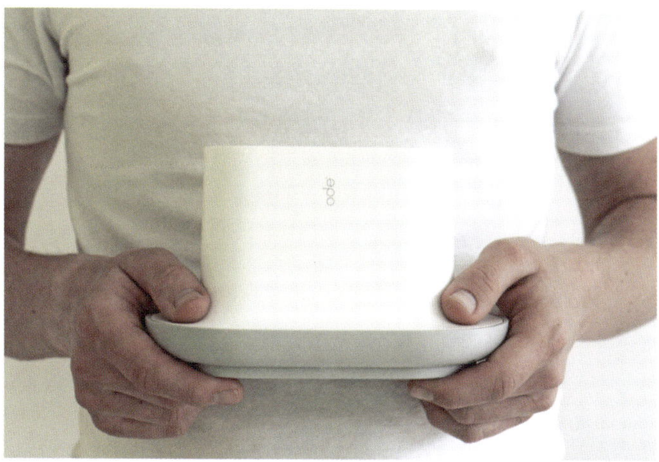

Ode, 2015; Ben Davies (British, b. 1973) and Lizzie Ostrom (British, b. 1982) from Rodd Design (Lyndhurst, UK, founded 2000) and the Olfactory Experience; Mixed materials; 20 × 12 × 12 cm (7 ⅞ × 4 ¾ × 4 ¾ in.); © Ode/Rodd

The Nostalgic fragrance menu includes pink grapefruit, meaty hot-pot, and chocolate cake. The Traditional menu offers fresh orange juice, cherry Bakewell tart, and homemade curry. Caregivers report stimulated appetite, stabilized weight, and improved well-being among their patients. The design harnesses a sensory process for well-being. Olfactory experience often has an agenda.

How does color pair with smell? Color influences how we identify a smell and how intensely we smell it.[11] We associate a cherry smell as red or an earthy smell as brown. Warmer smells like amber, patchouli, and caramel evoke warmer colors. Research shows that congruent color-smell combinations result in a more pleasant odor experience.[12] Packaging design often seeks to heighten these congruencies, tickling the eye in anticipation of the smell to come.

Malin+Goetz, a New York–based family-owned apothecary, coordinates color and smell in their scented candles. The packaging colors are narrative expressions of the fragrances they contain. The Tobacco candle's package is a burnt brown, like the color of tobacco leaves, evocative of velvety-hued cigar-rolling shops in Cuba or a tumbler of rich scotch. The scent of the candle blends bourbon vanilla and rye, chestnut honey, tobacco leaves, and the soft rosiness of guaiac wood. The package for the Cannabis candle is a deep, earthy, resonant brown, reflective of the seductive, spicy scent that is studded with notes of fig, pepper, sandalwood, and patchouli. The Mojito candle is packaged in Caribbean-sea blue, evocative of sun-saturated beaches, long holidays, and minty-lime cocktails. Color reinforces olfactory experience.

Smell is data. Among our most reptilian and ancient survival devices is our ability to scout danger through smell. A wildfire's pungently woodsy burn, a singed electrical wire, or the earthy dampness of an impending storm signals us to evacuate or find shelter. Yet we remain vulnerable to danger. We keep carbon monoxide detectors in our homes because our noses can't detect the odorless gas. When we sleep, olfactory processing is quiet and doesn't readily respond to the smell of

Malin+Goetz Tobacco candle packaging and color specs for scent collection, 2009; Andrew Goetz (American, b. 1962) and Matthew Malin (American, b. 1967), MALIN+GOETZ (New York, New York, USA, founded 2004); Designed by 2 x 4 (New York, New York, USA, founded 1994); Packaging: 10.8 × 8.6 × 8.6 cm (4 ¼ × 3 ⅜ × 3 ⅜ in.); Courtesy of MALIN+GOETZ

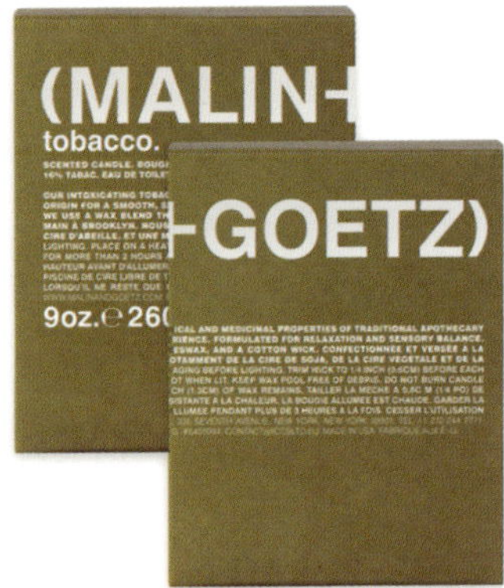

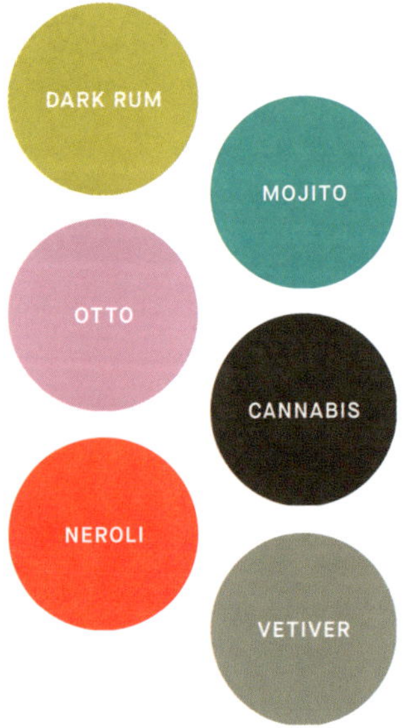

smoke, which is why fire alarms are installed near bedrooms. In fires, most deaths occur because people are sleeping or hard of hearing. The Wasabi Smoke Alarm offers emergency detection through nasal irritation. Researchers at the Shiga University of Medical Science in Japan discovered that an odor inducing a somatosensory response—burning irritation—will awaken us. After testing nearly one hundred smells, including mustard and rotten eggs, they landed on wasabi, waking users with its stinging pungency.

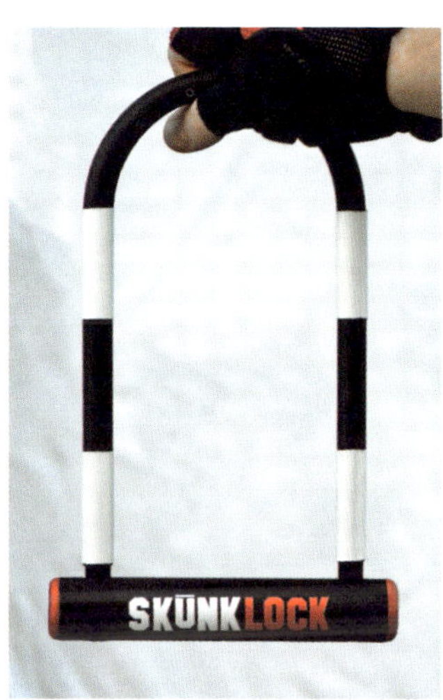

SkunkLock, 2016; Daniel Idzkowski (Polish and American, b. 1989), SkunkLock, Inc. (San Francisco, California, USA, founded 2016); Carbon hardened steel, plastic, rubber, ceramic; 1.9 × 13 × 23.8 cm (3/4 × 5 1/8 × 9 3/8 in.); © Daniel Idzkowski of SkunkLock, Inc.

Smell triggers involuntary reactions. Putrid stenches can make us gag and even vomit. This idea is behind Skunklock, a bike lock that releases noxious chemicals when broken, causing a would-be thief to vomit on the spot. Cofounders Daniel Idzkowski and Yves Perrenoud, avid cyclists based in San Francisco, were frustrated with bike thieves undeterred by even the strongest and smartest locks. The Skunklock uses smell as a crime deterrent. Other companies have sought the same, with more controversial results. Odortec is a company that weaponized smell with its noxious spray called Skunk, used by police and defense forces for nonlethal riot control. One journalist describes it, "Imagine taking a chunk of rotting corpse from a stagnant sewer, placing it in a blender, and spraying the filthy liquid in your face."[13] The spray is nontoxic and biodegradable, according to its developers. The product has been deployed by Israeli police forces against Palestinians. It is reportedly used not just during escalating protests but in peaceful demonstrations, aimed at homes and even funeral processions. Many see it as a tool used to humiliate Palestinians in the name of state-sanctioned crowd control.[14]

Various plants have chemical defenses that warn animals to stay away. Humans, however, learn to crave the bitter alkaloids in coffee or the metallic tinge of cilantro. Young children cling to bland foods, while adults seek sensory adventure. Concentrated oils of oregano and thyme will burn the hands and lungs if touched and inhaled.[15] In addition to flavoring a vat of pizza sauce, such oils can be used to poison and repel roaches.[16] Mint-X, made from mint, is added to trash bags to deter rats and raccoons. Repeated use trains animals to stay away. These animals are better sniffers than humans; a minty odor that smells mildly fresh to us puts them on toxic alert.

Animals also avoid capsaicin, the chemical that makes chili peppers hot. Humans, however, use heat to thrill the palate. Some cultures employ enough capsaicin to make the body run with sweat, which cools the skin with evaporation. Concentrated pepper sprays can cause temporary blindness, constricted breathing, and extraordinary pain.[17] The manufacturer Sabre makes multisensory tools of self-defense, including a line of products packaged in pink to appeal to women — pepper spray, a sonic alarm, and a kit for testing drinks for "date rape" drugs.

How can we protect ourselves from harmful smells? Smell happens with each and every breath, and just as we ingest odor molecules, our body ingests particulate matter from the air. Antipollution masks are on the rise, but trying to get a finicky kid to wear one is like wrangling a noodle. The Woobi Play is an antipollution mask designed for children by Danish firm Kilo with Airmotion Laboratories, a Singapore-based health-tech startup. Current models do not block smell, but odor filters may be developed in the future. The mask comes disassembled in its own cardboard carrying kit and translucent zippered pouch. An illustrated instruction manual tells a story about pollution with our hero (the mask) fighting off bad

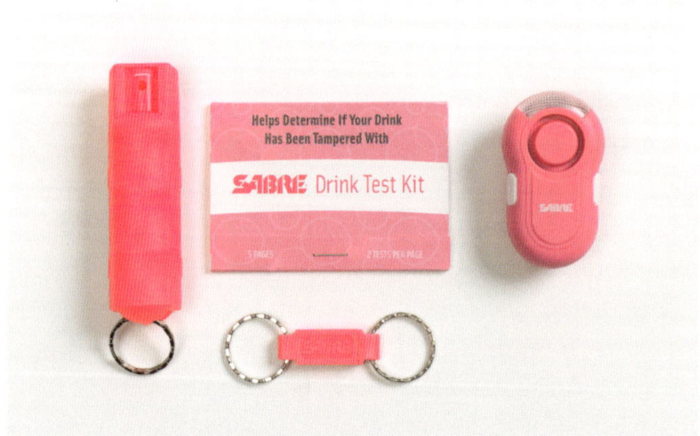

Sabre Pepper Spray and Personal Defense Kit; Plastic, capsaicin, electronic components; Photo by Matt Flynn © Smithsonian Institution

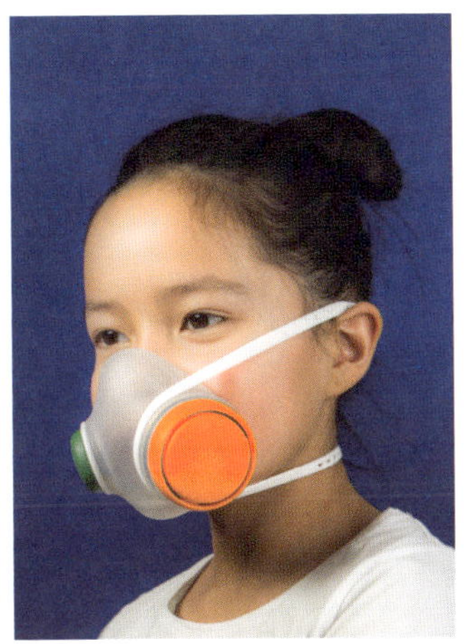

Woobi Play Anti-Pollution Mask, 2017; Kilo (Copenhagen, Denmark, founded 2005); Medical-grade silicone, plastic, hepa filter; 11.9 × 8.9 cm (4 11⁄16 × 3 ½ in.); Courtesy of Kilo

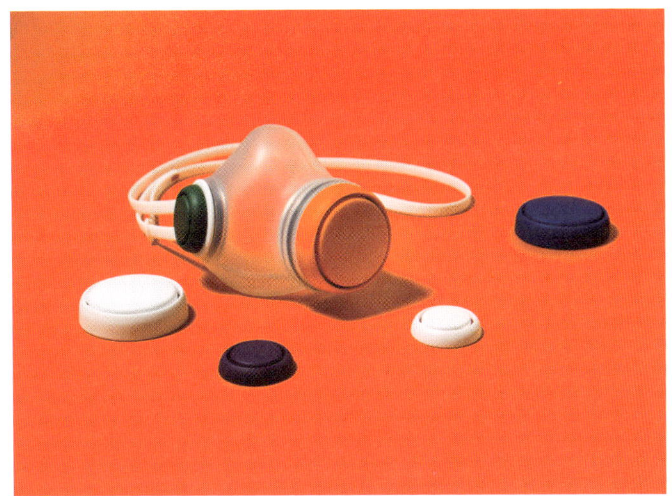

germy characters. Assembly instructions build on the mask's character. Colorful nozzles that look for bad germs are called "eyes"; the band that secures the mask around a child's head is called an "arm." Engage kids in play and they're hooked. But more than the mask's translucent material, bright colors, and contoured shape, consider the user—a child. The design enables the mask's user to be more accessible, approachable, and social. The mask repels pollution, not other people.

Smell is often considered an ancillary sense. Although smell has been guiding us since we were primitive organisms, it lost its urgency to the sense of sight and hearing in our pursuit of survival. We used to believe that humans could distinguish no more than 10,000 smells, but in 2014, scientists discovered that humans can perceive one trillion olfactory stimuli—vastly more than the half million tones and several million colors we can detect.[18] Our olfactory system constantly sends us cues about others, detecting disease, diet, health, and attractiveness, as much as it informs us about our environment and landscape, discriminating time of year, weather, activity, and culture. Olfaction is hardly a linear sense. Smell swirls around us, navigating us toward opportunity, tugging at a memory, moving us away from danger, like the coiling plume of an odor itself.

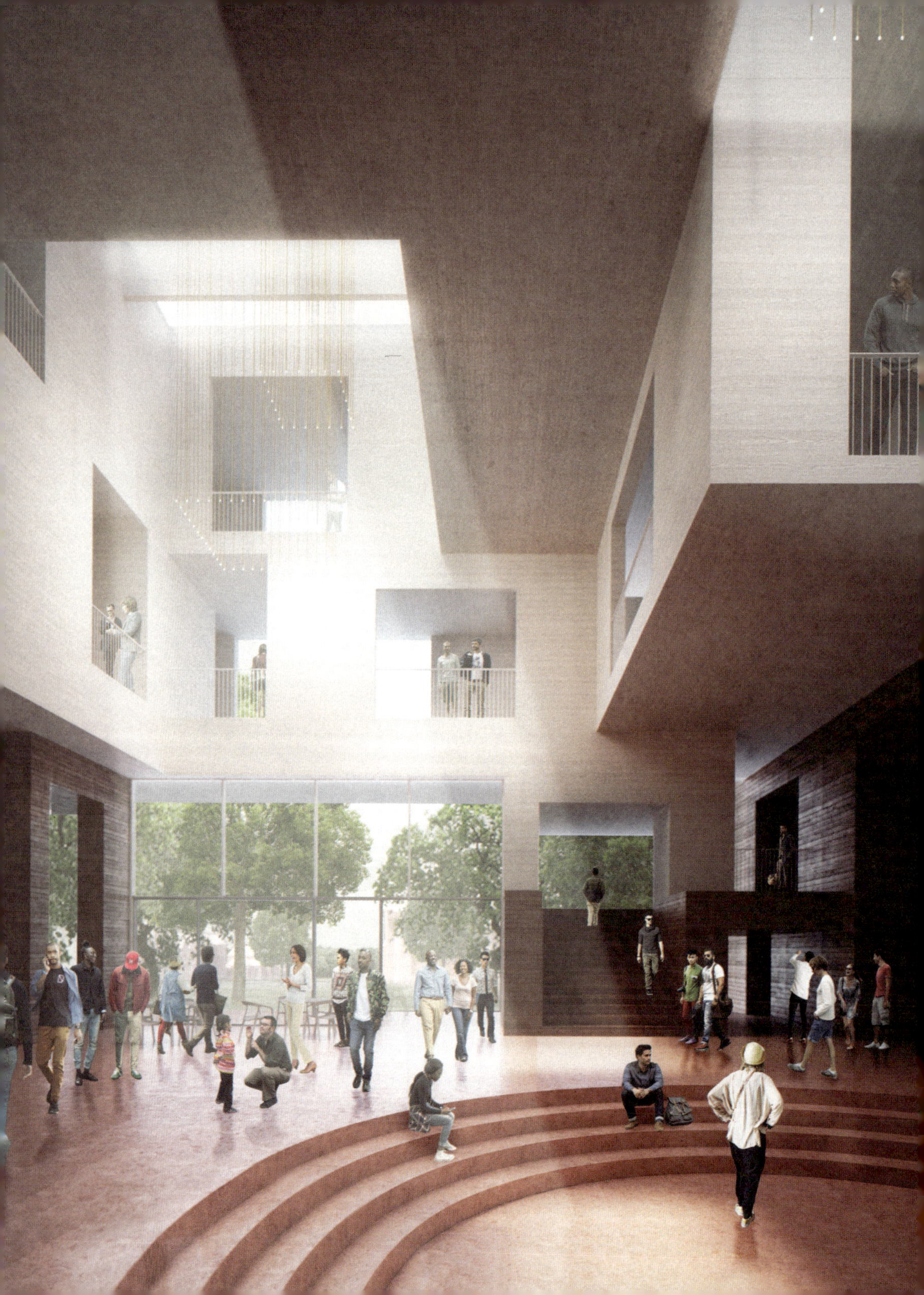

Sensory Environments Every human being has unique capacities to see, hear, touch, smell, and navigate the world. Sensory design offers people multiple ways to communicate, perceive the environment, and find their way through space. Sensory differences are an essential aspect of the human condition. By embracing these differences—which change across the lifespan of each individual—designers are contributing to inclusive design languages. Light, color, sound, texture, movement, vibration, and smell are ingredients of a full-bodied design vocabulary.

Rendering of Gallaudet University for Gallaudet University International Competition, 2016; Hall McKnight (Belfast, Ireland, founded 2003), AECOM (Los Angeles, California, USA, founded 1990); Courtesy of Hall McKnight

On the campus of Gallaudet University, a wide, gleaming hallway takes you through a Victorian building. At the end of this airy corridor, two glass doors open onto a small, bright room. Inside, two people are conversing in sign language. They stand and gesture to one another, their whole bodies in play. Lit by a bay window, these figures stand out like letters on a page. Glittering with life, this transparent chamber exemplifies the qualities of DeafSpace, a design philosophy formulated here at Gallaudet.

Founded in 1856, Gallaudet University is the only liberal arts institution in the United States created for people who are deaf or hard of hearing. Located in northeast Washington, DC, the campus has incorporated many design features over the course of its history that serve its unique community. The footpaths that wind through the campus grounds are unusually wide; the cobblestones bordering each walkway warn your feet that a curb is near. The corridors inside the campus's original buildings also feel wide and open. Reflections glimmer in the polished floors as people pass by. An open stairwell with multiple landings reveals people moving about on different levels, communicating visually. A light switch appears outside each faculty office. Rather than knock on the door, visitors flip the switch on and off to announce themselves.

DeafSpace is a theory and practice of design crafted for people who are deaf or hard of hearing. In DeafSpace, sensory details highlight human presence. Spacious passageways encourage gathering and conversation. Light and color clarify gesture and movement. Surfaces shimmer as bodies traverse

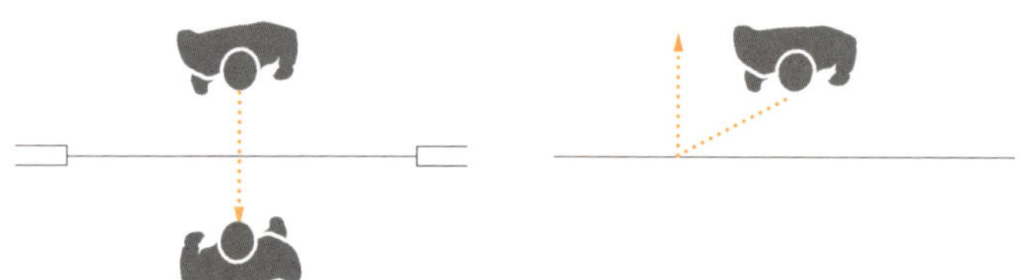

People who are deaf or hard of hearing use transparent and reflective surfaces to maximize their sensory reach. DeafSpace, 2015; Hansel Bauman; Courtesy of the designer

along them. Vibrations carry across wooden floors. Acoustic surfaces reduce noisy reverb. Circular seating arrangements allow people to talk together with their hands, eyes, and faces. Architect Hansel Bauman drafted the DeafSpace guidelines. Bauman, a hearing architect, was introduced to Gallaudet in 2005 by his brother, a professor of Deaf Studies at the university.[1] Through a series of collaborative workshops and courses conducted with students and colleagues at Gallaudet over a four-year period, Bauman and his colleagues distilled a body of sensory design principles.

"Air and light connect people," Bauman says during a walk through Gallaudet's grounds. "Reflections on a glass wall or a shiny floor alert you to your surroundings. Oak flooring vibrates. Concrete doesn't." As he talks, he lightly underscores his words with sign language, so that people passing by feel included. Bauman, who oversees campus design and works with international architects to create new buildings, sees himself not as the inventor or author of DeafSpace so much as its finder and keeper.[2]

A 14-month-old child who is deaf is touching a board-marked concrete wall in a building designed by Hall McKnight (Belfast, Ireland, founded 2003); Courtesy of Hall McKnight

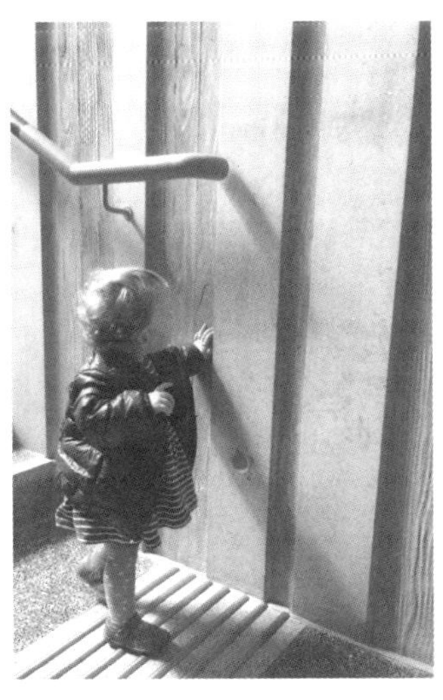

In 2016, Gallaudet awarded its latest commission to Hall McKnight, a prominent architectural firm based in Ireland, following an international competition. The new building will sit at the busy corner of 6th Street and Florida Avenue, replacing a heavy parking structure that squares its shoulders against the city. Different levels of separation connect the building to the outside world. The structure is more open to the neighborhood near 6th Street, and more private to the deaf community toward the campus interior. Hall McKnight conceived the building as a collection of planes and volumes—pierced with balconies—that open onto a central atrium. Recalling a Greek amphitheater, a low flight of circular stairs becomes impromptu seating in the round. Fins in the ceiling diffuse light. Rooms and galleries look down on the atrium, connecting people visually as they move through different parts of the complex. "We want to make places that offer a unique sensory experience conducive to, and expressive of, Deaf culture and people of all abilities," the architects explain.

DeafSpace builds on the instinctive adaptations of deaf people, who constantly design their own environments to maximize their sensory experience. Stephen Gorman, who holds degrees in nursing and anthropology, was born hard of hearing. He wears two digital hearing aids and spent nearly ten years in speech therapy learning to read lips. Learning to lipread, he explains, is about learning to vocalize as well as learning to understand the speech of others. Speech isn't just sound: it is a muscular activity involving lips, tongue, and throat. Speech is a tangible, physical process.

When Gorman enters a restaurant with friends, he looks for the best place to sit. He tries to find a spot that faces out (giving him a view of the space and his companions) and that has a wall directly behind him (blocking ambient noise). After taking his seat, Gorman adjusts his digital hearing aid with a smartphone app. The app's restaurant setting shuts out sounds coming from behind him. He thus uses assistive technology and the inherent architecture of the room to make sure he can see and hear everything that's important. He says, "My visual acuity is stronger than other people's. I am super-alert to movement in all directions." His partner, neurologist Richard Cytowic, laughs and says, "Steve can tell you what anyone in this restaurant is talking about, even if they're across the room, as long as he can see their faces."[3]

Bauman points out that while architects tend to approach design as a visual medium, they often fail to acknowledge the difficulties created by narrow, poorly lit spaces. The principles of DeafSpace include considering the distances between people as they move and communicate, extending the sensory reach of individuals by offering open views and visible destinations, and using light, color, and materials to enable communication and wayfinding.

Controlling acoustics is also important. A room bouncing with reverb is distressing for anyone, especially for those who use hearing aids or cochlear implants. Carpets and drapes change how rooms sound and feel. Imagine walking through an emptied-out apartment, just before the moving truck drives away. Perhaps you can sense your steps echoing in the void. Books, blankets, rugs, and chairs trap and scatter sound waves. The echoes in an empty room arrive a tiny bit later than sound waves heading directly to the ear; these late-breaking waves distort the pattern of the earlier ones, muddling the crisp sounds of speech.[4]

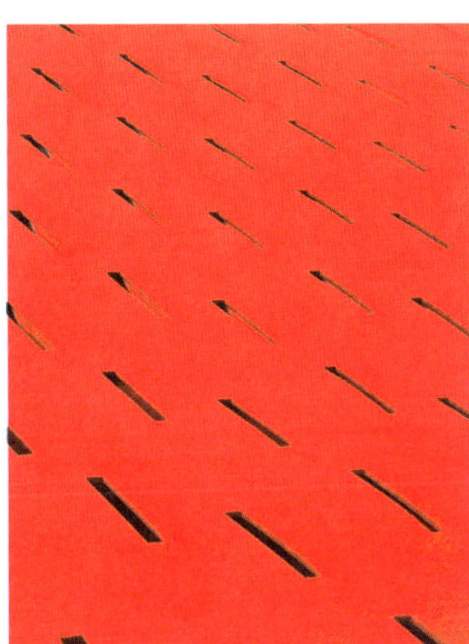

Hanging panels, 2014; Architecture Research Office (ARO) (New York, New York, USA, founded 1993), Manufactured by FilzFelt (Boston, Massachusetts, USA, founded 2008); ARO Array, 100% wool design felt; Courtesy of FilzFelt and Knoll

Brick, tile, glass, and plasterboard—the ubiquitous skins of modern architecture—make sounds bounce and echo. Drapes and carpets capture sound waves and keep them from springing back as echoes. Surfaces that are soft, perforated, or furrowed with grooves and gaps not only control the overall loudness of a room but also make speech more intelligible. Jonathan Hopkins, director of acoustics for DLR Group Architects, explains that absorptive materials make sound "decay" more quickly in the room, preventing individual syllables from blending together. "This makes the space more pleasant to be in," he says. "People will linger there longer when the loudness is controlled."[5] Wool felt is used in many acoustic architectural products as well as in the manufacture of audio equipment. ARO Array, a series of 100 percent wool felt panels designed for FilzFelt by Architecture Research Office (ARO), feature patterns of linear slashes inspired by the rhythm of rain showers. The perforations enhance the product's acoustic performance as well as producing an elegant surface.

In addition to absorbing sound, surfaces can diffuse or scatter it. The carved moldings and coffered ceilings often found in traditional interiors send sound waves off in different directions, enhancing the sound quality of a room. Acoustic diffusers disperse sound waves over a larger area, similar to the way a translucent lampshade can spread light from a single bulb through an entire room. Whether curved, faceted, or punched with holes, diffusers level out a room's acoustics while preserving the vibrant, "live" character of the space.

Sound interacts with space. A musical instrument sounds different when played in a vast auditorium instead of a small room. The history of architecture intersects the history of music. Musician and songwriter David Byrne explains that gothic cathedrals—with their narrow, soaring spaces—supported medieval chants, with long notes sung in a single key. Bach's music was performed in concert halls that were less cavernous than churches, supporting compositions of greater complexity and sonic differentiation. Mozart, who played in smaller, more sound-absorbing rooms than Bach, composed ornate, "frilly" pieces. In the twentieth century, the ability to amplify music in vast open arenas spawned stadium rock. To survive in this environment, stadium rock needs to make a big sound with a medium tempo. In contrast, musicians producing music for a car or an MP3 player can layer their songs with detail. From the cathedral to the Cadillac, environments set the stage for social interactions and musical creativity.[6]

Architecture's profound effect on sound is demonstrated in *The Wikisinger*, a video directed by Vincent Rouffiac for Touché Videoproduktion in 2015. Here, Joachim Müllner performs an original song in fifteen different locations, from an intimate bedroom and an underground tunnel to a soaring church nave and an open field. Moving from place to place, Müllner's voice can sound crisp or hollow or dipped in honey. Each surrounding can be heard in the song. Music producers often use reverb filters to add echoes and reflections to a piece after it has been recorded, creating an illusion of space. In *The Wikisinger*, those qualities are authentic to the spaces where the song was recorded.

Peaceful healthcare environments enhance wellness; it's tough to rest or recover in a noisy patient room.[7] Cacophonous hospitals or workplaces are distressing, but so are environments that are too still and too quiet. In a hospital setting, doctors, patients, and families need privacy to talk. To address this problem, many hospitals employ sound masking, a technology that distributes a pleasant, neutral sound throughout an environment to mask conversations.[8] For many people, the clatter of a café boosts concentration and creativity. Various smartphone apps pump social sounds of restaurants or parks into the headsets of urbanites craving escape from the lonesome muffle of a dorm room or home office.

Stills, *The Wikisinger*, 2015; Directed by Vincent Rouffiac (French, b. 1981); Produced by TOUCHÉ Videoproduktion (Vienna, Austria, founded 2015) for Joachim Müllner; Video; Courtesy of Vincent Rouffiac

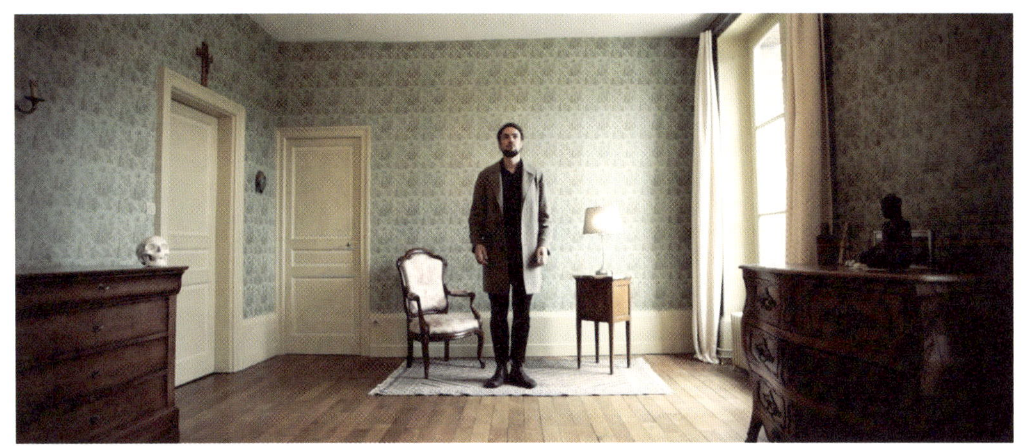

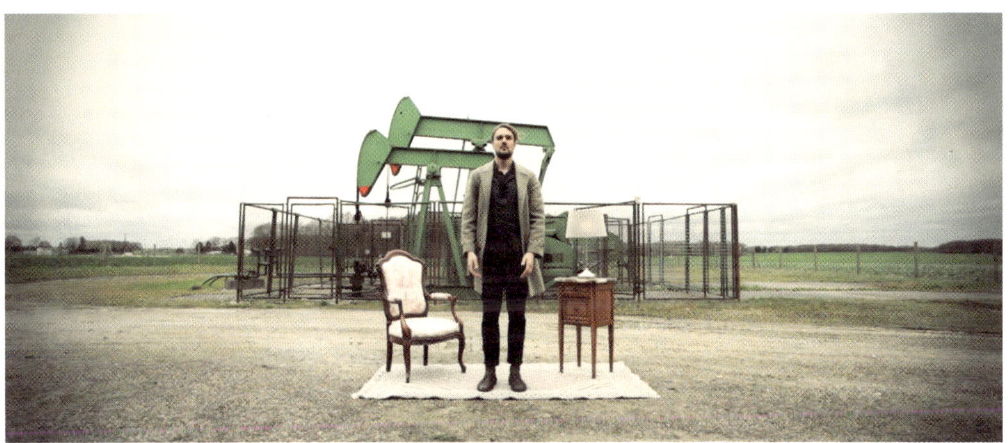

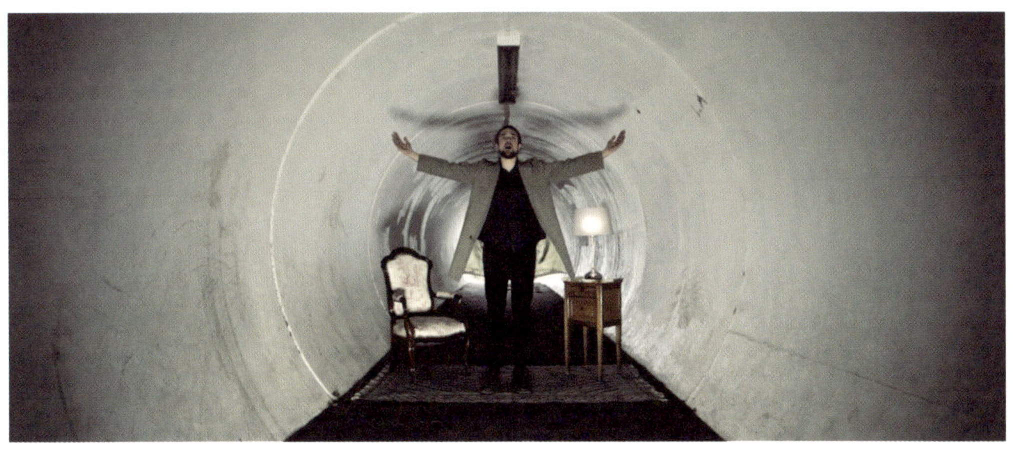

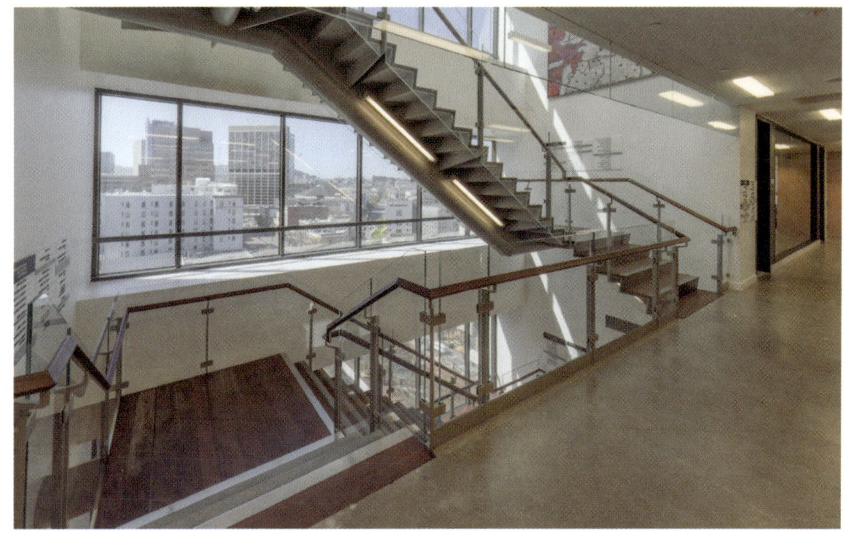

To experience a space designed for acoustic enjoyment and legibility, visit San Francisco's LightHouse for the Blind and Visually Impaired, occupying several upper floors of an urban office on Market Street. As you move from the elevator to the LightHouse lobby, you might hear people moving up and down the stairs and in the hallways. A carpeted area around the reception desk creates a quiet zone, enabling conversation with the staff. The wide passageways are designed for people walking with mobility canes, guide dogs, and human companions. Natural and artificial light work together to create consistent illumination, maximizing visual clarity without reducing people to mere silhouettes when viewed with low vision conditions. The LightHouse interior was designed in 2015 by Mark Cavagnero Associates in consultation with Chris Downey, an architect who became blind after surgery for a brain tumor. Downey says, "I'm interested in how to convey delight in architecture whether it is seen or not."[9]

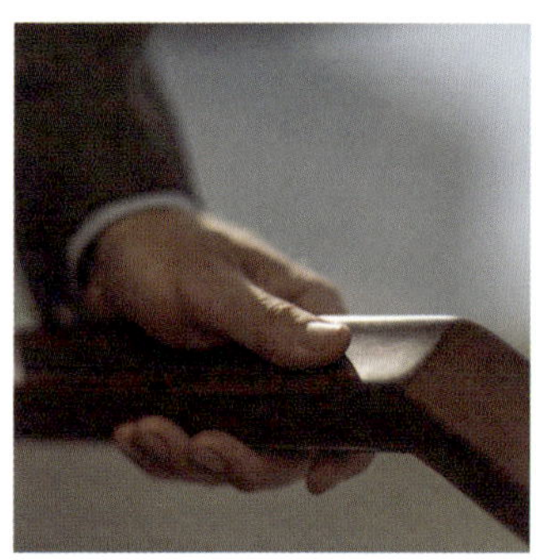

Stairwell and stairwell railing, 2015; Chris Downey (American, b. 1962), Mark Cavagnero Associates (San Francisco, California, USA, founded 1988) for LightHouse for the Blind and Visually Impaired (San Francisco, California, USA, founded 1902); Photo by Don Fogg

The staircase at LightHouse engages sight, sound, and touch. The railing feels good in the hand, and it is mounted with brackets that aren't sharp and angular. Downey explains, "When you are blind and you grab a handrail, you might not know when a bracket is coming." Downey creates tactile

Tactile Drawing for Stairwell Railing, LightHouse for the Blind and Visually Impaired, San Francisco, 2015; Chris Downey (American, b. 1962); Wax sticks on paper; Photo by Don Fogg

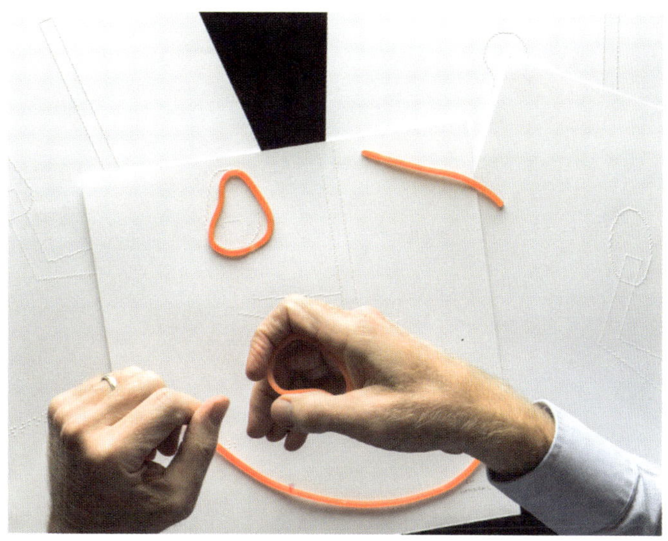

drawings with thin wax sticks that he presses onto sheets of paper. For the LightHouse project, he made a series of these tactile drawings to suggest different profiles for the railing. The design team produced 3D prints to test how the railing would feel. The stair treads employ hard, tropical ipe wood and a textured front edge that is legible to a mobility cane. "The stair's acoustic attributes animate the space," Downey says. "We intentionally didn't carpet the stair. If you carpet the stair it disappears to a blind user. We used wood not metal, because metal cane tips on the metal stair would be too loud."[10] Concrete floors in the hallways and public spaces make the sounds of canes and footsteps audible.

Downey worked with Shane Myrbeck at the engineering firm Arup to simulate and test the building's sound. Together, they sought to capture the blind experience of architecture. There is no way to draw or share an acoustic design until it's built—unless you can model it in Arup's sophisticated sound lab. Downey and Myrbeck created a "tap-through" of the space, based on recordings of Downey's cane tapping on comparable materials. Myrbeck added these sounds to a digital model that captures the sonic reflectivity of materials and their interaction with the architecture.

NEXT SPREAD
Tactile Architectural Drawing, 2015; Chris Downey (American, b. 1962), Mark Cavagnero Associates (San Francisco, California, USA, founded 1988) for Lighthouse for the Blind and Visually Impaired (San Francisco, California, USA, founded 1902); Embossed digital print; Photo by Don Fogg, Courtesy of LightHouse for the Blind and Visually Impaired

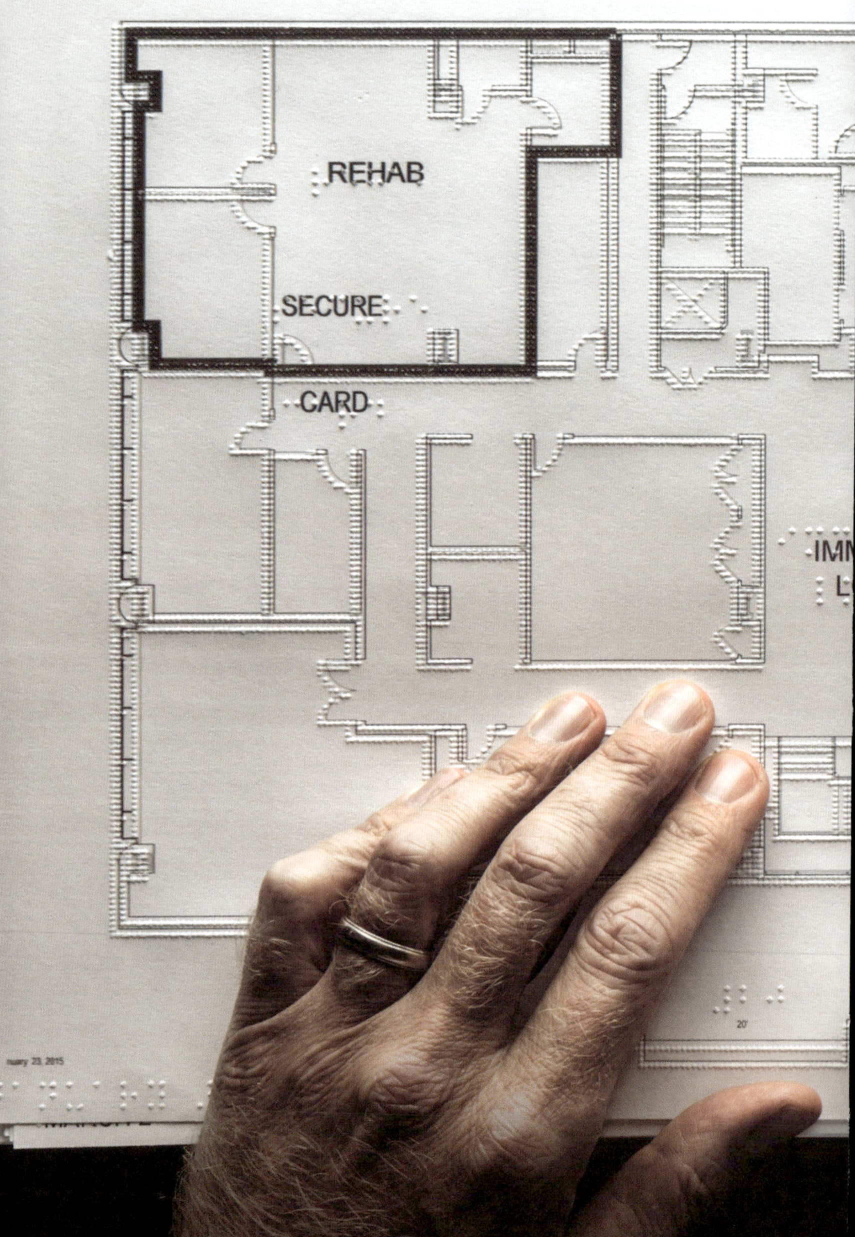
REHAB
SECURE
CARD
20'

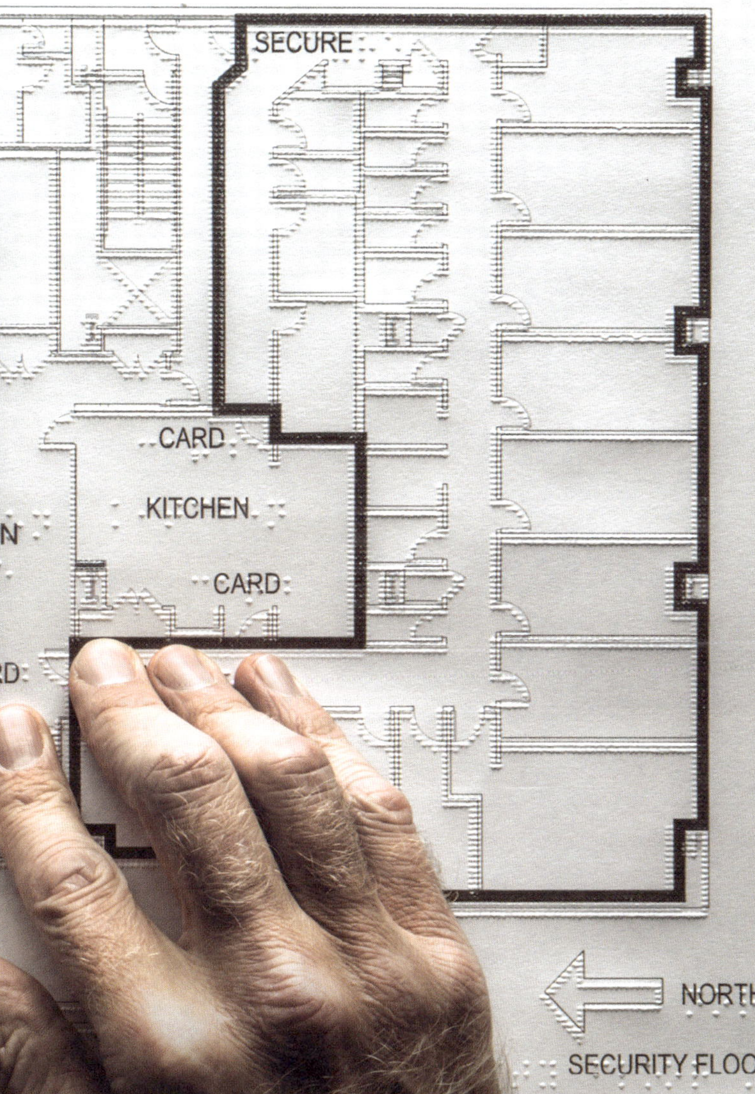
CARD
SECURE
CARD
KITCHEN
CARD
NORTH
SECURITY FLOOR 11

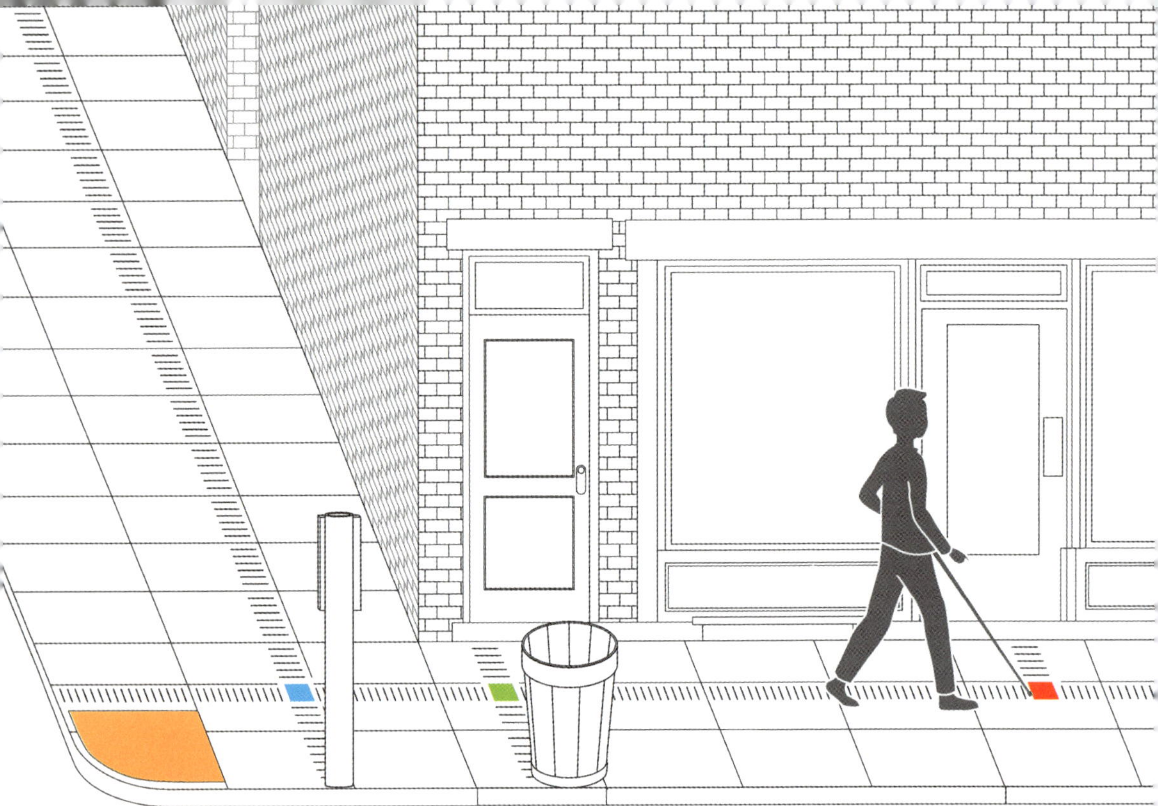

Tactile City is an experimental proposal for a citywide tactile communication system for visually and cognitively impaired pedestrians. The project was conceived by a group of Cooper Union students, led by faculty member Theodore Kofman, in response to a challenge posed by the NYC Department of Design and Construction and the Mayor's Office for People with Disabilities. The Tactile City concept expands on existing tactile paving systems. Different textures would indicate points of interest, such as a bus stop, trash receptacle, building entrance, or signage post indicating the street address and the major public facilities nearby. Different textures would be used to identify different street amenities. After identifying a texture change, a user can turn accordingly to locate the object. Tactile City is conceived as a standard system that can be learned.

Tactile City, 2015; Project Instructor: Theodore Kofman, Students: Charlie Blanchard, Chris Taleff, Thomas Heyer, and Ratan Rai Sur, Alumni team: Emilie Gossiaux and Wai-Jee Ho; The Irwin S. Chanin School of Architecture, The Cooper Union (New York, New York, USA, founded 1859), with support from the New York City Department of Design and Construction; Courtesy of Theodore Kofman

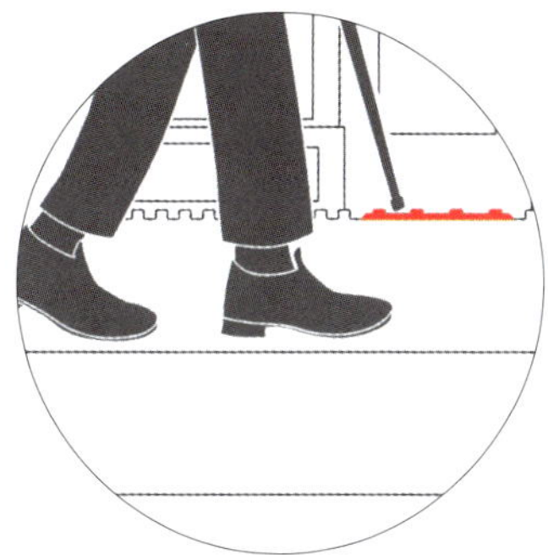

Tactile City also addresses urban construction sites, which generate countless pedestrian detours throughout New York City. For short-term detours, Tactile City proposes to install tactile aids on existing barriers. Along the upper edge of a barrier, text in braille or raised letters could be felt by hand. Along the base of a barrier, tactile aids could be felt with a mobility cane. For long-term construction detours, Tactile City proposes adding ramped, elevated platforms throughout the detour. Here, when the tactile path reaches a construction site, a large textured surface would announce the upcoming detour. The textured surface shape would correspond with the

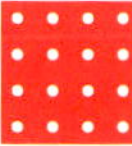

BUILDING ENTRANCE

Interviews with visually impaired pedestrians revealed that marking building entrances is crucial to navigating the city.

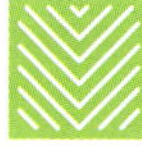

STREET FURNITURE

Benches and seats will be marked on the tactile path.

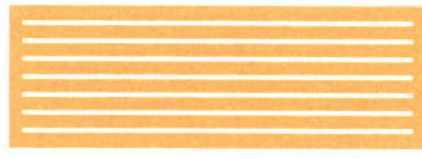

BLOCK SEGMENT

A "tactile" address will divide the block into four segments, each identified by words, letters, and numbers. For example: "block x, third segment, first door."

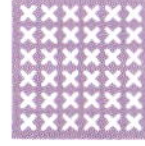

TRANSIT STOP

With no tactile signifiers, stations are tough to identify. A tactile indicator will make public transportation more accessible.

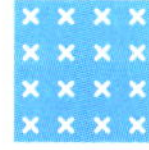

INFORMATION PANEL

Indicates the address in braille as well as providing useful information about the block.

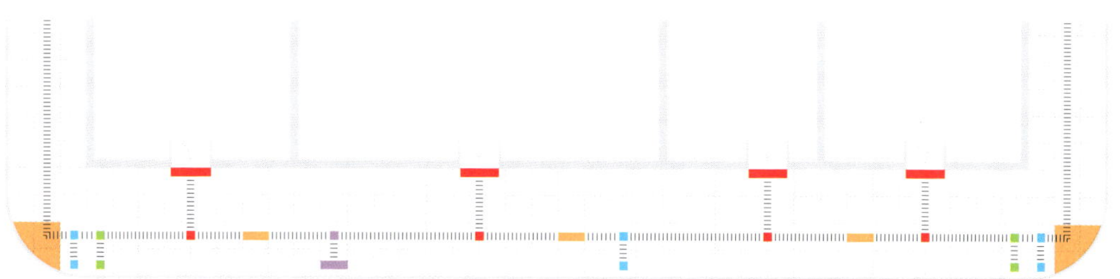

direction of the turn. An additional motion-activated sound device placed on the barriers would show users which way to turn. This noise-sensitive device would be louder when the environment is loud, and quieter at night and other quiet times. Braille placed at railing height would indicate the distance to the next turn, as well as the distance to the end of the temporary path.

Seiichi Miyake invented the concept of tactile paths in Japan in 1967. His patterned yellow paths were first adopted by Japan National Railways and then mandated for broader use in Japan in 1985. Their bright color is visible for people with low vision or cognitive impairments. Although similar paths have been used in other countries, the paths have been constructed inconsistently over time.[11] Tactile paths and textured paving blocks are controversial. The commonly used truncated-dome pattern can cause pain and discomfort to wheelchair users. Some people argue that tactile paths separate blind pedestrians from other citizens, imposing a strict rectilinear movement in a context where others are moving around organically. In response, Kofman says, "The tactile path system offers an option, an alternative. It doesn't mandate anyone following it or walking along it. In this regard, a person might feel more comfortable walking with a guide dog instead." The creators of Tactile City (Theodore Kofman, Emilie Gossiaux, Charlie Blanchard, Thomas Heyer, Christopher Taleff, Ratan Rai Sur, and Wai-Jee Ho) believe their concept should be further developed and tested, in a process that would account for its potential benefits and shortcomings.

Every city is a brew of sensory stimulants. Streets and sidewalks teem with life. Sensory design can shape the beauty and function of a place—and address dangers and obstacles. A busy café could jangle the nerves or buzz with energy. A museum layout could encourage sustained looking or trigger a mad rush to the gift shop. An urban park could flicker with breeze and birdsong or roar with traffic under a hard sun. A room or a landscape that tingles with sensory energy gives everyone something to feel.

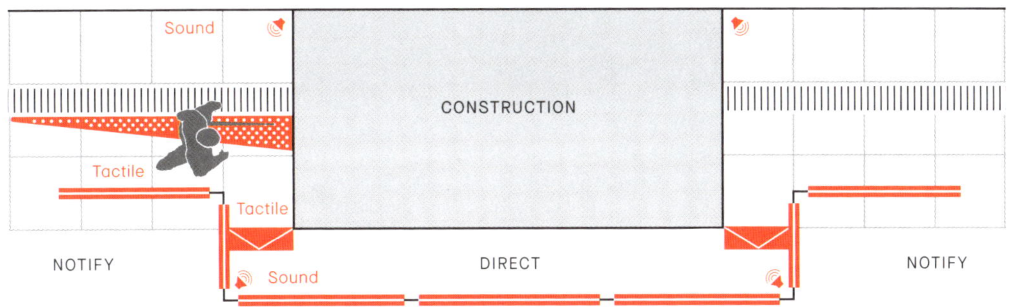

When pedestrian movement is interrupted by a temporary construction barrier, it is necessary to convey information about the interruption to multiple senses simultaneously. The proposed solution uses both sonic and tactile markers to identify barriers in advance and guide pedestrians through them.

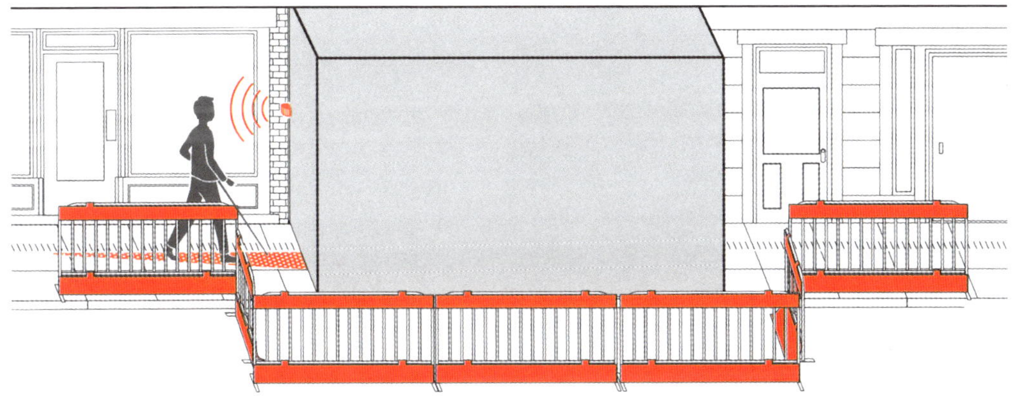

Tactile City, 2015; Project Instructor: Theodore Kofman, Students: Charlie Blanchard, Chris Taleff, Thomas Heyer, and Ratan Rai Sur, Alumni team: Emilie Gossiaux and Wai-Jee Ho; The Irwin S. Chanin School of Architecture, The Cooper Union (New York, New York, USA, founded 1859), with support from the New York City Department of Design and Construction; Courtesy of Theodore Kofman

Hansel Bauman

DeafSpace

Many in the deaf community identify with Deaf culture, which is built around a shared language, shared life experiences, and common cognitive sensibilities. DeafSpace is one way in which Deaf culture, in all its diverse dimensions, can thrive. DeafSpace cultivates the unique cognitive, cultural, and creative dimensions of deaf experience.

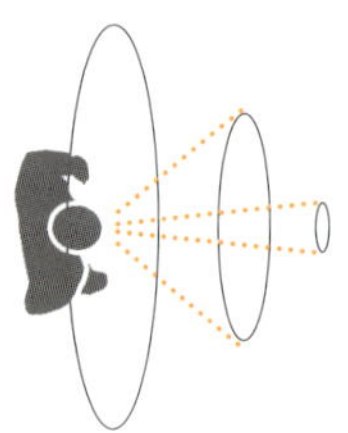

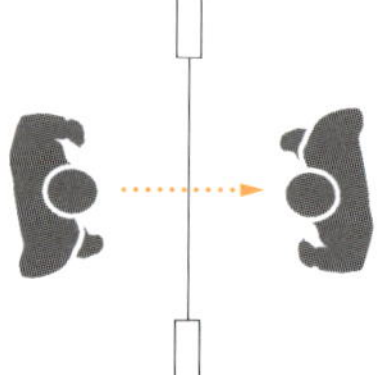

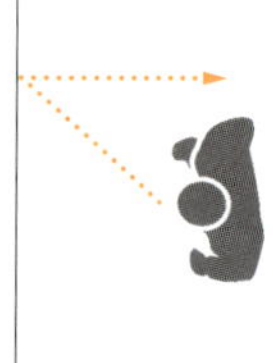

PERIPHERAL

The first means for extending sensory reach is the use of rhythmic, repetitive, and intuitive visual cues to allow a deaf person's peripheral vision to work more effectively in orientation. As a design element, this can manifest itself as a large scale wayfinding strategy or as the simple legibility of building or room uses. Such cues offer multiple points of reference to people seeking to orient themselves visually.

+ TRANSPARENCY

Visual connections, openness, and transparency serve to extend sensory reach. This complex endeavor must be carefully balanced with privacy and comfort concerns. The degree of enclosure needs to reflect the situation and assure a balance of visual connectivity, privacy, and safety.

+ REFLECTION

Reflection can extend vision, allowing deaf individuals to see behind themselves and around corners, as well as helping them gauge depth. By using strategically placed reflective surfaces, individuals can carry on signed conversations while monitoring their environment in 360 degrees. Reflective surfaces can also be used in corridors to avoid collisions around corners and alert individuals when someone is approaching from behind.

Sensory Reach

Sensory reach consists of the interrelated modes of perception (hearing, seeing, smelling, feeling) that are used to orient oneself in space. Although deaf individuals do not hear sound, they have developed ways to extend their sensory reach and successfully sense the world around them. Although vision is one means by which deaf individuals gain information about their surroundings, they also utilize vibratory, tactile, and social cues to achieve the 360-degree sensory reach that hearing typically provides.

Extending sensory reach is a primary goal of DeafSpace, a set of sensory design principles that support physical and emotional well-being. In this space one's own unique identity as a deaf person can be explored and nurtured. Deaf experiences offer insight about people's sense of disconnection and connection with others and with their environment. The deaf experience foreshadows a broader cycle in society of lacking and desiring connection.

HANSEL BAUMAN is Executive Director of Design and Construction at Gallaudet University, the world's only university designed to be barrier-free for deaf and hard-of-hearing students. He is the creator of the DeafSpace guidelines. These sensory design principles have been applied to projects on the Gallaudet campus and other public institutions.

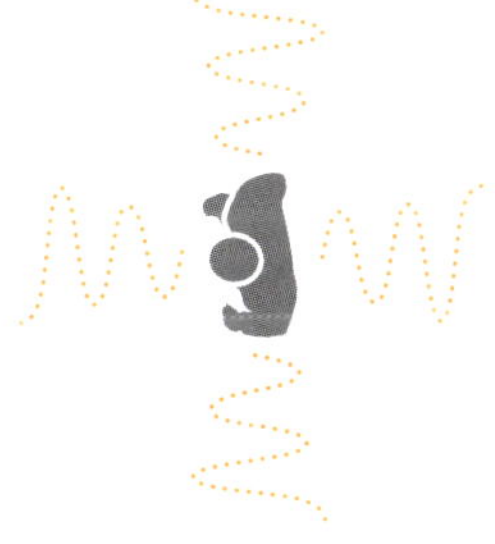

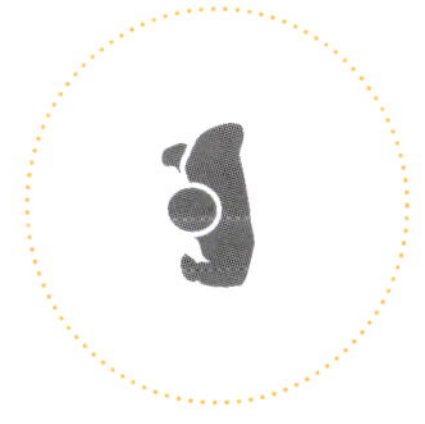

\+ **VIBRATION**
Floor surfaces that allow for some degree of noticeable vibration should be used in defined spaces where deaf occupants may desire to initiate contact with one another through a tap on the floor or furniture. Such spaces may include meeting rooms, classrooms, and living spaces within a residential setting.

\+ **SHARED SENSORY REACH**
When deaf individuals navigate their environment, they depend on one another to extend their sensory reach. For example, if two people are walking down a sidewalk, one person might point out children playing behind his companion while the other might warn the first about an approaching car. Shared sensory reach is deeply rooted in the Deaf community.

= **360 DEGREES**
A sense of self—or "personhood"—for deaf individuals is reinforced through eye-to-eye contact and a sense of shared sensory experiences and creative endeavors. Buildings for the deaf community should foster a sense of community by providing multiple opportunities to view peers engaged in creative endeavors and to display this work with others.

Cognitive Sensibilities

Spatial orientation, wayfinding, and the awareness of activities within our surroundings are essential to maintaining a sense of personal safety and well-being. Visual cues seen through openings to adjacent spaces, or subtle images seen in reflected surfaces or felt through structure-borne vibrations, happen through the fundamental aspects of architecture—form, material, and light. Primary building uses, especially interior social spaces like lounges, conference rooms, and large assembly spaces, should be made legible from the outside whenever possible. This legibility aids in wayfinding within buildings and their broader context. The built environment, from the city scale to the scale of a room, should be planned and designed with a coherent and intuitive set of cues indicating destinations and signifying important places. These should be visually accessible from multiple vantage points and along circulation pathways.

VISIBLE DESTINATIONS & VIEW CORRIDORS

Major destination points should be visible from multiple places within a building. When entering a building or public space, destinations should be immediately apparent and their access unobstructed. Circulation routes and layouts should be clear and intuitive.

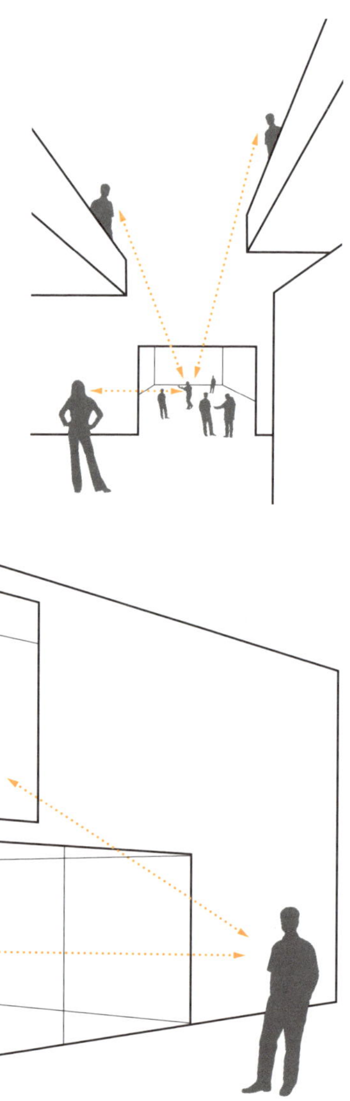

Legibility of building

TRANSPARENCY & REFLECTION

Bay windows allow individuals a wider range of view and connection to the outdoors. This increased range provides greater visual access to activities taking place outside of the building and increases connection to a building's grounds and the neighborhood context. Reflective surfaces should also be used in movement spaces to prevent collisions around corners and alert individuals when someone is approaching from behind. Glass elevators lessen the feeling of confinement, increase actual and perceived safety, and allow visual connection to adjacent spaces.

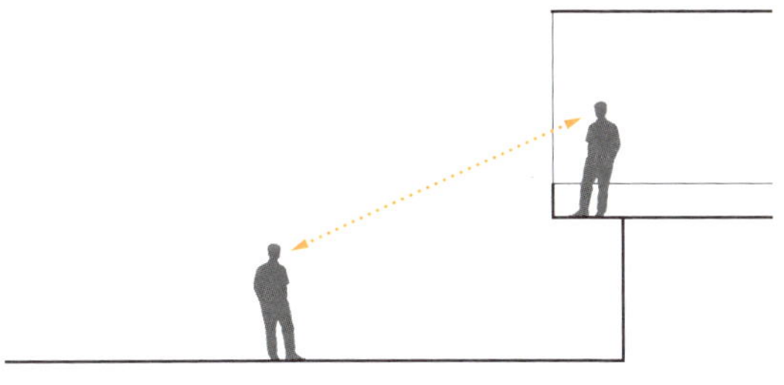

Bay windows

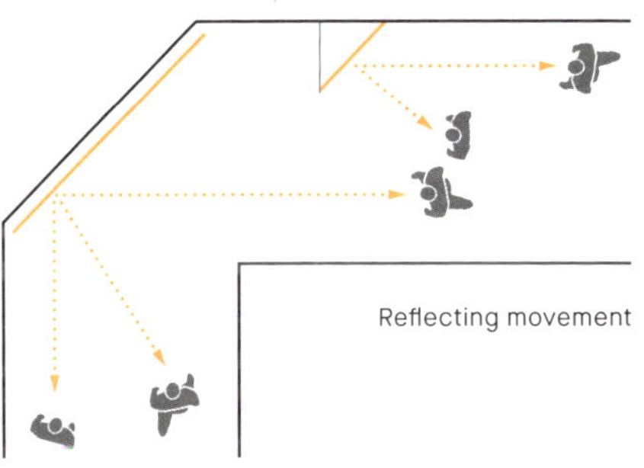

Reflecting movement

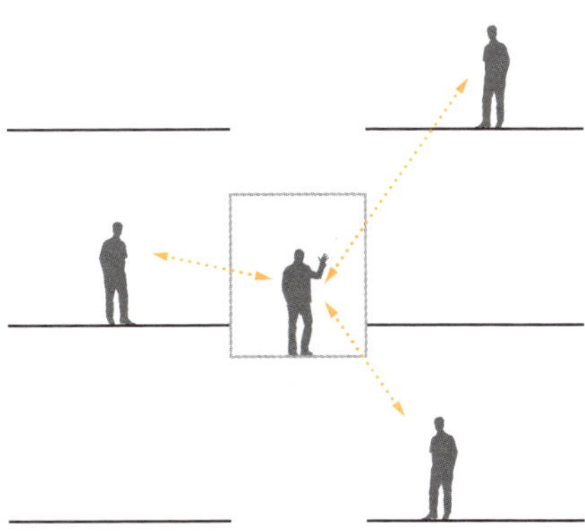

Glass elevators

VIBRATION

Floor surfaces that propagate perceptible vibrations allow deaf occupants to tap on the floor or furniture to initiate communication. The edges of these areas should be well defined and buffered from undesired sources of vibration. Zones of floor surfaces that transmit vibration can serve as wide thresholds between public circulation areas and private spaces, providing a subtle cue of approaching visitors.

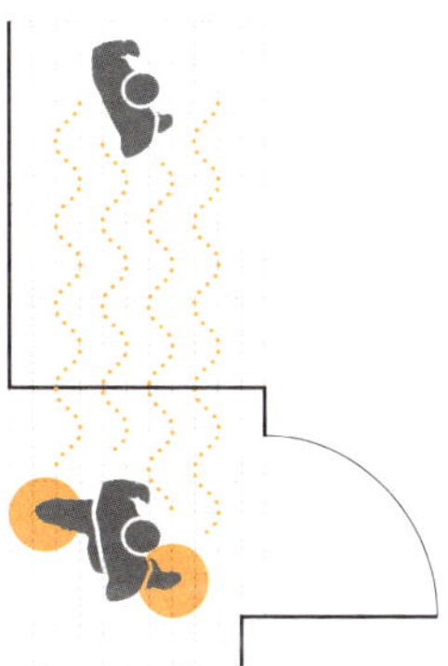

Vibration zone: approaching visitor can be sensed

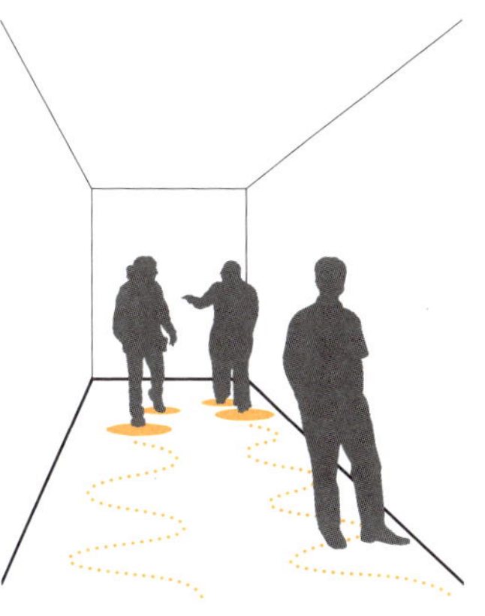

Vibration within room

Cultural Expression

Deaf culture is collectivist. Fundamental architectural elements of form, material, color, and light can be used to encourage sustained social interaction. Within Deaf culture, the built environment takes on anthropomorphic characteristics. The deliberate openness and visual connection between spaces introduces building occupants to one another so they are able to interact socially.

Buildings can serve as "the third person"—the one within a group of signers walking together who scans the path forward and warns the group of hazards or a change in direction. Like the third person, buildings can enhance personal safety and wayfinding. Building spaces can also be designed to care for social interactions. By balancing visual connection and privacy, interior spaces help sustain a sense of spatial and social connection. The "sensory threshold," for example, creates a wall or zone between spaces that allows subtle cues of movement to pass between the spaces—in other words, to draw the attention to the movement of others without startling interruption.

VISIBILITY THROUGH GLASS

Making activity spaces, conference rooms, labs, and offices transparent to circulation areas stimulates interest in what's going on and creates a connection that is vital to Deaf culture.

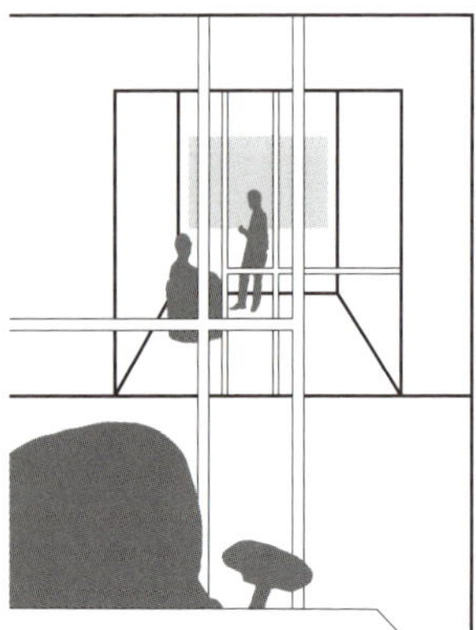

WIDE WALKWAYS

Sidewalk/path width allows several groups of signers to pass one another easily. Textured surface demarcates the edges.

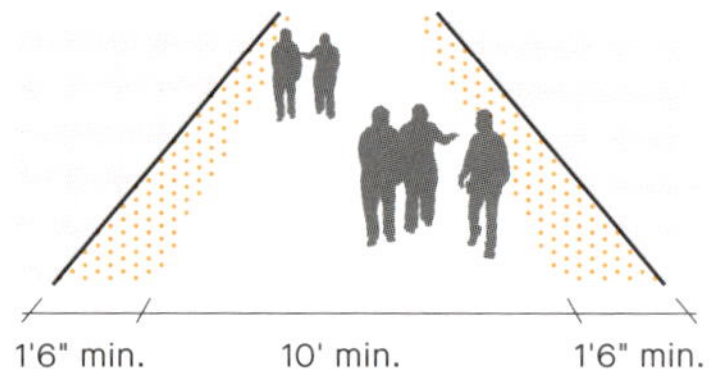

SEATING ARRANGEMENTS

Seating and tables accommodate seeing the faces of, and making eye contact with, all participants.

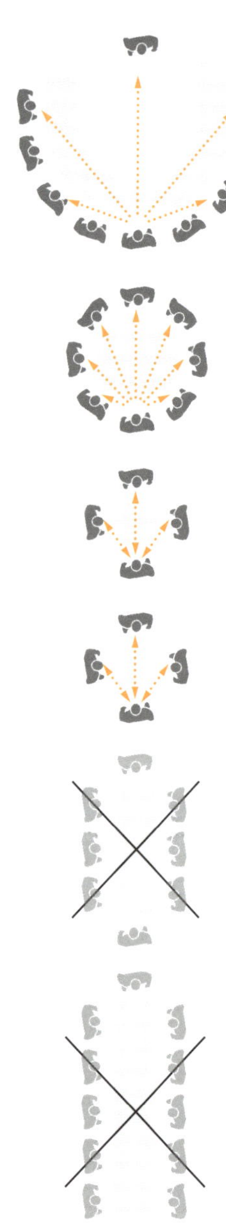

CASUAL SEATING

Architectural elements with multiple functions can encourage gathering and conversation. These elements should be located in casual indoor and outdoor social spaces and configured such that a group of two or more individuals may sit within 1'-6" to 3'-0" of one another.

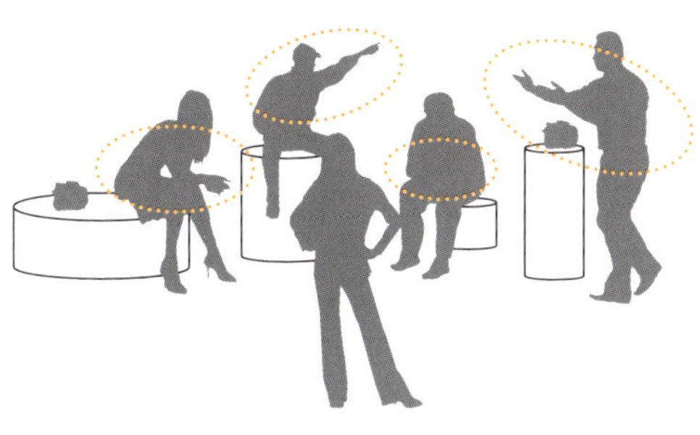

NODES

Encourage spontaneous social interaction by locating collective spaces at "nodes" along the way to other locations. This can be achieved at the scale of the campus, building, and city. Openings inside buildings allow deaf individuals to see their colleagues at work and in social situations while satisfying privacy requirements.

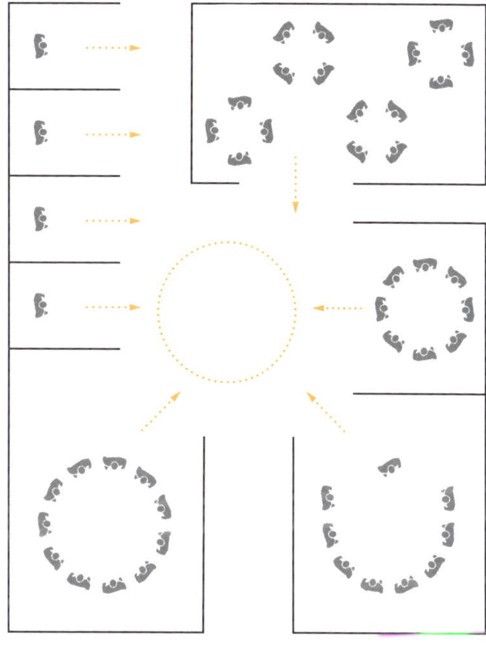

VISIBLE ARRANGEMENT OF FURNITURE

Maintaining visual accessibility while working enhances productivity and collegiality.

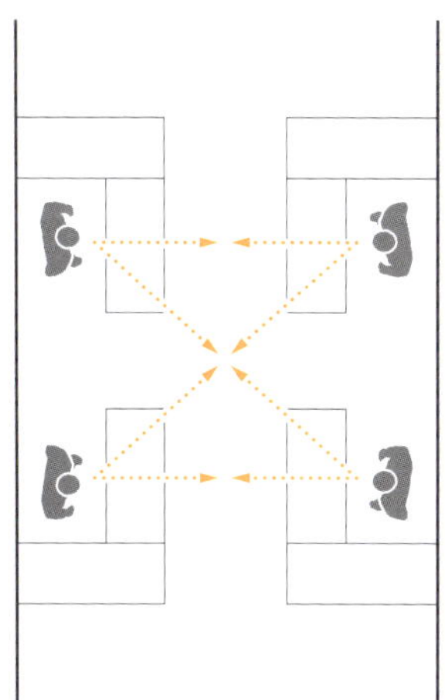

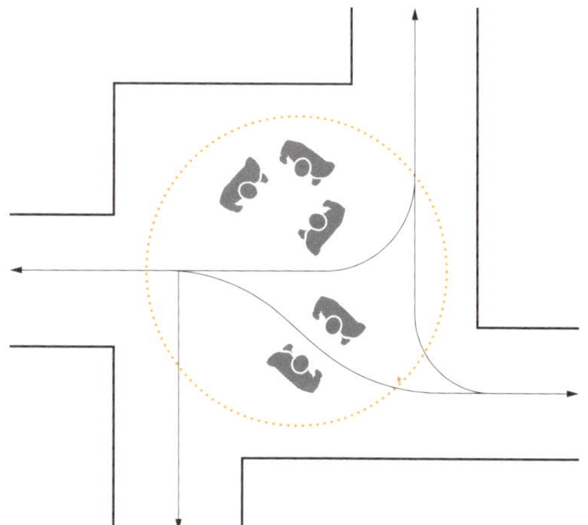

Light and Color

Light, color, and surface texture are intertwining elements that can all be used to shape DeafSpace. In the visual-centric Deaf culture, color is more than just a fashionable or aesthetic feature. It is an important way to shape space and aid in orientation and wayfinding. In addition, signing conversations require a clear contrast between the background environment and the details and movements of the signers' hands and faces. Color can set up a relationship between background and signer that encourages participation and ease of communication. Color-based systems of wayfinding aid the movement of individuals who are signing. Color and light should be considered together. Light colors tend to reflect light. Diffusing light minimizes glare and reflections, which deaf individuals find distracting. Dark colors can absorb this strong reflective light.

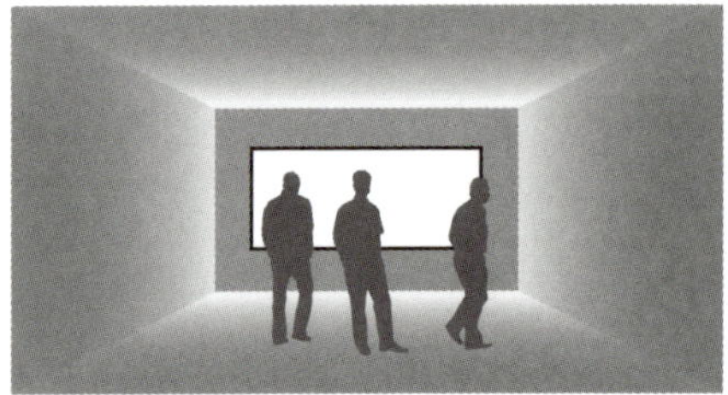

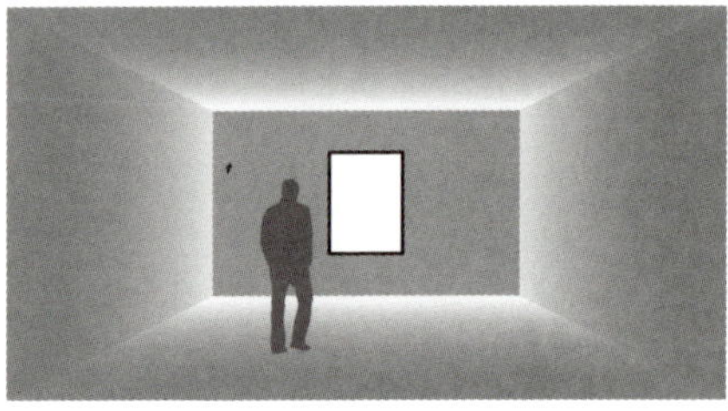

AVOID BACKLIGHTING

Bright windows located behind people or focal points in spaces cause high contrast between subject and environment. A person standing in front of a bright window will be silhouetted, causing difficulty in reading facial expressions and making eye contact.

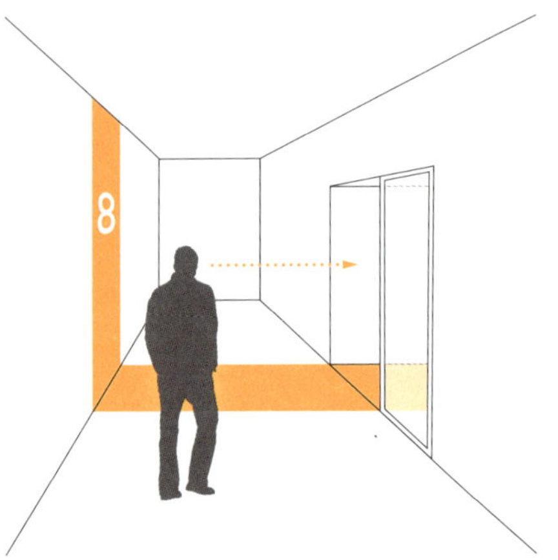

COLOR: ORIENTATION AND WAYFINDING

Color should be used to create simple, easy-to-navigate visual orientation systems. Color should be used consistently and repetitively for orientation at major thresholds and to mark vertical changes, street and sidewalk edges, and other situations that normally cause a pause in signed conversation due to navigation issues.

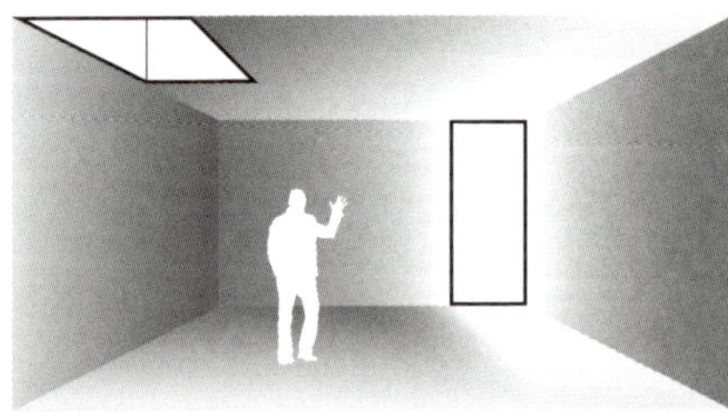

WASH SURFACES WITH LIGHT

Lighting surfaces rather than spaces helps avoid hot spots and shadows that can compromise visual communication. Windows and skylights should not be located in the middle of rooms, but should be located so that they wash walls, floors, and ceiling surfaces with natural light.

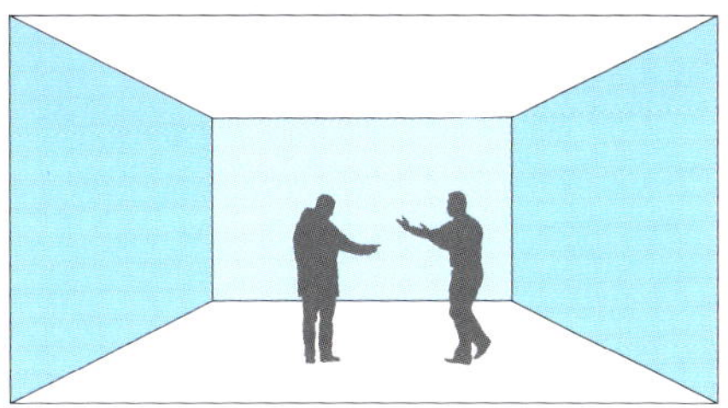

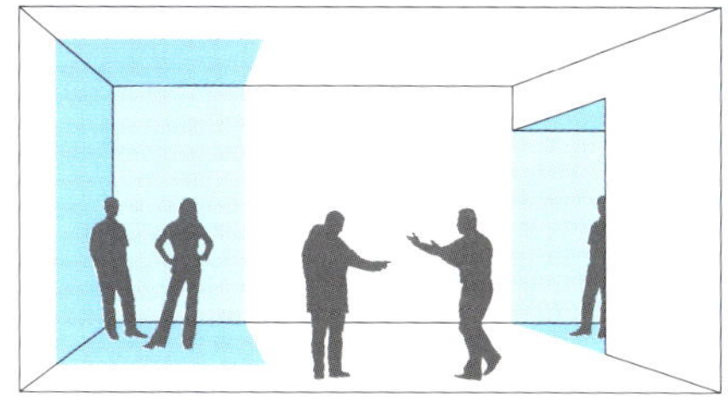

COLOR: CONTRASTING SURFACE AND VISUAL LANGUAGE

Since communication between deaf and hard-of-hearing individuals is so dependent on visibility, colors that contrast with skin colors are ideal backgrounds for signing. Blues and greens contrast with most skin colors. In addition, blues and greens promote visual calm. These colors do not overstimulate the eyes, and they provide a restful backdrop for movement and signing. In large and active spaces, painting surfaces blue or green will help deaf and hard-of-hearing individuals communicate.

SHAPING SPACE: COLOR EDDIES

Intimate areas for signed conversations should be created off of main spaces. Darker colors applied to surfaces in select smaller spaces can create an intimate feeling of being enveloped. Color and floor pattern can create feelings of closeness for smaller conversations while maintaining a sense of connection to a larger space.

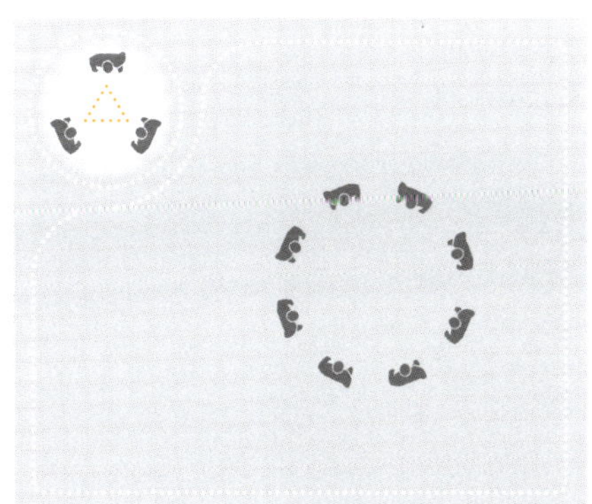

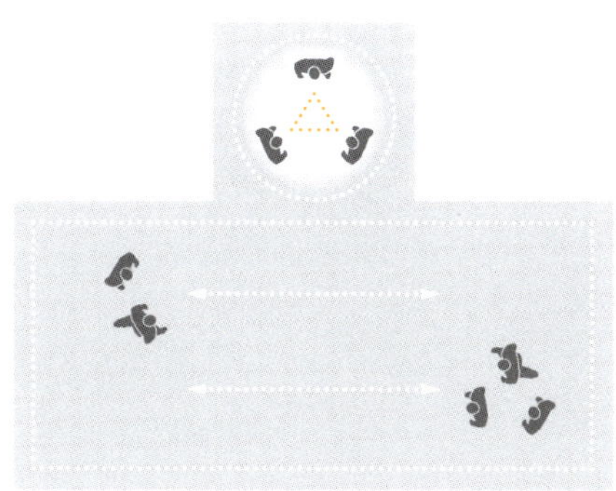

Sorenson Language and Communication Building
Gallaudet University, completed 2008; SmithGroupJJR Architects (Washington, DC, USA, founded 1818) and MEP Engineering (Denver, Colorado, founded 2004); Photography © Prakesh Patel and Ken Wyner.
Courtesy of SmithGroupJJR

SmithGroupJJR Architects were the first designers to apply the principles of DeafSpace to a complete campus building. The central atrium allows inhabitants to see one another and communicate from different floor levels. A seating area in the shape of a horseshoe enables group conversation. Glass walls reveal the building's activity from the outside and provide abundant natural light inside, screened by a colonnade that reduces glare. Wide interior hallways and exterior walkways enable people to walk together while signing. The building connects individuals to nature, light, and the history and context of Deaf culture.

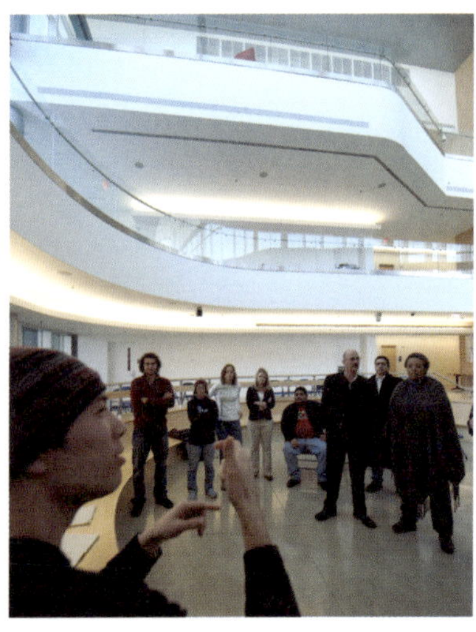

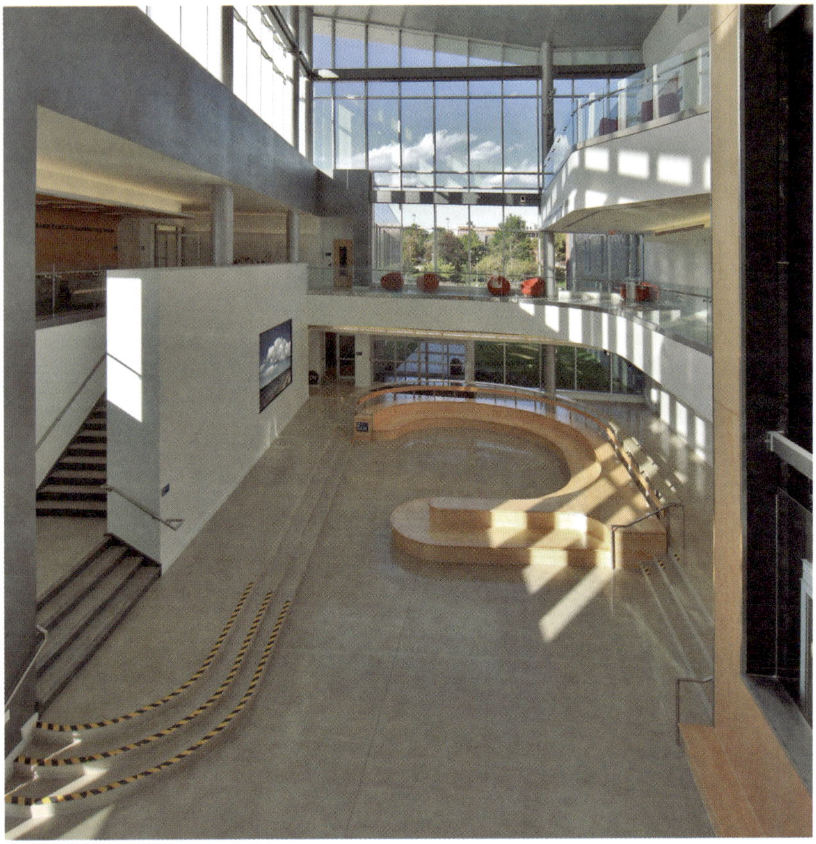

Rocky Mountain Deaf School, completed 2014; Anderson Mason Dale Architects (Denver, Colorado, USA, founded 1960); Photography © Frank Ooms

The Rocky Mountain Deaf School serves deaf and hard-of-hearing children and young adults. Classrooms, science labs, art rooms, audio testing rooms, and numerous public spaces emphasize visibility and social interaction. The wide corridors support the movement of people walking and signing, as well as offering places to stop and study, read, work, or converse. Color defines pockets of space off the main thoroughfare.

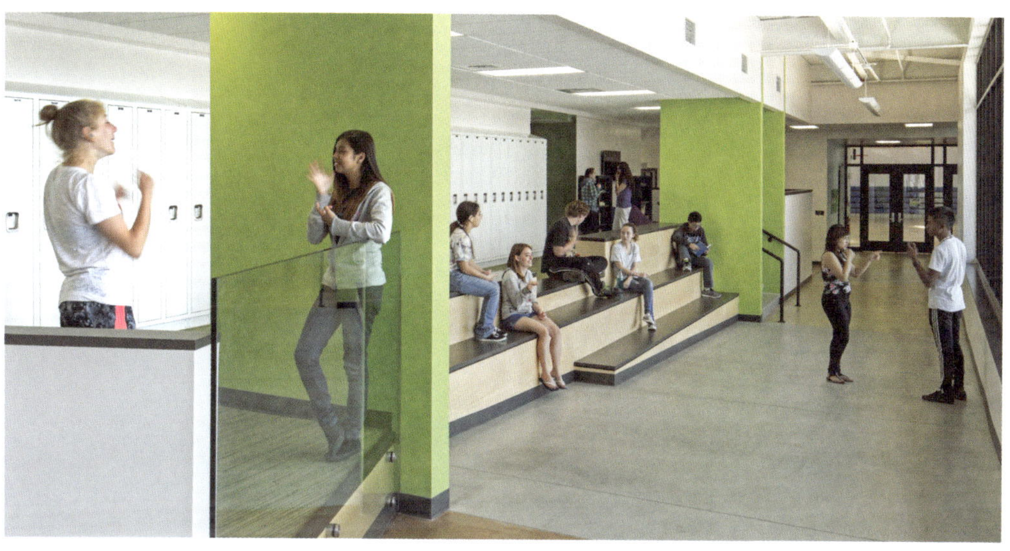

Hall Memorial Building, Gallaudet University, completed 2016; Studio Twenty-Seven Architecture (Washington, DC, USA, founded 1999); Photo by Anice Hoachlander, Hoachlander Davis Photography, LLC.

This interior renovation of Gallaudet University's science, technology, and math laboratories transformed a dreary facility into a thriving campus hub. The open staircase penetrating the central atrium enables visual communication. The architects removed walls and exposed columns and beams to create fluid, interconnected spaces. Reflective glass panels enhance sensory reach, allowing people to perceive others approaching behind them.

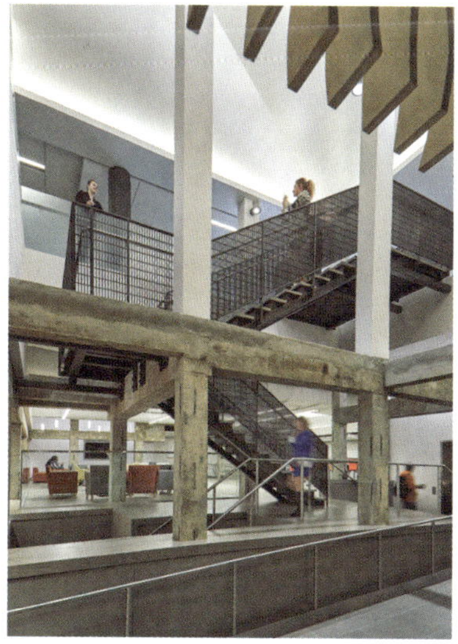

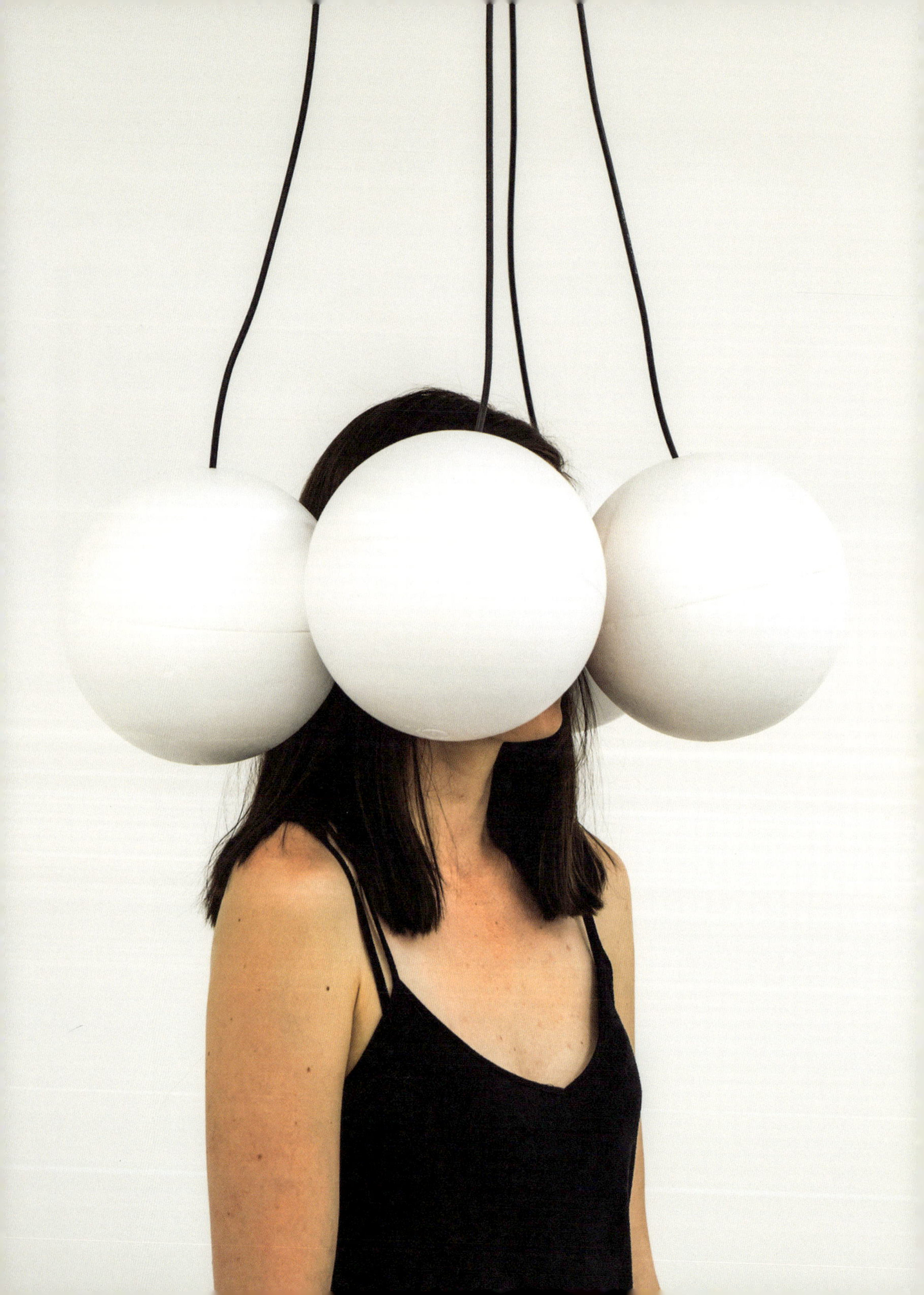

Adèle Bourbonne

Tactile Sound

Sound reminds us of the vitality of the world and tells us what is happening outside and inside our bodies. Whether sound transports us to a thrilling bubble, wraps us in a zone of concentration, or pings us with annoying intrusions, it can trigger a physical and emotional response. Sound startles us, alerts us, orients us, and riles our skin with shivers and goose bumps. People experience sound differently. Hearing people apprehend sound through their ears, but people can also feel sound with their bodies. Designers are creating products and visualizations that translate sound into tactile vibrations and graphic images, allowing us to understand it in multiple ways.

Tactile Headset, 2014, revision 2017; Alessandro Perini (Italian, b. 1983), executed by Rossella Siani, VAHA (Naples, Italy, founded 2015); Wooden spheres, metal chains, vibration speakers, ceiling mount; Spheres: 22 cm diam. (8 11⁄16 in.); Photo by Michela Benaglia

Sound is vibration. Hearing occurs when incoming sound waves vibrate against the eardrum and pass through our middle ear bones to the cochlea in our inner ear. There, delicate hair cells—a few micrometers long—convert the vibrations into electric signals. The brain processes and interprets these signals as sound.[1] Individuals with impaired hearing may lack the ability to transfer sound waves from the outer to the inner ear. Damage may have occurred to the inner ear (frequently to the hair cells) or to the auditory nerve leading to the brain.[2]

Music is experienced beyond hearing. Writer and scholar Rachel Kolb explains how she enjoys music in multiple dimensions—visually, by watching a performance or music video; haptically, from vibrations; kinesthetically, by dancing; and via auditory stimulation with a cochlear implant. Jason Johnson, a music fan who was born deaf, delights in experiencing his local marching band. While dancing in the front row, he can tell which sounds came from the brass instruments and which come from the drums, using his ability to feel sound waves. Research shows that deaf people can feel music in the same part of the brain that hearing people use when melodies get stuck in their heads.[3] Sean, a non-hearing musician working today, creates music for hearing-impaired individuals. The German composer and pianist Ludwig von Beethoven continued composing music after losing his hearing.[4]

Objects, as well as our own bodies, can vibrate and produce sound; thus listening experiences are physical ones. Our brain can make sense of vibrations that are touched, seen, or felt. When talking, our vocal cords vibrate. When tapping a table or clapping our hands, we cause air particles to vibrate, thus initiating sound waves. Each disruption produces a different sound wave. The vibration of a smartphone makes a different sound sitting on a tabletop than buried in a pocket. The sound waves travel differently, undulating and rippling, bouncing off of and being absorbed by surfaces on their way to our ear. These waves have differences in amplitude, from high to low volume, as well as differences in frequency, from a high "treble" pitch to a low "bass" pitch.[5]

ADÈLE BOURBONNE earned an MA in the History of Design and Curatorial Studies in 2018 from Parsons School of Design and Cooper Hewitt, Smithsonian Design Museum. Born and raised in France, she is passionate about modern and contemporary design as well as 18th-century French furniture and interiors.

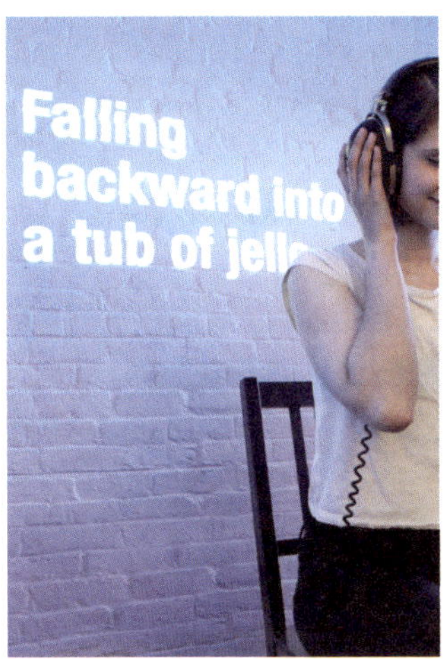

A Seated Catalog of Feelings, 2012–18; Eric Gunther (American, b. 1978), Sosolimited (Boston, Massachusetts, USA, founded 2003); Wooden chair, transducers and electronics, headphones, projectors; Sizes vary; Courtesy of Sosolimited

Designers are using data visualization and 3D-printing technologies to enhance and explore our experiences with sound on our body, enabling us to see, hold, feel, and transform sound. The word "haptic" refers to the physiology of touch. Receptors in the skin and nerves shuttle information back and forth between the central nervous system and the point of contact. Haptic technologies use motion and vibration to create different qualities of touch.[6] The haptic interfaces used in smartphones stimulate the skin surface, while devices that use force feedback, such as a 3D mouse, engage sensations in the fingers or limbs, engaging body position and movement.[7] Such technologies exploit the close relationship between sound and tactility. We hear with our ears and feel with our skin, but our brains combine this information to create integrated experiences. Interactive devices such as Lofelt's Basslet and Liron Gino's Vibeat bring sound and tactility together. They help us feel sound with our skin and bones.

Eric Gunther's project A Seated Catalogue of Feelings is a set of vibrating chairs that pair unique patterns of vibration with verbal descriptions of unusual experiences. The descriptions are whispered in the ear and projected on the floor. A phrase such as "falling backward into a tub of Jello" is paired with a rippling motion travelling through the seat and back of the chair to stimulate the user's body. The full sensation compresses together language, expectation, and haptic experience.

Sound artist Alessandro Perini creates installations that use vibration in place of audible sound. His Tactile Headset consists of four spheres designed to vibrate against a user's head. Each sphere vibrates with a unique pattern, just as four audio speakers in a musical installation would play different sounds coming from different directions. The space of music becomes localized on the skin.

At a concert or club, the energy of the sound spreads through our minds and bodies, sometimes releasing us from consciousness. The low, bass frequencies produced by a club's sound system pound against our skin, creating a powerful experience. Our understanding and appreciation of music

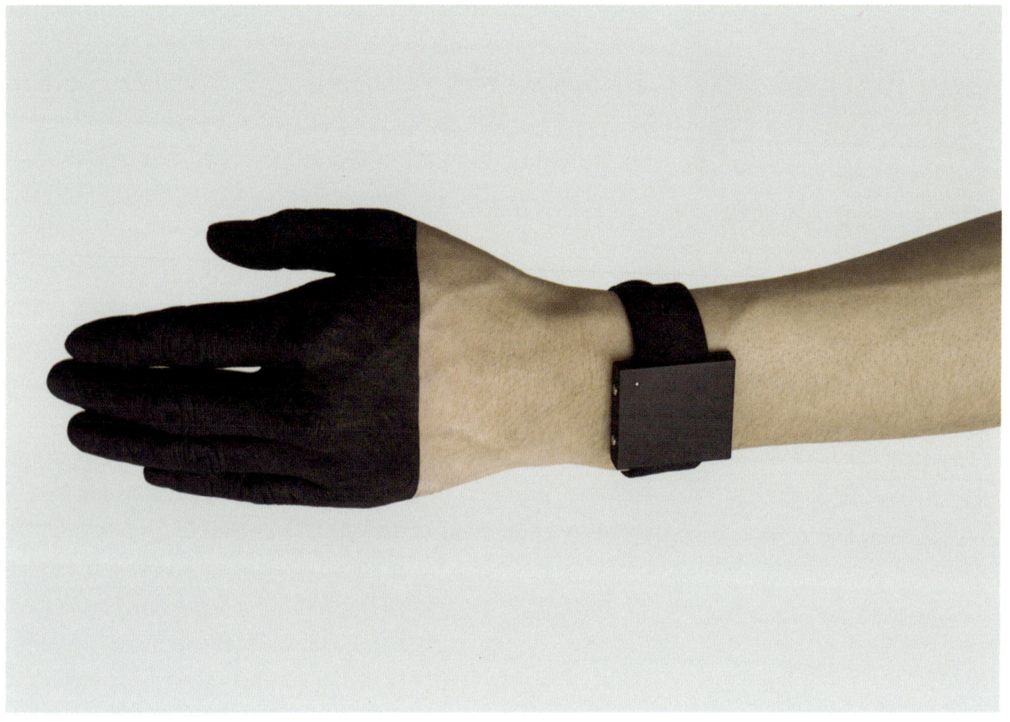

The Basslet, 2016; Lofelt (Berlin, Germany, founded 2014); Polycarbonate; 3.6 × 4 × 0.9 cm (1 13⁄32 × 1 9⁄16 × 11⁄32 in.); Courtesy of Lofelt

changes based on how we hear it. The creators of Basslet (rhymes with "bracelet") wanted to enhance the physicality of music for people wearing earbuds or headphones, bringing the tactile energy of a music concert or club to individual listeners. Launched in 2016 by the German company Lofelt, this watch-size wearable subwoofer delivers the bass frequencies of soundtracks straight to the skin. The sleek black bracelet communicates wirelessly with the "sender," a small case that also serves as a charger. The user puts on the bracelet and plugs a headset into the sender's mini-jack output. Lofelt created their own high-definition haptic engine, called the LoSound engine, which is housed inside the Basslet. The haptic engine translates sound frequencies into vibrations and delivers them to the body. The Basslet is designed to enhance the experience of music, gaming, and virtual reality. The Basslet brings sound and music to the body, transcending the experience of being stuck in the mental space of a headset.

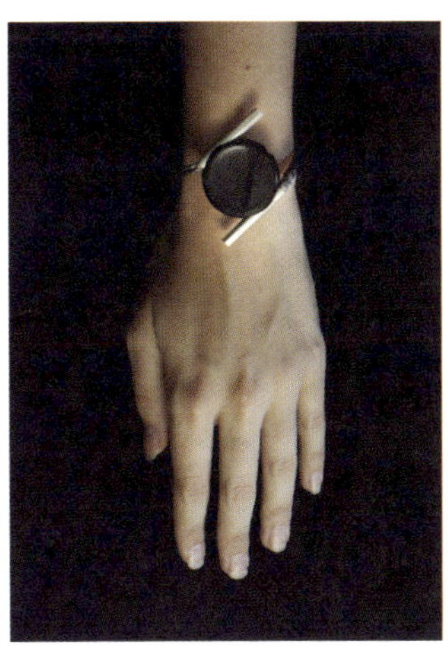

Vibeat: Bracelet, 2016; Liron Gino (Israeli, b. 1989); Metal, plastic; 3.6 × 7.1 × 6.1 cm (1 3/8 × 2 13/16 × 2 3/8 in.); Photo by Alexandra Yakovleva

Vibeat is another wearable device that converts sound into vibrations perceptible on the skin. Vibeat was designed by Liron Gino, a graduate of Jerusalem's Bezalel Academy of Arts and Design, Israel. She conducted research with deaf and hard-of-hearing people, including a club DJ. She spent time talking with people about their daily lives. She recalls, "One of the recurring topics during these conversations was, to my surprise, music. Curiosity, as well as my own love for music, sparked the interest in how one can feel music in ways other than hearing it." Her jewelry-like pieces can be worn as a bracelet, brooch, or necklace. Two users can share an experience by each clipping a module to their clothes. Designed with elemental beauty, Vibeat promotes accessibility and allows music to be experienced without ears. The device can be used both with a headset (i.e., listening and feeling simultaneously) and by itself. The vibration complements the experience of hearing. For those who do not hear, the vibrations provide a unique sensory experience.

Ultrahaptics is a UK-based company that lets users touch sound. Imagine controlling technology with "buttons" and "dials" that we can feel, but aren't there. The technology employs transducer boards that emit ultrasonic audio waves, a sound frequency inaudible to the human ear. The ultrasound vibrations are projected onto a user's hand as distinct sensations. We can feel and interact with solid yet invisible objects. It is sound as tactile interface. For our *Senses* exhibition, we invited Marcelo Coelho to develop an experience with Ultrahaptics. Coelho, a Cambridge-based computational designer, often works with emergent technologies, media, and processes to imagine how they will enhance our interactions.

Potential applications of Ultrahaptics include an invisible slider for pumping up the bass on a home stereo or a virtual knob for an induction cooktop. Museums could let visitors handle fragile objects. In 2017, the German electronics company Bosch introduced a concept car that features haptic controls. Instead of touching a screen, drivers can move their hands in the air. The sensors "see" the gestures, and the driver

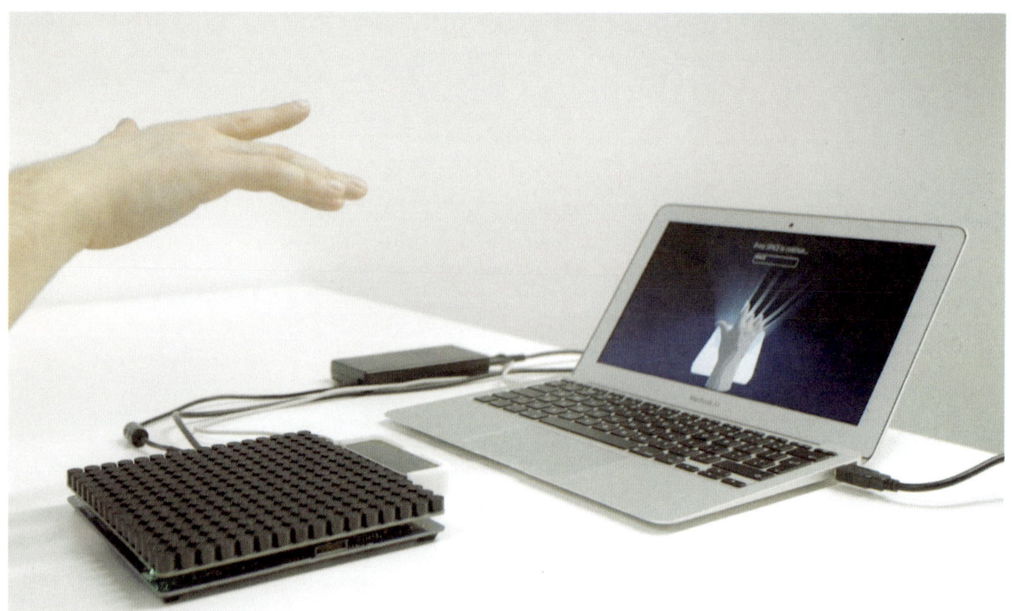

Ultrahaptics, 2017; Ultrahaptics (Bristol, UK, founded 2003); Ultrasonic transducer array: 2.5 × 16.7 × 16.7 cm (3 1⁄32 × 6 9⁄16 × 6 9⁄16 in.); Courtesy of Ultrahaptics

Vibeat: Necklace, 2016; Liron Gino (Israeli, b. 1989); Metal, plastic; 0.7 × 15.2 × 20.1 cm (1⁄4 × 6 × 7 7⁄8 in.); Photo by Alexandra Yakovleva

can "feel" the controls, swiping to the right to skip to the next music track or swiping left to adjust the air conditioning. Such features could allow drivers to keep their eyes on the road.[8] Universal design applications are also promising.

Each of these projects deepens—and broadens—our connection with sonic vibrations. They leverage sound as something we feel as well as hear. Sound resonates through the body. It tickles the surface of our skin with subwoofers designed like jewelry. It offers new forms of tactile interfaces. It heightens the realm of sensory knowledge. Psychologist Theodor Reik said, "Something of the poet lives in all of us and expresses itself not only in our dreams, but also in the daydreams, fantasies, and associations when we listen to music."[9] Sound activates sensory channels that make us think and feel, listen and touch, see and imagine.

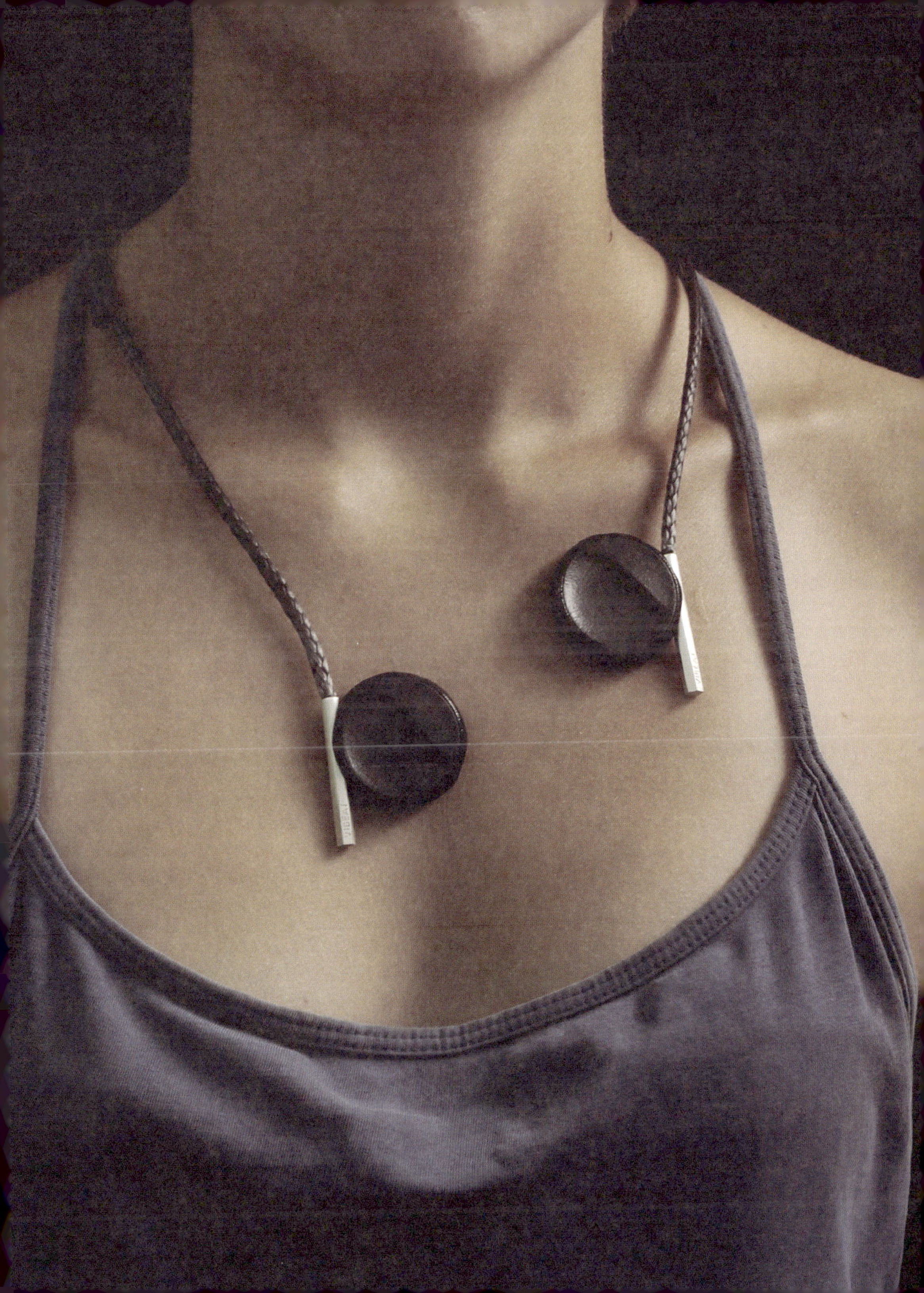

Joel Beckerman

Sonic Branding

Short sounds are all around us all the time. These sonic triggers can be the sparks that lead to physical actions or memories or feelings. You've probably responded to one in the past few minutes. Close your eyes for a minute if you're outdoors or in a crowded environment, and you'll probably hear one again within a few seconds.

These triggers are defined by their ability to convey a lot of information in an instant. Memory is a big factor here—what experience, recent or distant, do you associate with that short sound? New moms and dads will tell you they suddenly have heightened reactions to the sounds of babies crying—they hear it everywhere and it almost always startles them. The chirp of certain birds—a whip-poor-will or loon, for example—can call to mind particular times of year at specific places, probably by a lake or other body of fresh water. The sudden symphony of the wings of cicadas or locusts in the middle of the day can conjure memories of hot climates and summer months.

When sound is working at its highest potential, it surprises the ear. Have you ever been to a concert where the band has been playing all night, and then, just as they are nearing the natural peak of a song, it happens: wham! One note or beat radically changes the experience in a rapturous way, and you soar off into a completely unexpected musical direction.

Sonic surprise is one of the oldest sonic tricks in music, movies, entertainment, and even advertising. You hear it whenever an actor's voice is intentionally replaced by the voice of someone from the opposite gender or someone younger or older than him or her. Or when an expected animal sound is replaced with a human one. It gets your attention. But getting someone's attention is the easy part. Effective sonic branding often involves creating or facilitating sonic triggers that break expected patterns, get the listener's attention, and then use that attention to call to mind positive experiences with the brand or story.

We already recognize these kinds of snippets in the real world, and we pull information from them all the time. Think about the satisfying sound a golf ball makes when you sink it or the clean successful swish of a perfect three-pointer in basketball. Each of these causes a thrill while confirming something or telling you what you need to know in the moment. They're almost Pavlovian, except they're initiating something far more complex than physiological reactions. This is bigger than drooling.

It's easy to use sonic triggers to turn a forgettable experience into something memorable and meaningful. In fact, you already do. You yell "Surprise!" to make a birthday party boom. You clap louder and shout "Bravo" when a performer is especially inspirational or above and beyond the expected. Sonic triggers can also be deployed as effective functional sounds. They can be a welcome or a reminder, provide vital information, or help you understand where you are. When you think about the short sounds cars make, you probably think about revving engines, horns, or squealing tires. You most likely don't think about the purr of an idling or near-idling engine—but you'd think about it if it weren't there and you suddenly found yourself in the middle of an intersection staring at the grille of an oncoming electric car that you didn't hear coming.

In 2009, the National Highway Traffic Safety Administration (NHTSA) found that when slowing, stopping, backing up, or leaving a parking space, a hybrid-electric vehicle was two times more likely than a vehicle with an internal-combustion engine to hit a pedestrian. In January of 2013, the agency proposed new rules requiring electric vehicles going less than 18.6 miles per hour—that's the speed at which the sound of an electric car matches the sound of an idling internal combustion engine—to emit warning signals that walkers, cyclists, joggers, and blind people could hear over typical background noise. The NHTSA said these warnings didn't have to sound like the annoying beeps of reversing commercial vehicles. Carmakers would get to choose their own signals—rarely does government regulation present such opportunities for brands to have boom moments. Audi found one with its e-tron electric sports car; its engine-rev noise sounds like the light cycle in the Disney movie *Tron*.

A Danish audio software company called AM3D markets its binaural headwear apparatus to firefighters; it allows them to know, in smoke-filled, nearly blind environments, where their team members are. They hear three-dimensional, spatially accurate sound cues. The company also markets the tech to the defense industry. It's used in some A-10 and F-16 fighter aircraft. Pilots receive audio alerts about missiles or enemy fighters through speakers in their helmets, and in addition, the sound tells them, in an instant, what direction threats are coming from (including above, below, or behind them). Reacting to a visual warning takes about a second or so longer than reacting to an audio cue, and in a situation where a pilot has about five seconds to react to an incoming missile or enemy jet, that extra second is potentially lifesaving.

When used in gadgets, short sounds are typically called user-interface sounds. In my business we call them brand-navigation sounds. The term reminds us that they must be both emotional (the brand part) and functional (the navigation). The sound has to work harder, creating a sense of identity with the brand and making the technology more intuitive for the user.

The creators of one of the most popular games on the planet, *Call of Duty*, made short sounds work harder and become essential in gaming—gamers use the sounds to recognize surroundings and advance through levels. The makers of *Angry Birds* created a satisfying crunch and squawk to make you crave endless rounds of play, then used those sounds to trigger the same cravings in an endless array of toys and products and media. Product engineers and designers such as Jim Reekes created short sounds for Apple's early Macintosh machines—most notably, Reekes's Zen-like start-up sound, which lives on in the Macs we know and love today. All of these pioneers know a secret: we're entering an era of hardworking short sounds that help guide our experiences with everything.

JOEL BECKERMAN is founder of Man Made Music, a company specializing in sonic branding. Essay excerpted from his book *Sonic Boom: How Sound Transforms the Way We Think, Feel, and Buy*, with Tyler Gray (Boston: Houghton Mifflin Harcourt, 2014); by permission of the publisher.

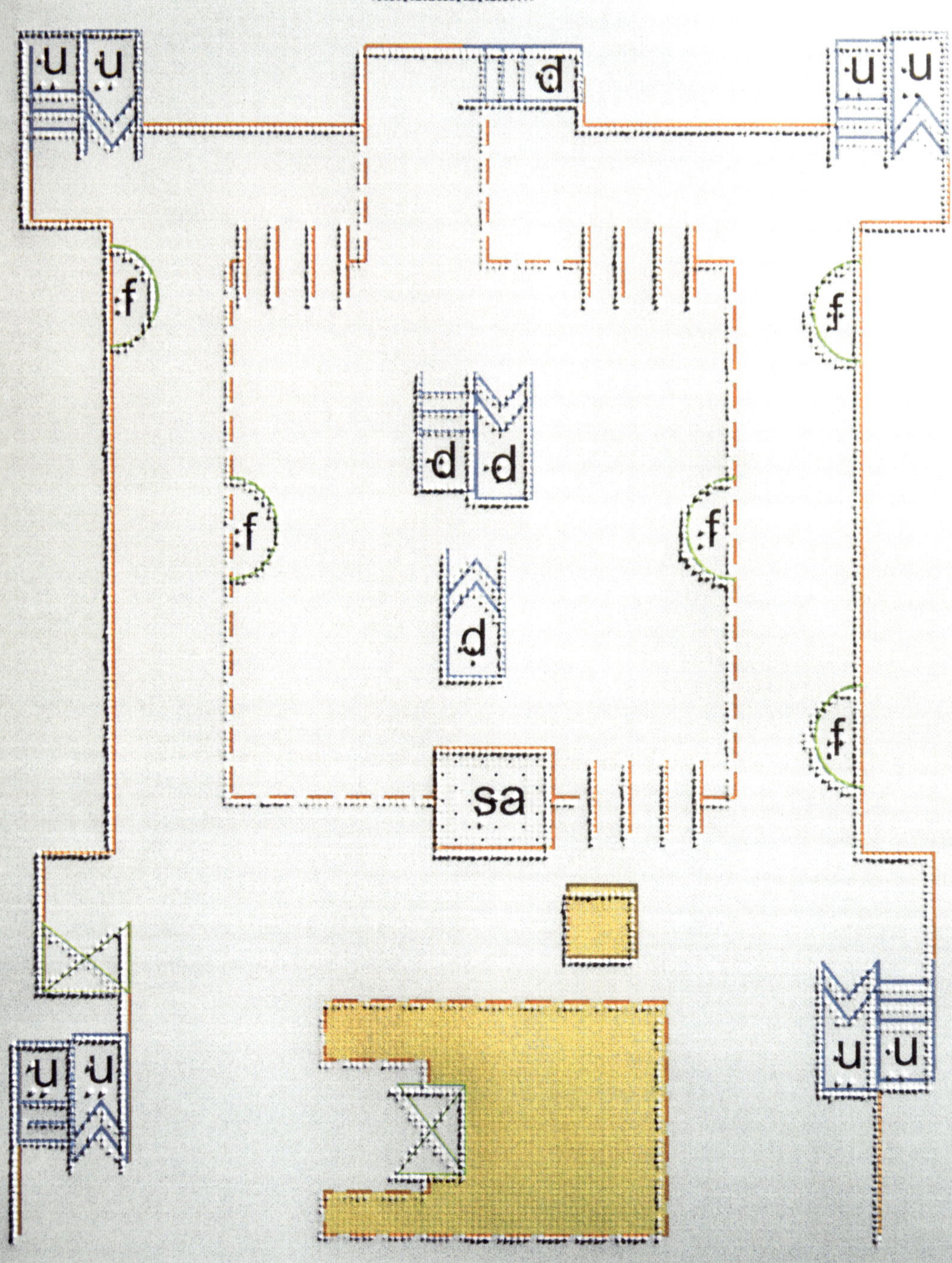

u
u
d
u
u
f
f
d
d
f
f
d
f
sa
u
u
u
u

Tactile Graphics

What is writing? What is drawing? What is a map? What is paper, ink, or printing? Graphic designers attend schools of visual art, where they work with colors and fonts, pictures and patterns. Yet not all graphics are made from visible lines and shapes. Ancient forms of communication used tangible materials—such as knotted twine, a networks of sticks, or hatch marks carved in wood—to represent objects, numbers, and space. Today, designers are using embossed lines, textured inks, 3D-printed surfaces, and audio-tactile interfaces to activate the capacities of touch.

BART Station Map (detail), 2011; Joshua Miele (American, b. 1969), with Greg Kehret and BJ Epstein, LightHouse for the Blind and Visually Impaired (San Francisco, California, USA, founded 1902); Embossed print; Photo by Matt Flynn © Smithsonian Institution

Joshua Miele is a designer, scientist, and educator whose work challenges assumptions about maps and graphic communication. He runs a lab at the Smith-Kettlewell Eye Research Institute in San Francisco and has a PhD in psychoacoustics (the study of sound perception and its physiological effects) from the University of California at Berkeley. When Miele was four years old, a mentally ill neighbor threw acid on his face in the doorway of his family's home in Brooklyn, burning his eyes and skin.[1] As a child, he attended mainstream classrooms and used braille to master reading, writing, math, and science. Today, he is an activist and innovator dedicated to expanding access to information.

In 2003, Miele and Smith-Kettlewell designed the first generation of TMAP (Tactile Maps Automated Production). TMAP uses online geographic information systems (GIS) to create "on-demand, user-centered tactile maps for blind pedestrians and connoisseurs of the environment."[2] The TMAP system generates schematic maps of local neighborhoods, using lines of embossed dots. When Miele began developing this mapping system, the science of the day had concluded that blind people simply aren't able to use maps for navigation. Tactile maps existed, but they were designed to depict big geographic areas—a continent or a country—in broad outlines with minimal details. What didn't exist were local maps that functioned as tools for getting around a neighborhood.

Miele knew, instinctively, that the current assumptions about blind people and maps were wrong. As a child, Miele had discovered a braille book about maps on a bookshelf in his elementary school classroom. The book was illustrated with embossed diagrams exploring simple fictional journeys—such as how to get to Grandma's house—by depicting roads and landmarks with embossed shapes and lines. Fascinated, Miele studied the book for hours. These maps were hypothetical, but he knew they could work.

That revelatory book stayed with him as he became a leading expert in communication for the blind. When Miele successfully prototyped his TMAP system with San Francisco's LightHouse for the Blind and Visually Impaired in 2003, users were stunned. Some wept. For the first time in their lives, they could picture the streets around their homes. They could understand, in spatial terms, the places they went every day as well as the prospect of exploring new places with the aid of useful maps. The LightHouse has partnered with Smith-Kettlewell and Raizlabs on a project—now in beta testing—to enable LightHouse to quickly generate TMAPs based on nearly any local street address in the world. (The TMAP system draws data from OpenStreetMap, a GIS platform that maintains data about roads and streets around the world.) The team addressed numerous graphic design problems. They figured out how to fit braille street names on the page while preventing the names from overlapping, and how to create a web tool that would allow both sighted and non-sighted LightHouse staff to create maps for users.

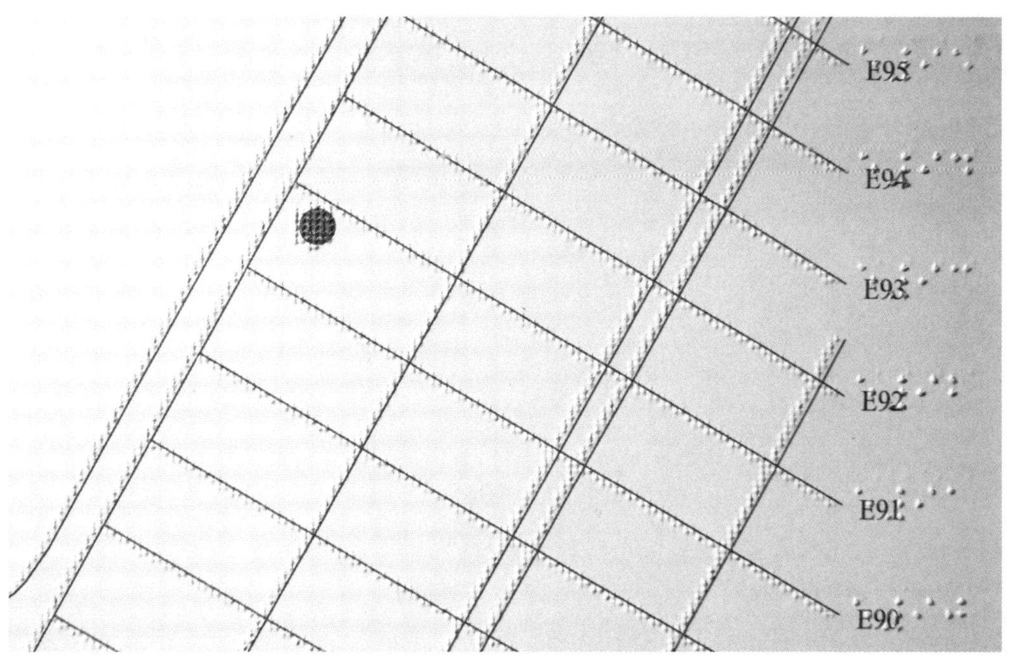

TMAP (detail), 2017; Joshua Miele (American, b. 1969), with Scott Blanks, Greg Kehret, and Naomi Rosenberg, LightHouse for the Blind and Visually Impaired (San Francisco, California, USA, founded 1902) and Brian Vogelgesang, Raizlabs (Oakland, California, USA, founded 2003); Embossed print; Photo by Matt Flynn © Smithsonian Institution

The dot at the center of the map is Cooper Hewitt, Smithsonian Design Museum, 91st Street between Madison and Fifth Avenues, New York City.

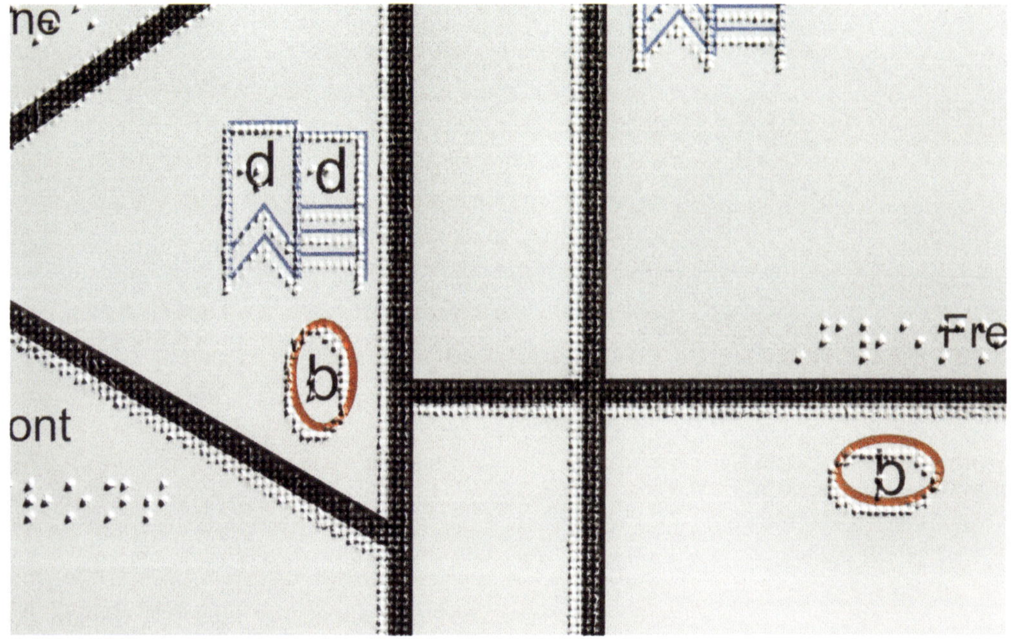

Miele also helped design station maps for San Francisco's BART subway line in 2011. He and a team of designers and volunteers—some blind and some sighted—documented every useful landmark in BART's forty+ stations. The maps represent features that a blind person can use to plan a detailed route—such as spatial relationships between a street, a stair, and a bus stop—without concern for exact location or dimensions. The BART maps have no uniform scale. "In my maps, space is elastic," says Miele. "This drives my sighted collaborators crazy, but it works for blind users." Blind people, says Miele, don't need to know whether a wall is fifty feet or eighty feet long; they just need to know that they can move from one landmark to the next by tracking along that wall with a cane (a mobility technique called "shorelining").

Blind people rely on stored mental understandings of space to a greater degree than sighted people.[3] Miele's maps help expand and annotate those mental pictures. His approach to mapmaking adds a new chapter to "psychogeography," the practice of urban wandering promoted by Guy Debord.

BART Station Map (with detail), 2011; Joshua Miele (American, b. 1969), with Greg Kehret and BJ Epstein, LightHouse for the Blind and Visually Impaired (San Francisco, California, USA, founded 1902); Embossed print; Photo by Matt Flynn © Smithsonian Institution

Debord, who founded the Situationist movement in Paris in the 1950s, presumed a seeing subject, yet his urban theories were open to multiple sensory realms. Psychogeography, he wrote, is the "study of the specific effects of the geographical environment, consciously organized or not, on the emotions and behavior of individuals."[4] His methods relied on landmarks and "ambiances" rather than on strict measurements. To create *The Naked City* in 1957, Debord chopped a map of Paris into chunks of experience and rearranged them on the page without regard to geographic fact.

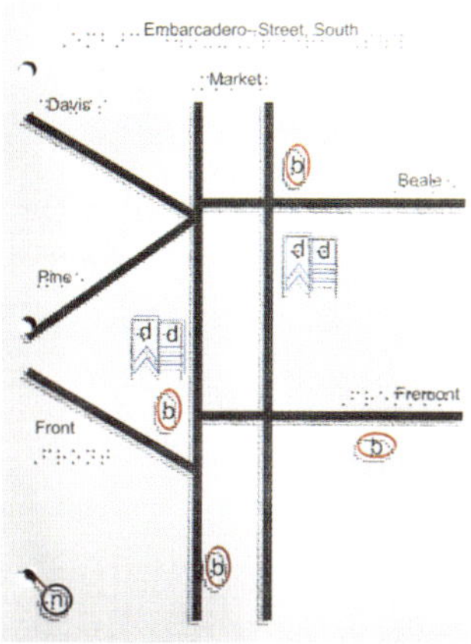

In a more systematic, science-based manner, Miele's maps enact an embodied, fluid conception of space. Miele resists the idea of setting fixed standards for designing tactile graphics. "Standards dampen creativity," he says. "And they make you think that because you are following the standards, you are doing it okay." Methods for printing tactile graphics vary in cost and richness of detail, from low-resolution, dot-based embossers to thermography, a method suited to longer-run printing that generates smooth lines in rich colors. (Thermography, which employs a powder that swells when heated, is commonly used to simulate the feel of engraving on low-cost business cards.) Each tactile printing method affords different sensory qualities and different levels of detail. Context and purpose matter, too. Some graphic content requires more text labels than others, while a handheld map for personal use will be different from a large map or 3D model installed in a public place. Every design problem, like every user, is unique.

Miele's BART maps are audio as well as tactile. A faint pattern of marks printed across the surface can be accessed with a digital pen that delivers an audio message explaining what's on the map. Thus the user reads the map with a combination of touch and sound. The designer of this pen device is Steven Landau, a pioneer in the field of audio-tactile graphics. Landau, a sighted designer who studied architecture at the Harvard School of Design, is founder of Touch Graphics, an innovative producer of tactile maps, graphics, and artifacts for schools, museums, and city governments.

Landau is especially interested in creating audio-tactile displays for museums. "Clutter," he explains, "is the enemy of tactile graphics." A tactile map needs labels to be understandable, but its surface quickly gets overwhelmed with braille and Latin text. For Cooper Hewitt's *Senses* exhibition, Landau prototyped an audio-tactile map of the Smithsonian Castle and nearby buildings, gardens, and monuments. Users can explore the map with both hands, a method of touching preferred by many blind people. To play audio text, users tap a building once to hear its name, and double-tap to hear additional content. 3D-printed models of buildings are installed on top of a touch screen. The models are painted with conductive materials that—when touched—transmit electrical charges to the screen, tricking the computer into thinking the screen was touched directly by a finger.

For decades, graphic designers have argued about what to call themselves. To some, "graphic design" (a term coined

Smithsonian Castle Interactive Touch Model, 2018; Steven Landau (American, b. 1960), Touch Graphics (Elkton, Maryland, USA, founded 1997); Touch monitor, UV-printed tactile graphic overlay, translucent 3D prints, brushed aluminum bezel, stainless-steel mount, Android Mini PC; 7.6 × 60 × 40 cm (3 × 23 5/8 × 15 7/8 in.); Courtesy of Steven Landau

SMITHSONIAN CASTLE
Touch anywhere and follow the tone to find Smithsonian Castle.

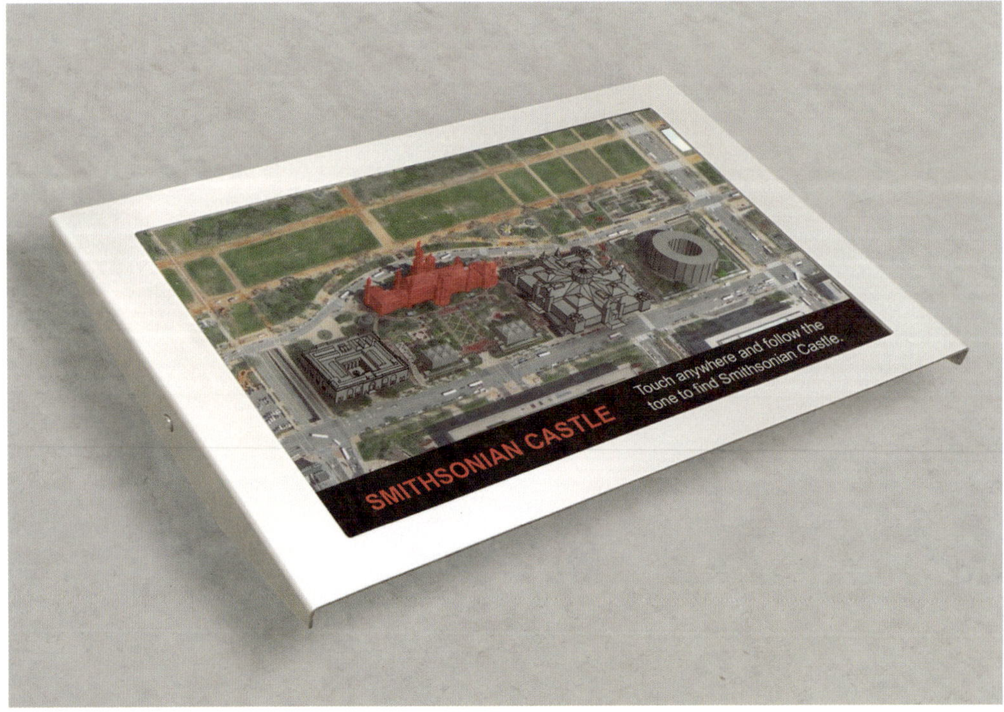

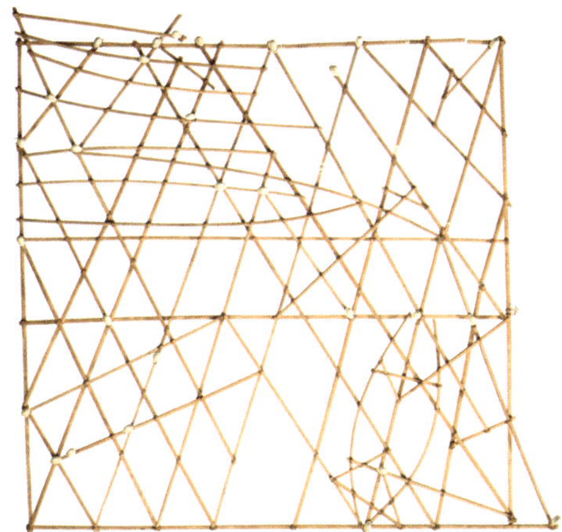

Stick Navigation Chart (Marshall Islands), before 1950; Carved wooden sticks, cowrie shells, twine lashing; 99.4 × 101.9 × 4.4 cm (39 ⅛ × 40 ⅛ × 1 ¾ in.); Department of Anthropology, National Museum of Natural History, Smithsonian Institution, E432083; Photo by Donald E. Hurlbert © Smithsonian Institution

in the 1920s) seems dated and old-fashioned, entrenched in a world of printing presses and rubber cement. In contrast, the term "visual communication" sounds rather sleek and businesslike. It turns out, however, that graphic communication isn't always visual. Early traders and herdsmen counted goods by carving lines into sticks of wood. Ancient Sumerian cuneiform was produced with a tiny wedge-shaped stylus, yielding intricate, repetitive indentations in clay. The rows of beads in an abacus are tangible numbers, felt and manipulated with the fingers. For centuries, sailors in the Marshall Islands have made maps of islands and ocean swells by tying together sticks and cowry beads. These tools embody the oceanic knowledge of the community.[5]

A web of sticks or a string of beads can be touched as well as seen. The dominance of print culture, however, has glorified vision and downgraded the other senses. Many people were barred from the kingdom of the alphabet, including the blind. In the early nineteenth century, advocates for blind education in Europe and the United States began designing touchable alphabets. Tactile fonts are an overlooked chapter in the history of typography. Samuel Gridley Howe designed his Boston Line letters in 1835. Howe, a Harvard-trained physician who directed the first school for the blind in the United States, was a pioneer in special education. He believed every student had the capacity to learn, including those who were

Boston Line Embossed Typeface, 1835; Samuel Gridley Howe (American, 1801–1876); Digitized by Harold Lohner (American, b. 1958); Courtesy of Harold Lohner

samuel gridley howe designed this tactile font in 1835. because each letter has unique features, the font achieves what modern type designers call legibility—the distinctiveness of individual characters in a typeface.

blind, deaf, deaf-blind, or developmentally disabled.[6] Each character in his Boston Line alphabet has strong differences from others in the system. The bowl of the *p* is curved, while the bowl of the *d* is diamond-shaped. The font has no ascenders or descenders, and no lowercase and uppercase characters. Thus, users need to learn only one character set. The resulting alphabet is quirky and strange—for a purpose. It achieves what modern type designers call "legibility"—the distinctiveness of each individual character in a font. Similar ideas about differentiating letterforms are used today in experimental typefaces for people with dyslexia.[7]

Howe's Boston Line typeface rejected the uniformity of Latin typography. Breaking from the alphabet more radically, however, would lead to a far more effective alphabet for the blind. In 1821, a twelve-year-old student in Paris began designing a tactile writing system made from raised dots. Louis Braille had lost his sight as a young boy and attended the National Institute for Blind Youth. The school's founder, Valentin Haüy, had created an embossed typeface employing uppercase roman letters. Although sighted people could easily read Haüy's typeface, blind people found it cumbersome. Furthermore, blind people who could read Haüy's letters still had no way to write letters of their own. Louis Braille knew that true literacy requires the freedom to write as well as to read.

Writer and performer Vincent Bijlo wrote the text that appears on the following pages for the Dutch magazine *Plain Paper*, where it is printed in braille on rich red paper.

Louis Braille based his tactile code on a system of dots and dashes developed by a French Army officer for communicating at night. Braille translated the alphabet into a six-dot grid, yielding an elegant set of symbols that are easier to read by touch than raised roman letters. He devised an inexpensive stylus and frame for writing; a similar "slate and stylus" is still in use today for writing braille by hand. Braille spread among blind users after its inventor's death in 1852. The system gained traction more quickly in Europe than in the US, where sighted educators resisted the idea of having to learn a system so different from the alphabet.[8]

Braille alphabet, Louis Braille (French, 1809–1852)

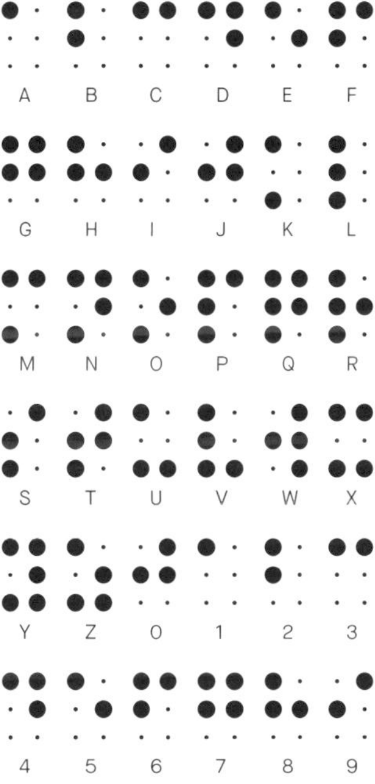

NEXT SPREAD
Trompe Le Doigt (Fool the Finger), from *Plain Paper*, 2016; Vincent Bijlo (Dutch, b. 1965), Philip Stroomberg (Dutch, b. 1967), and Esther Krop (Dutch, b. 1974); Offset lithography and braille press on Curious Matter Désirée Red

Today, braille is used around the world in many languages for signage and publications. Braille is not truly universal, however. In the US, only a small percentage of blind and visually impaired people (between 1 and 10 percent) have learned to read braille. Chancey Fleet, assistive technology coordinator at the Andrew Heiskell Braille and Talking Book Library in New York City, is an advocate for braille literacy. She told us that braille literacy correlates with employment, enabling independence. Yet media reports commonly pronounce that braille is dead or dying, being swept aside by new technologies. Why do so few blind children and adults learn to read braille? According to Fleet, the reason is not a problem with braille but a problem with access to education. The cost of state-of-the-art tools is an issue, too. Fleet, a fluent reader and writer of braille, uses a Vario Ultra note taker. This portable networked device is equipped with a keyboard and a tactile braille display. With this device, she can read any text that is available on her smartphone in braille, and she can quickly type braille and store the text digitally. Fleet says, "The note taker is expensive because the market is small. Every blind person should have access to this device."[9]

Although digital technologies are providing new ways to access text in audio formats, tactile writing remains a crucial

Nothing is as patient as paper
Like a sheet can lie waiting
For thoughts written down
Emptiness begging for making sense
Sentences, words, letters
There is something else that can keep
Fingers, eyes hooked.
I put my hand down, skin onto paper
I feel quietness.

Let's just keep it
Like this, this calm
A deep slumber, free from language
No expression today
No layout
No comma
Semicolon
No full stop.

tool. Visual impairment is not a single condition. Nor does it define the totality of a person's needs and desires for perceiving the world. Some people are blind from birth, while others lose their vision gradually, often late in life. A person who is legally blind might be able to make out rough patterns of light and dark. Some blind people call themselves "visual thinkers," because they prefer thinking in terms of spatial structures rather than linear paths. A visual thinker may enjoy reading braille more than listening to audio books and text-to-speech readers. Some blind people rely on braille for public signs but prefer audio for longer texts.

The Elia Frame system is a contemporary counterpart to Howe's Boston Line letters. This modified Latin alphabet was initially conceived by Elia Chepaitis in 1988, after her 74-year-old mother was diagnosed with macular degeneration.[10] Like many people who lose their vision later in life, she felt unable to master braille. At the time, Elia Chepaitis was studying industrial design. While reading about human factors, she noted that a well-designed control panel has a frame around each symbol, separating symbols from one another. (Picture a row of buttons with engraved markings.) Thus was born the Elia Frames concept: a series of modular symbols made from raised rectangular boxes. Each character has distinctive gaps and ticks that reference the letters of the Latin alphabet.[11]

Elia Chepaitis's son Andrew Chepaitis, a college student at the time, helped his mother design some of the characters. The invention went unrealized, however, until over a decade later, when Andrew founded ELIA Life Technology, dedicated to making Elia Frames a functioning tool. Over a period of years, he and his team tested the system with different groups of users, including sighted people over the age of sixty-five (blindfolded) and people with visual impairments. They found that the Elia Frame system was easier to learn than braille and could be read with greater accuracy by new users. It could also be read at multiple sizes, whereas braille typically is implemented at a single standard font size. With sixty hours of training, a person could achieve a level of literacy gained after

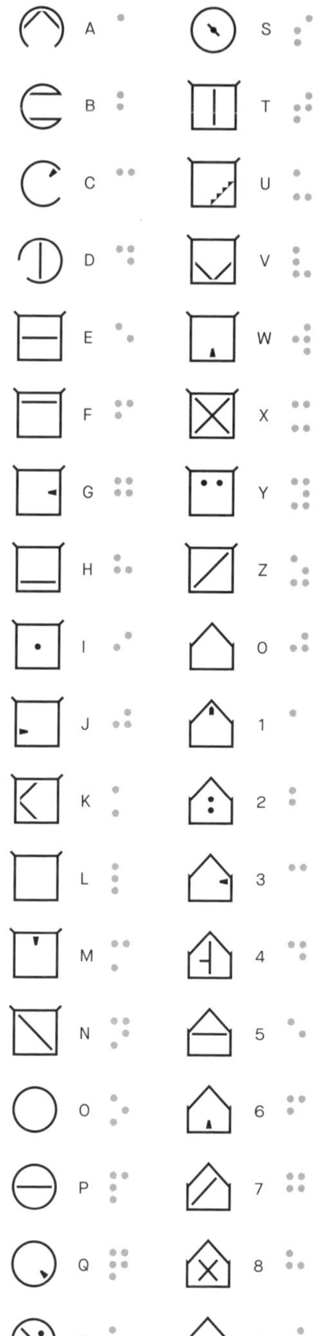

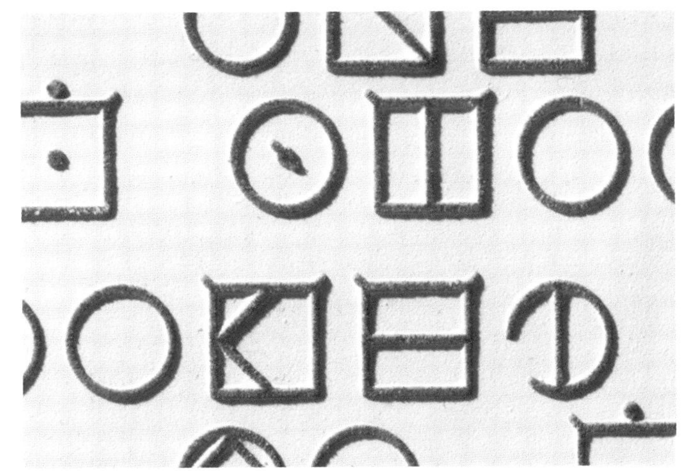

Elia Frame system (2000–16) and text converted to Elia Frames; Elia V. Chepaitis, Andrew Chepaitis, Reed DeWinter, and Hosea Jan Frank, ELIA Life Technology (Brooklyn, New York, USA, founded 2000); Embossed print, Courtesy of ELIA Life Technology

four to five years of studying braille. ELIA Life Technology is now developing an economical tactile printer useful not only for printing Elia Frames but also for printing braille and tactile illustrations, maps, and graphics. The tactile printer requires no special software, and Elia Frames is a standard font file.

How has the braille community reacted to Elia Frames? According to Andrew Chepaitis, some advocates for braille literacy are opposed to introducing new systems that might dilute the relevance of braille. Instead, they argue that more effort should be exerted on spreading and supporting braille literacy. Others, however, recognize that Elia Frames offer a potentially useful alternative for people who are not willing or able to learn braille.

Designing nonvisual wristwatches is another communication problem with multiple solutions. The most familiar and widely used solution is the talking watch. These timepieces speak the time when the user presses a button. Such watches are inexpensive and require little effort to learn. The sound, however, can be a drawback; many users don't want the whole room to know every time they check the time. The Bradley Eone tactile timepiece features two channels, each containing a small ball bearing. Magnets attract the ball bearings to raised markings defining the clock face. The inner ring represents minutes; the outer ring represents hours. Beautifully crafted from durable materials, this elegant, high-end product can be read both by sight and by touch. It is useful for anyone who wants to be able to check the time without looking at or listening to a device.

Another ingenious tactile timepiece is the Dot Watch, which has a dynamic pin display. The tactile pins move up and down to depict numbers. In braille mode, the watch displays the time in digital format using braille numbers. In tactile mode, a simpler set of dots represents the time for non-braille users. Employing a Bluetooth connection, Dot Watch can also receive text messages in braille from a user's smartphone. Designed by cloudandco, Dot Watch is the basis of an ambitious series of products with revolutionary potential. The Dot Mini and the Dot Pad are handheld tablets designed for reading and writing braille text as well as tactile maps and graphics. Dot Public is a system of information screens for use in public facilities.

From transit maps to tactile timepieces, such products show the rich possibilities of tangible graphics. Consider the

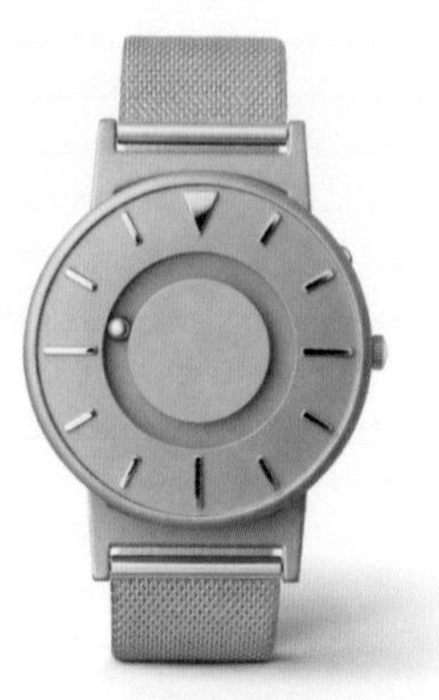

Bradley Mesh Silver, 2017; Eone Timepieces (Washington, DC, USA, founded 2012); Titanium, stainless steel; 24 × 7 × 1.1 cm (9 7⁄16 × 2 3⁄4 × 7⁄16 in.); Courtesy of Eone Timepieces

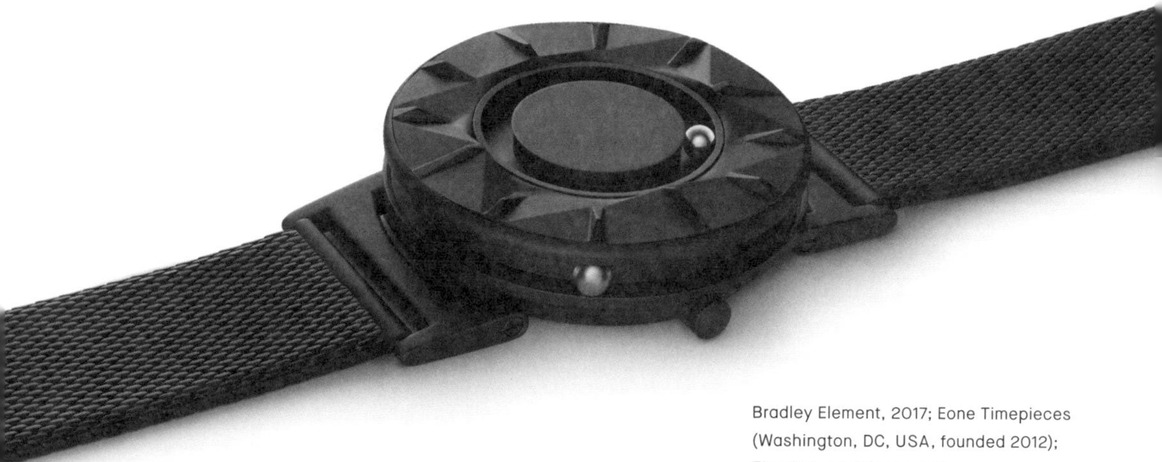

Bradley Element, 2017; Eone Timepieces (Washington, DC, USA, founded 2012); Titanium, stainless steel; 24 × 7 × 1.1 cm (9 7⁄16 × 2 3⁄4 × 7⁄16 in.); Courtesy of Eone Timepieces

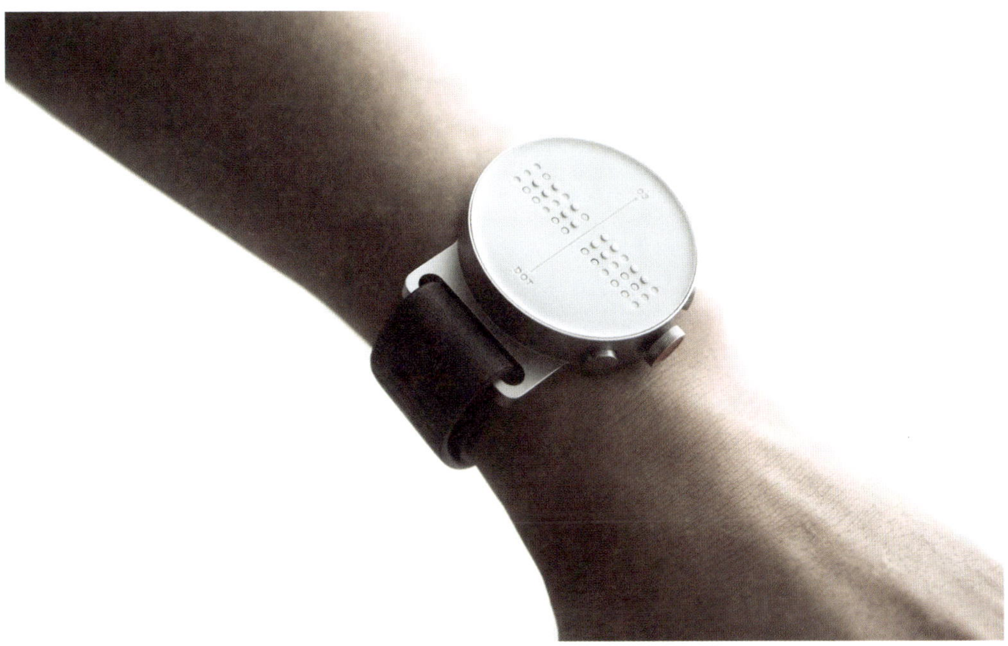

Dot Watch, 2017; Dot Incorporation (Seoul, South Korea, founded 2014); Designed by cloudandco (Seoul, Korea, founded 2010); Creative Director: Yeongkyu Yoo (Korean, b. 1971); Industrial Design: Yeongkyu Yoo, Kihwan Joo, Youngwoo Choi, Jaesung Joo; Graphic Design: Yeongkyu Yoo, Nara Ok; Concept Editor: Michelle JY Park; Anodized aluminum case, gyroscope, touch sensors, wireless MCU platform, leather; Watch: 4.3 × 1.25 cm diam. (1 11⁄16 × ½ in.); Courtesy of Dot Incorporation

art of drawing, the foundation of the visual arts. Drawing is more than a visual medium. It is a physical act using physical tools. For a sighted person, drawing from observation requires harnessing hand to eye. The classic DIY text, *The Natural Way to Draw*, by Kimon Nicolaides, explains that people are best equipped to draw objects and places that they know through touch: "Merely to see, therefore, is not enough. It is necessary to have a fresh, vivid, physical contact with the object you draw through as many of the senses as possible—and especially through the sense of touch."[12]

Low-relief tactile illustrations star in the Tactile Picture Books Project, launched by Tom Yeh at University of Colorado, Boulder. This digital library offers public access to files for books that users can print themselves. Users can customize pages and create their own books from a collection of 3D models representing nouns, verbs, and textures. Jeeeun Kim, a PhD student in computer science, is a member of the project team. Her tactile edition of the classic book *Goodnight Moon* represents complex objects such as light shining from a lamp.

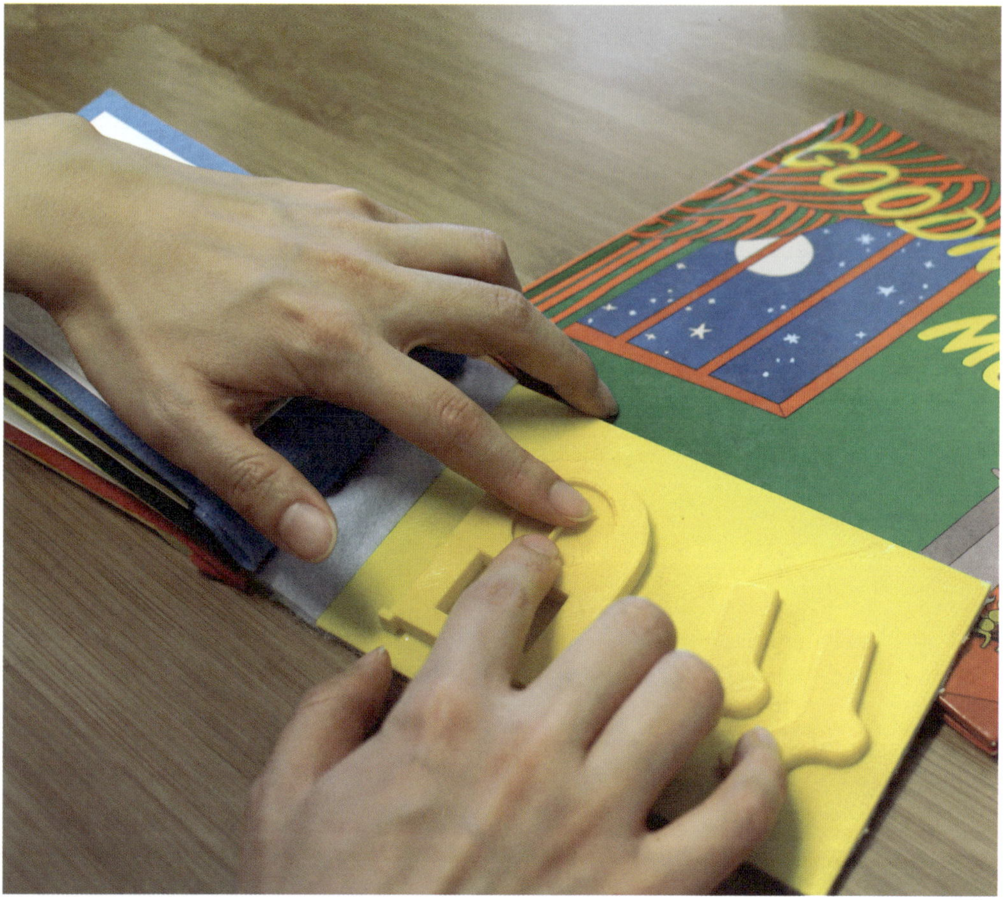

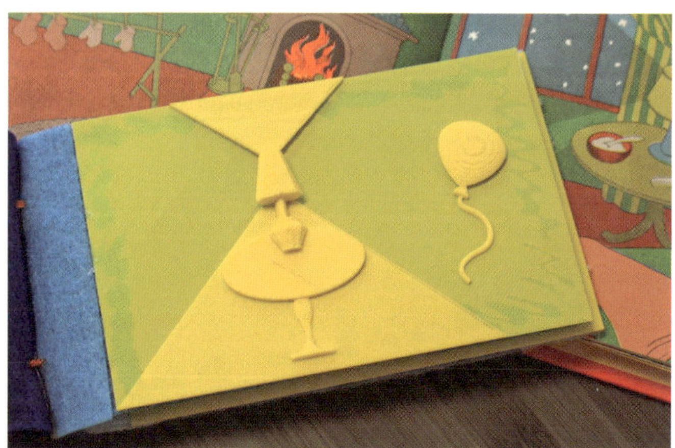

Tactile Picture Books Project, 2017; Jeeeun Kim (South Korea, b. 1986) and Tom Yeh (b. Taiwan Province of China, 1977), Sikuli Lab, Computer Science Department, University of Colorado Boulder (Boulder, Colorado, USA, founded 2012); 3D-printed illustration with braille text; Courtesy of Jeeeun Kim

While braille is traversed with the tip of a finger, tactile pictures and maps typically are explored with both hands.

Artists who are visually impaired create tactile sculptures as well as drawings with raised tactile lines or images in low relief that express concepts such as figure/ground, overlapping forms, and the use of diminishing size to represent depth.[13] Artist Emilie Gossiaux, who has no light perception, has experimented with numerous tools, from BrainPort, a device that stimulates the tongue with patterns the brain interprets as images, to a rubber drawing board that creates tactile lines.

Writing and drawing are physical acts. Letters take root in mind and hand through gesture and repetition. Sensory design celebrates our bodily experience of text and information. Sighted and nonsighted designers are helping users navigate space and content. A book, map, or city designed for inclusion takes different forms—print, audio, braille, and beyond. Diagrams and alphabets, street signs and web menus, are landmarks along the paths of our collective consciousness.

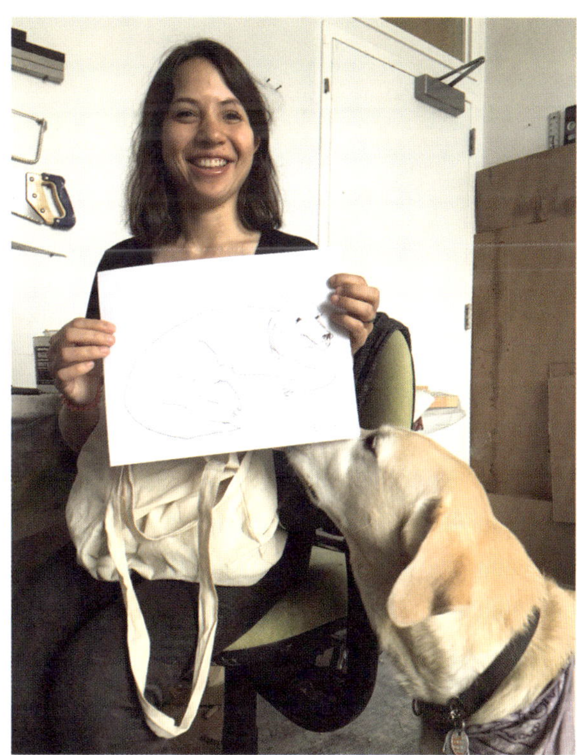

Artist Emilie Gossiaux holds up her sketch of her guide dog, London, as London pokes her nose up into the photo, bottom right. The drawing has raised lines, created with the Blackboard tactile drawing board from Sensational Books (sensationalbooks.com).

Steven Landau

Drawing by Touch Artist Emilie Gossiaux explores new modes of self-expression through touch. One of her tools is a rubber drawing board that provides real-time tactile feedback as she draws.

STEVEN LANDAU, founder of Touch Graphics, Inc., designs and produces tactile maps and models for use by visually impaired students, scholars, and museum visitors. Touch Graphics recently collaborated with Emily Gossiaux to create a large-scale tactile drawing board.

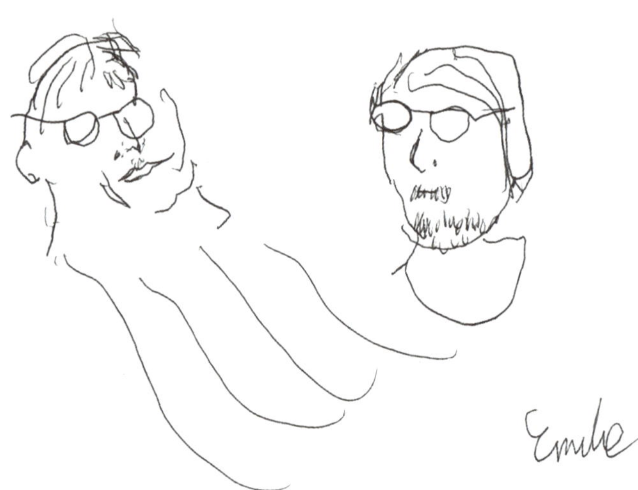

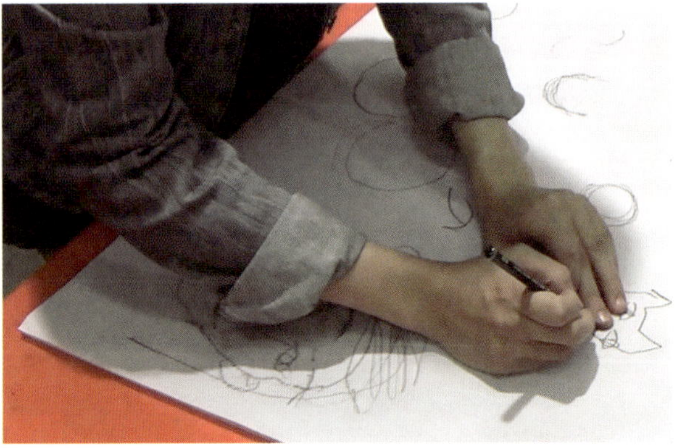

TOP
Mom and Dad, tactile portrait by Emilie Gossiaux. Ball point pen on copy paper, 2017

BOTTOM
Emilie Gossiaux demonstrates the tactile drawing board in her studio. She holds the pencil in one hand and feels the lines she is making with the other hand.

A Tactile Drawing Board

A person can learn to draw without seeing, by replacing visual perceptions with tactile feedback. In pioneering experiments in the 1970s, psychologist John Kennedy at the University of Toronto taught adults who had never had sight how to draw using a rubber mat placed under a sheet of drawing paper. Their pencils created raised furrows in the paper as they pressed down into the resilient surface, and the artists could feel these furrows with one hand as they drew with the other hand. When they weren't drawing, they were using both hands to scan the emerging tactile composition, so they could comprehend and plan the overall picture, placing each new mark in the right location to create simple, recognizable figures.

A Power User

Sculptor Emilie Gossiaux, who has no light perception after a bike accident seven years ago, uses a tactile drawing board like the one in the earlier study to sketch and illustrate ideas about her artworks. After years of practice, the experience feels to her like visual drawing, which is not surprising, since fMRI studies at Harvard in the 1990s showed the same parts of the brain lighting up during both activities. Gossiaux's pictorial explorations using this simple tool are pushing the boundaries of tactile portraiture, showing us a new level of expressiveness and mastery of this form of sensory substitution.

Design of Tools

To achieve these results, Gossiaux experiments with different surfaces, stylii, and paper, to optimize the tactile drawing experience and find the "sweet spot," in which she receives the most accurate tactile information, capturing not only the placement of lines, but also visual characteristics like darkness or thickness. Pressing a little harder with the stylus should result in a barely perceptibly higher raised line; this requires a rubber pad with just the right resiliency, and paper that stretches a bit but does not rip when you really bear down. A good analogy is a singer who listens to herself through the highest-quality headphones during recording sessions: the more precisely she can hear herself, the more accurate and steady her pitch and timbre.

Tactile Mindfulness

While Gossiaux's work reveals exceptional artistry and skill, probably anyone with good fingertip sensitivity can learn to use the tactile drawing board to make simple figures. The key to developing these abilities is temporary or permanent lack of vision. Just putting on a blindfold causes us to switch our focus from vision to touch, bringing tactile sensations to the perceptual foreground. Because vision is effortless, operates at a distance, and can take in an entire scene at once, it always supplants touch as the dominant sense. Sighted people can learn tactile mindfulness with training but as soon as their blindfold is removed, vision takes over and their newly-acquired tactile skill will probably start to fade.

Mastery

But for those living without vision for many years, tactile ability can become highly refined through constant use and the absence of visual distractions. The tactile drawing board is a low cost, low tech, portable tool for non-visual self-expression and communication that builds tactile mindfulness through its continued use, leading to some extraordinary artistic accomplishments, and highly developed manual skills that probably carry over into every aspect of the artist's life. As with any skill, the key to achieving mastery appears to be intensive practice and access to appropriate tools, adapted to one's specific needs and preferences.

Adapted from an essay first published in *Cooper Hewitt Design Journal* (Fall/Winter 2017)

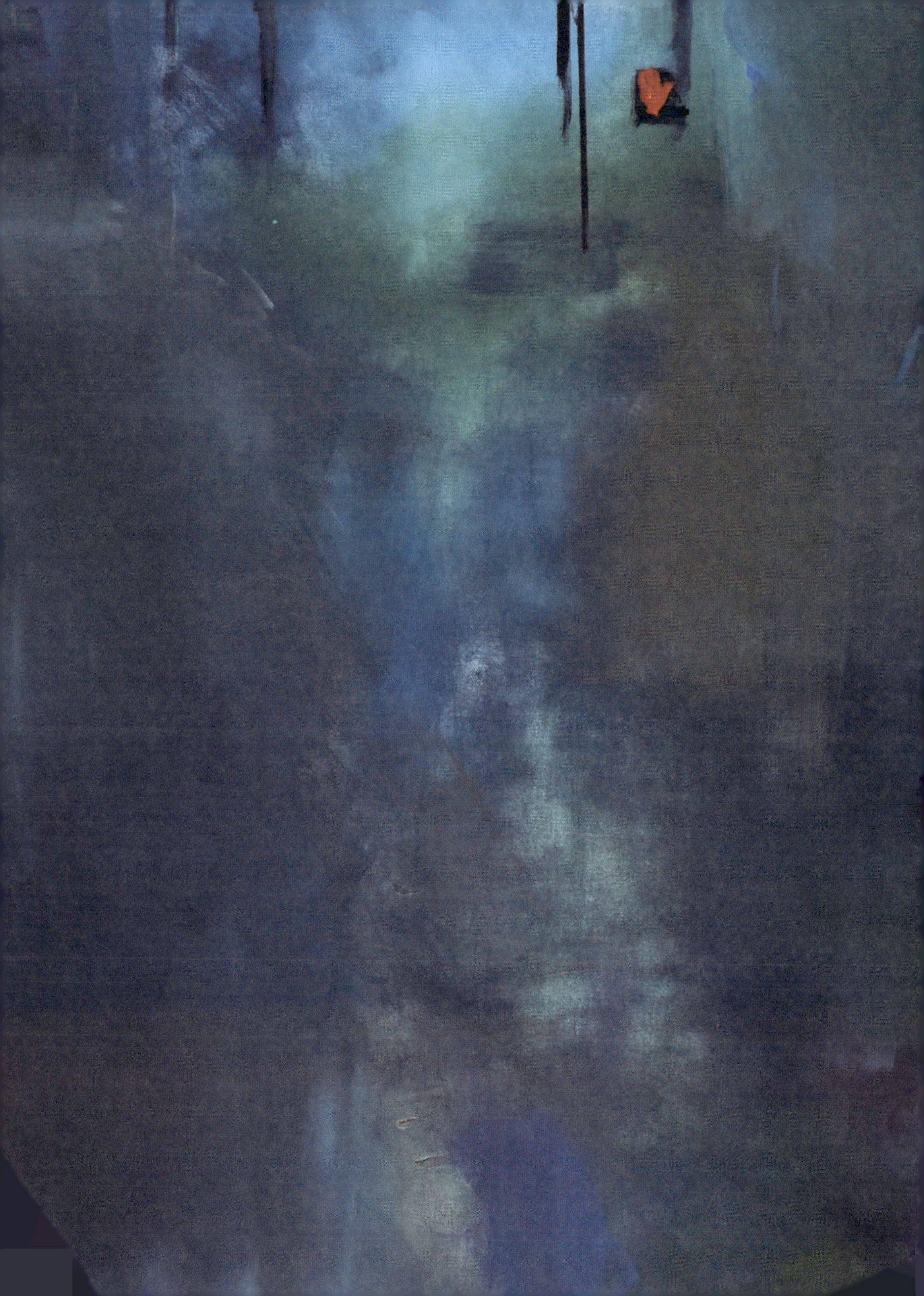

Color & Cognition Blue sky, green grass, red apples, and yellow bananas. Children fill their coloring books with crayons and markers as a way to identify and explore the world. Everyone sees color differently, however. For people with color blindness, the colors red and green or blue and yellow look similar. (Color is in the eye of the beholder.) Some people see no light (and thus no color). Those with low vision rely on strong contrasts to navigate places and use products. Employed strategically, strong colors can become wayfinding elements that help people understand and remember their surroundings.

Painting (detail), Beacons: Red Hand 1, 2006: Annie Leist (American, b. 1974); Oil on canvas; 101.6 × 152.4 cm (40 × 60 in.); Courtesy of the artist

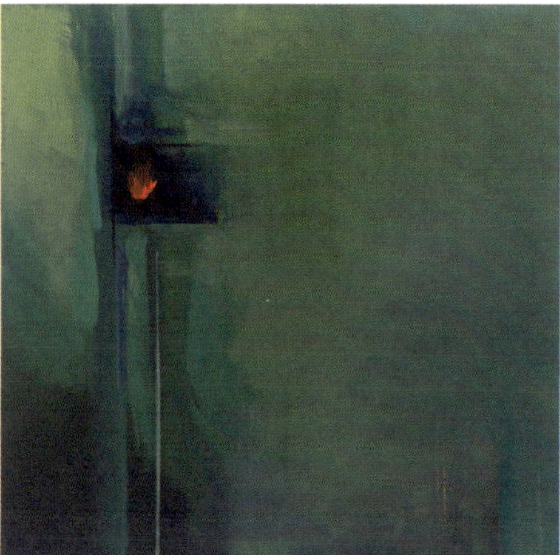

Painting, Beacons: Red Hand 6, 2010; Annie Leist (American, b. 1974); Oil on canvas; 40.6 × 40.6 cm (16 × 16 in.); Courtesy of the artist

Painter Annie Leist creates richly colored depictions of crowds. Sharp halos of light reveal the silhouettes of passersby, their individuality and presence revealed by postures and body language. Leist is legally blind and doesn't experience depth perception. She says, "I do have a particular sensitivity to the unruly, deceptive, and beautiful elements of space and light, especially where they confront humanity and its need for orderly systems."[1] In a series of paintings called Beacons, Leist depicts crosswalk signs in New York City. In each image, the form of a red hand emerges from the luminous blur of the surrounding street. The red hand signals "don't walk," but for Leist, the sign is more than that. It is a nonverbal anchor pulling her through the city. She says, "In a chaotic environment if I can find the red hand then I know I can be safe. Red hands are more significant for me than the white man walking, which doesn't stand out enough for me to see clearly. So instead of looking for the 'walk' sign, I look for the 'don't walk' sign. When it blinks off, that's my signal."[2] Leist has also used photography and oil sketches to track the life of orange traffic cones. Her work shows how colors and signs can guide the flow of people and become means of knowing and acting.

Globally, 285 million people experience different forms of visual impairment. Vision loss can occur at birth or as a consequence of accidents, illness, and aging. How can color

BINGLEI YAN earned an MA in the History of Design and Curatorial Studies in 2018 from Parsons School of Design and Cooper Hewitt, Smithsonian Design Museum. She co-curated the exhibition *Objects of Dispute* (2017), in which she explored gender issues in design. She has researched the role of women in 19th- and early-20th-century design.

improve the lives of people who see the world differently? As a child in Portugal, Filipa Nogueira Pires learned reading, writing, and mathematics from her great aunt Du, who was blind in one eye. Pires's early encounter with visual impairments, together with months of contact with students at the Helen Keller Center in Lisbon, Portugal, in 2009, inspired the invention of Feelipa, a system that translates colors into shapes that can be felt by touch. Feelipa represents the three primary colors with the basic geometric shapes: red is a square, yellow is a triangle, and blue is a circle. Using basic color theory, the Feelipa system represents additional colors by combining shapes. Since orange is a mix of red and yellow, its shape is a square combined with a triangle (a trapezoid). Horizontal lines express shades of gray. Three lines indicate black, two lines mean gray, and one line means white. Thus dark red is created by placing three black lines over a red square; pink (light red) is a square underscored with a single line. These different combinations of shape and line generate twenty-four colors, yielding shapes and lines expressed with tactile symbols.[3] For someone who can see some color, the shapes and colors reinforce one another. Although Feelipa has not been widely adopted, this simple system could enable people to add tactile stickers to various products, from clothing to food packages and pill bottles.

A system similar to Feelipa is ColorADD, also developed in Portugal. ColorADD was created by Miguel Neiva to address color blindness. This modular system translates the six primary and secondary colors (plus black and white) into simple marks, each based on a part of a square. The shapes for the primary colors (red, yellow, blue) can be combined to create secondary colors (orange, green, purple). The system has been applied to art supplies, tourist maps, healthcare products, and the popular card game UNO, which for decades has used colored backgrounds to depict the different suits in the game.

Psychologist Lawrence E. Marks explains that all senses can be traced back to a single primitive sense—touch. Vision, hearing, taste, and other senses gradually differentiated from

Feelipa Color Code

PRIMARY COLORS

SECONDARY COLORS

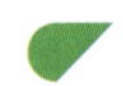

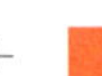
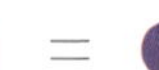
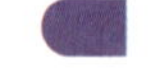

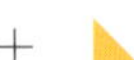
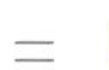

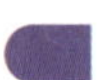
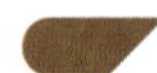

ACHROMATISM

Black Gray

SHADES & TINTS

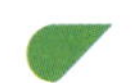
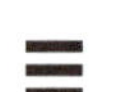
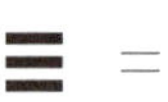
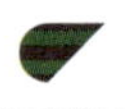

Dark Green

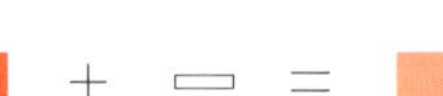

Light Red

Feelipa Color Code, 2009; Filipa Nogueira Pires (Portuguese); Graphic system, redrawn from original design

ColorADD System

PRIMARY COLORS

SECONDARY COLORS

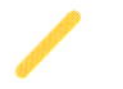

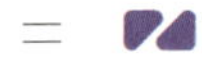
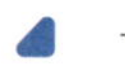
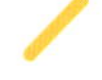
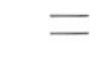

ACHROMATISM

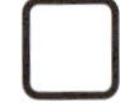

Black White

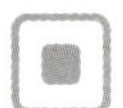
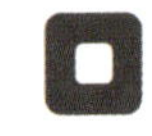

Light Gray Dark Gray

SHADES & TINTS

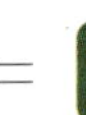

Dark Green

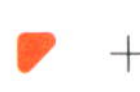
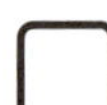
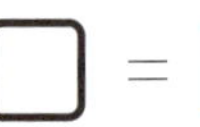

Light Red

METALLICS

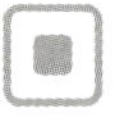
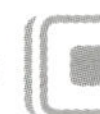

Silver

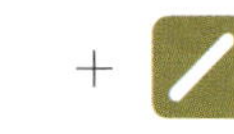
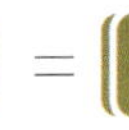
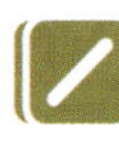

Dark Yellow Gold

ColorADD system; Miguel Neiva (Portuguese, b. 1969), ColorAdd (Portugal, founded 2008)

one another and became distinct modalities. The course of embryonic development reflects this process, as different senses emerge individually from ectodermal tissue.[4] Architect Juhani Pallasmaa asserts that all senses, including vision, extended from the sense of touch.[5] Considering medical evidence, anthropologist Ashley Montagu confirms that "touch is the parent of our eyes, ears, noses, and mouths. It is the sense which became differentiated into the others, a fact that seems to be recognized in the age-old evolution of touch as 'the mother of the senses.'"[6] Likewise, psychologist Richard L. Gregory proposed that "the earliest visual system—the first eyes—emerged out of a tactile system."[7] Touch is the ancestor and prototype of vision. Martin Jay remarked, "'Through vision we touch the sun and the stars.'"[8]

Simon Kinneir, a product designer from the UK, is partially sighted in one eye. For his graduate degree project at the Royal College of Art, Kinneir designed products for people with impaired vision. He conducted research on vision loss, which occurs gradually for many people, and he spent a day simulating total blindness himself. Leaven is a set of prototypes for kitchenwares that exploit tactile cues as well as extreme color contrast to support "self-confidence in the kitchen."[9] Each piece of cutlery bears a graphic mark on its handle: the spoon features a raised horizontal line, the fork has a raised vertical line, and the knife bears an indent. These distinctive markings help users recognize each piece and to know by touch the right way of holding it.

Kinneir also applied tactile cues to his Leaven chopping board. A grid of black grooves runs across the surface in horizontal, vertical, and diagonal directions. The visible and textural contrast between the dark grooves and the smooth white surface of the cutting board guides users as they cut. The Leaven mug features thumb-shaped indentations that invite touch. The mug is thinner at these indented areas, allowing the user to feel the temperature change and know when to stop pouring. A thin black line provides a visual target. Kinneir explains that his Leaven products give passive tactile

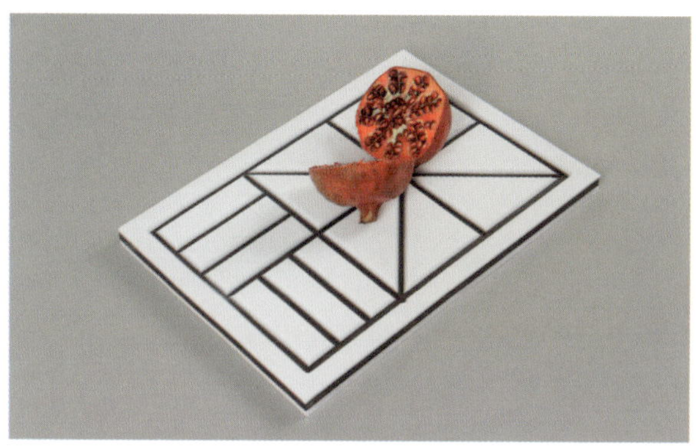

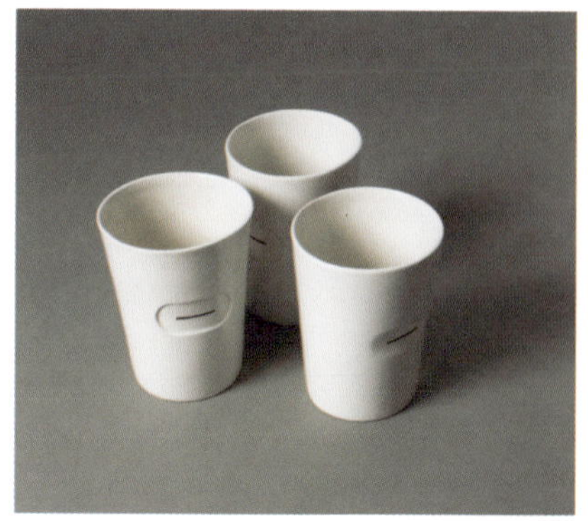

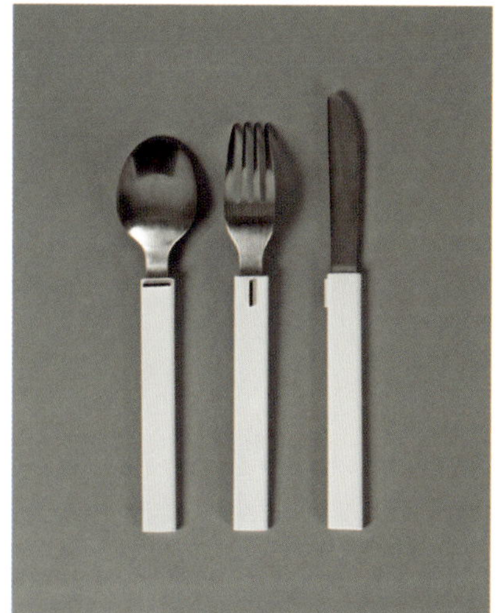

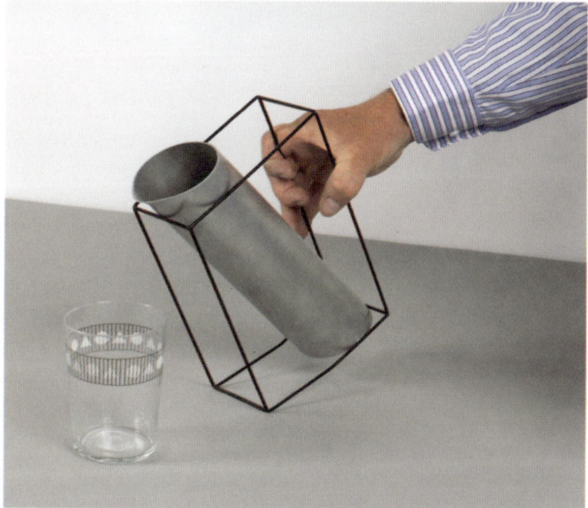

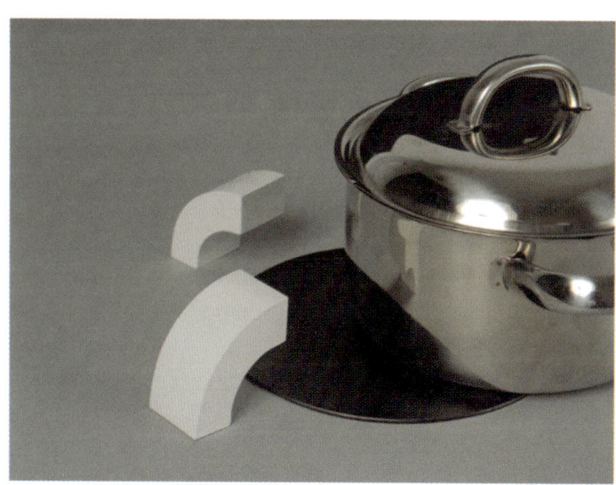

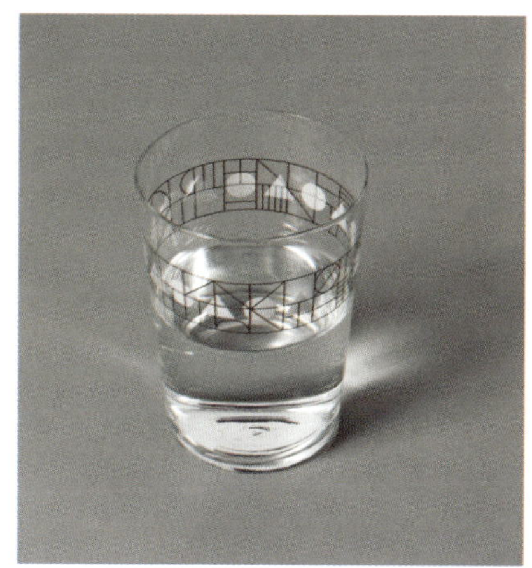

Leaven Range collection, 2013; Simon Kinneir (British, b. 1984), The Everyday (London, UK, founded 2013); Porcelain, stainless steel, aluminum, powder-coated steel, brass with rare earth magnet, glass, resin; Chopping board: 1.7 × 30 × 21 cm (11⁄16 × 11 13⁄16 × 8 1⁄4 in.), Mug: 12 × 9 cm diam. (4 3⁄4 × 3 9⁄16 in.), Jug: 24 × 17 × 8 cm (9 7⁄16 × 6 11⁄16 × 3 1⁄8 in.), Pot holder: 3.2 × 5 cm diam. (1 1⁄4 × 1 15⁄16 in.), Glass: 12 × 9 cm diam. (4 3⁄4 × 3 9⁄16 in.), Cutlery, each: 1.7 x 2.5 × 14 cm (11⁄16 × 1 × 5 1⁄2 in.); © Simon Kinneir, James Cartwright

pointers and sensory feedback during tasks to free people from having to be constantly "watching what you're doing."[10]

Impaired vision is a consequence of several common illnesses, including dementia. Although dementia often occurs among older people, it is not a consequence of normal aging but is associated with disease affecting the brain. People with dementia encounter deterioration of memory, language, and judgment as well as diminished sensory functions.[11] The ability to recognize and position objects also is affected, because dementia impairs semantic memory, "the central conceptual system in which information from the various sensory modalities is ultimately processed and... thinking occurs."[12] The breakdown of semantic memory causes people to respond erratically to their visual environment.

In Germany, approximately 1.5 million people have dementia, a number that increases by 300,000 each year.[13] The German company HEWI designs continuous systems of hardware and fixtures for use in sanitary areas and public facilities. A well-designed handrail is a visual guide as well as a physical support. Color contrast and appropriate lighting helps fixtures stand out from their surroundings and clearly signal their function. HEWI provides a wide range of colors for door levers and railings. To make a horizontal push bar on a door less confusing to use, HEWI highlights one end of the bar with a bright color, signaling to users where to push the lever. HEWI uses strong colors to highlight the functional elements of a washbasin, soap dispenser, handlebar, and other bathroom fixtures, facilitating perception and use.

Color can enhance object recognition. A study published in 1985 explored the effects of color on naming and recognizing objects. By measuring the reaction time required for subjects to name fruits and vegetables on colored and black-and-white slides, researchers found that objects shown in color were named more quickly.[14] Another experiment presented images of food to subjects in either full color or black and white. In the study, people with normal vision obtained higher accuracy and had shorter reaction time when looking at colored images. For low-vision subjects, color substantially boosted object recognition.[15] Another study shows that objects become more memorable when experienced with multiple senses. A garment that consumers can physically touch is recalled more vividly than one seen only online. Because sensory acuity diminishes with age, older people benefit from multisensory design.[16] For example, strong contrasts in color, texture, shape, or hardness can help users distinguish the lid on a bottle or the zipper or buttons on a jacket.

Color plays a powerful role in Eatwell Assistive Tableware, designed by Sha Yao from Taiwan Province of China. Yao was inspired by the experience of her grandmother, who had Alzheimer's disease. 50–60 percent of all dementia patients have Alzheimer's.[17] Meals should be a time of enjoyment and social connection, but for Yao's grandmother, they were predicaments. Her cognitive and sensory impairments caused her to eat less than she should.[18]

Yao's Eatwell design is based on research conducted by Boston University. The Massachusetts study found that 40 percent of people with severe Alzheimer's had significant weight loss due to insufficient food intake. However, when patients were served with brightly colored plates and cups,

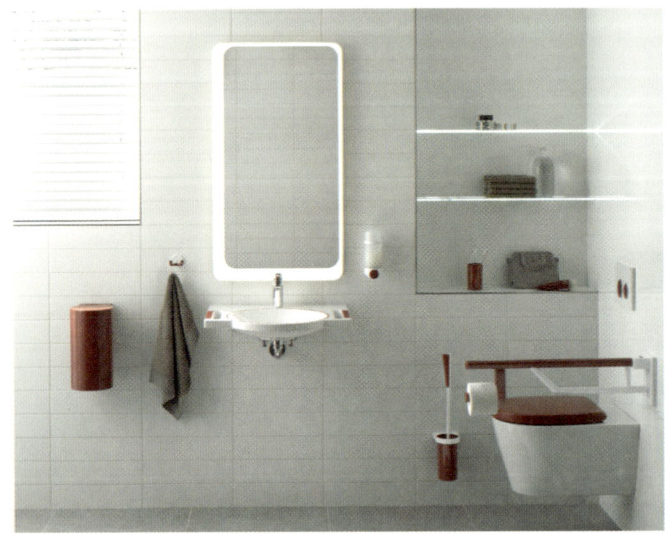

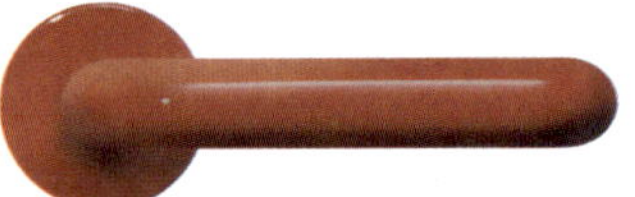

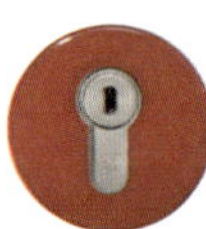

Dementia Care Bathroom Setting; HEWI (Germany, founded 1929); Courtesy of HEWI

Door Lever, from the Dementia Care Bathroom Fixture collection; HEWI (German, founded 1929); Polyamide, corrosion-resistant steel insert; 2.3 cm diam. (7/8 in.), handle: 15 × 6.7 cm (5 7/8 × 2 5/8 in.); Courtesy of HEWI

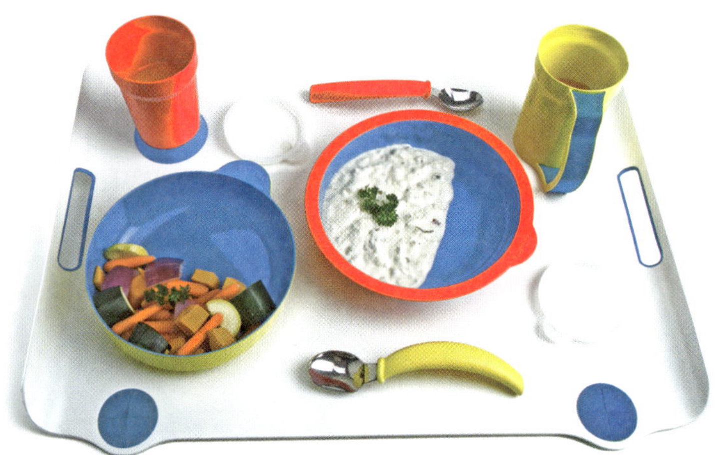

Eatwell Assistive Tableware Set, 2015; Sha Yao (b. Taiwan Province of China, 1983), Sha Design LLC (Redwood City, California, USA, founded 2013); PP, TPE, silicone, stainless steel; Sizes vary, up to 4.5 × 19.5 cm diam. (1 ¾ × 7 11⁄16 in.); Courtesy of Sha Yao

they ate and drank more than when served meals on white or stainless-steel wares. The participants in the experiment "ate about 24 percent more food and drank almost 84 percent more liquid with the red tableware compared with the white tableware." In general, people with Alzheimer's have trouble seeing contrast, making it hard for them to distinguish "a plate from a table setting, food from a plate, or liquid from its container (e.g., milk from a white cup)."[19] Hence vision difficulty is a factor in patients' willingness to eat.

Yao's Eatwell products use blue, a color that does not appear in food, for the bowls' interiors, helping Alzheimer's patients distinguish food from the dish. The exteriors use red and yellow to stimulate appetite. The same concept is applied to the rest of Eatwell tableware. All pieces stand out prominently from the table setting to enhance visual cognition.

Designers like Pires, Neiva, Kinneir, and Yao, and companies like HEWI, offer tools for engaging with the world through color and touch. Such products are beacons and guideposts, illuminating purpose and meaning. People can use them to bring pleasure, independence, dignity, and beauty to daily life.

Karen Kraskow

Insights Beyond Vision

"Cities are fantastic places for the blind," says Chris Downey, an architect who lost his sight after designing buildings for twenty years. He continued to design and build, vigorously redesigning his way of working and using all his senses in their unique power.

Downey makes drawings with flexible wax sticks; these are the basis for discussions with architects and collaborators. His design practice addresses the tactile, olfactory, and acoustic experience of users. Architects like Downey, and others who experience blindness, are expanding the frontier of design holistically.

Barbara Apel, a former fine jewelry designer (for 22 years) describes how she uses her senses today. Her observations are the wellspring from which designers can draw to make accessible products that utilize multiple senses. "I use smell very differently now than I did when I was sighted," she says, "because it's part of seeing. Going in an elevator, through smell, I can sense another person's presence, regardless of their perfume. Touching is part of seeing: when I cook I gently touch a hamburger to test its doneness. Listening is a part of seeing: when I go to museums and listen to the curator describe sculpture or painting, I visualize their images. If I am given the opportunity to touch the sculpture I get a better sense of its proportions and the artist's concept." Smell, touch, hearing, and taste are ways we take in information about our environment. Each is an option. Some use one best, others have strength in another.

KAREN KRASKOW studied industrial design at Rhode Island School of Design and Pratt Institute. Through personal interviews, she researches universal design and shares users' insights through writing, design school presentations, and research for museum exhibitions. She reviews disability film festivals (including ReelAbilities) and was an Interviewer for *Visible Lives: Oral Histories of the Disability Experience* (New York Public Library). She is a member of the Design for Aging Committee of the American Institute of Architects.

Illustrations by Jennifer Tobias

In this essay, we will discuss design solutions proposed (or recommended) by users who capitalize on four of our senses—those beyond sight. We will point out existing products and spaces on the market that function for all, or at least are a step in that direction. By highlighting what our users with blindness or low vision create, purchase, or use every day, we hope to stimulate creative thinking. We will learn from users I've interviewed what design limitations they encounter, and what they would like to see improved. We will meet with them in the home, the workplace, the city, the marketplace, etc. The following individuals have generously granted their time and insights: Chancey Fleet, a technology consultant; Chris Downey, an architect; Frank Senior, a jazz vocalist; Joan Reveyoso, a professional singer; Barbara Apel, a former fine jewelry designer and currently an avid museum afficionado; Annie Leist, an artist; and Christine Ha, 2012 winner of the television competition *MasterChef* and producer of the television cooking show *Four Senses* (AMI). All these consultants delve into their work in private and public spaces, using sound, touch, smell, and taste. Some have been blind or visually impaired since birth, and some have lost eyesight later in life.

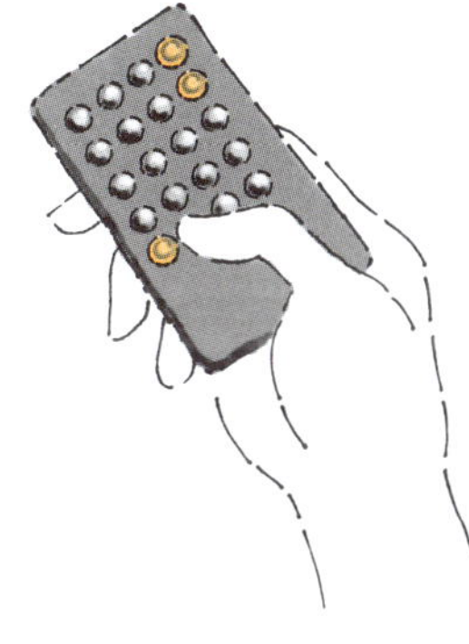

The drawing shows a remote control that has been customized by the user with silicone dots. The dots make it easy to find important functions.

The expert users I interviewed aim to accomplish their goals with independence and self-direction, in a well-designed environment. Desiring healthy relationships, they do not want to rely on others unless truly necessary. They also would prefer not to count on memory where the other senses—if mobilized in the design of objects and spaces—could successfully communicate information needed for use. The people I spoke with think about themselves in different ways. Some call themselves "sightless," to indicate that they have rich capacities in other senses (these abilities may vary, of course, from individual to individual). Others use the word "blind," "low vision," or "visually impaired" to directly and openly name a factor in their lives. Not all the solutions we will discuss have achieved the goal of universal design (accessibility for all), but they suggest milestones, or stepstones, along the path to that goal as seen in the day-to-day lives of these individuals.

Navigating the environment is our starting point. Chris Downey listens acutely to the sound of traffic—such as a person stepping on a metal plate on the sidewalk or the footsteps of other pedestrians. These cues contribute to his sense of direction. Chancey Fleet crosses a street by listening for the "parallel surge" of traffic going in the same direction as she is, which indicates it's okay to cross in that direction. If traffic is traveling perpendicular to her line of travel, she must wait. When she goes to a place that is unfamiliar, she prepares by printing out a TMAP (tactile map) on an embossed printer. The map, with its raised dotted lines and street names in braille, provides her with a mental model of her journey. If the crossing is especially difficult, because a market has recently been set up in the street, for example, she uses the app Be My Eyes on her smartphone. With this app, she can scan the environment with her phone's camera and talk with a volunteer who views her images and can suggest directions.

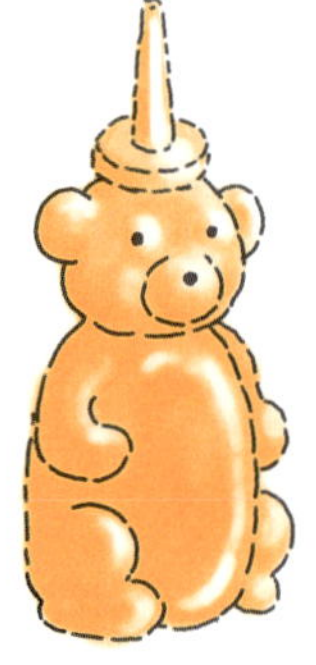

The illustration shows a plastic honey bear package, whose shape can be recognized by touch.

It should be noted that not all who navigate using the four senses we are highlighting are tech-savvy. Some grew up before technology reached the mainstream; others prefer simple, personally devised solutions. For example, a friend of Chancey's brings a supply of braille labels as her shopping list; she places them on the objects she picks up at the store so she knows what is in the packages when she gets home. She may have picked them off the shelf herself (honey bears or foil-topped Pellegrino cans can be identified by feel) or found them with assistance. Some people are quite comfortable with technology and use digital devices in many aspects of their lives. Similarly, some designers develop their ideas using traditional methods and materials, creating elegant, simple products, while others focus on digital solutions. All avenues are worth exploring.

A much-lauded tool on smartphones harnesses sound. Screen readers, like VoiceOver (on iOS) and TalkBack (on Android), turn text into voice. When the user passes a hand across the home screen, for example, the device speaks the names of the icons they touch. When the user hears the one they are seeking they double tap it, and the application opens. This touch-sound technology has been applied to (or recommended for) many devices—in the kitchen, in taxis, etc.

Frank Senior is a tech maven. He uses BlindSquare, a smartphone app, to guide him in getting around New York and other cities. BlindSquare is similar to the GPS systems used in cars. GPS plus third-party navigating apps (e.g., Open Street Map and Foursquare) allow it to determine your location and give you oral directions to your destination. He speaks his starting location into the phone, and it responds with step-by-step voice directions. "Seventeenth and Seventh Avenue," he says to his phone, as he disembarks the bus to Manhattan. "Turn right," the phone responds. "Walk two blocks straight...," and so on. At intervals, BlindSquare lets him know how close he is to his destination: "One hundred feet... fifty feet..." and so on. The closer he is, the more the app talks. If he wishes, Frank can set it to tell him about places of interest he is passing, should he like to stop by. When he arrives at his destination, a ring will sound. Frank also uses BlindSquare when he travels internationally to perform. Once, when walking to his performing venue in Denmark, BlindSquare (the English version) had some trouble pronouncing the Danish street names—a tech problem that is solvable. Frank says that BlindSquare would be even more useful if, in addition to helping him find his way to streets and building locations, it could tell him in a park or other open area that "the footpath is four feet ahead... when you get there, turn left." Paths are not yet describable by location in the same way as buildings located on a street are.

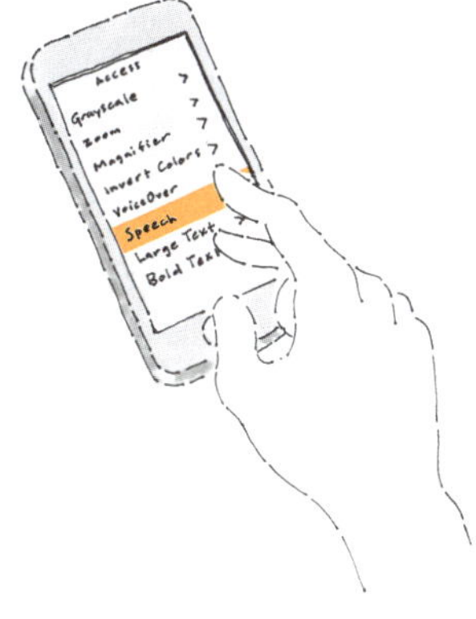

In the image, a user is selecting from a menu of accessibility features, which are built in to Apple's iPhone, including VoiceOver, Zoom, Magnifier, Invert Colors, Grayscale, Speech, Large Text, and Bold Text.

An innovation found at a number of street corners in the United States is the Audible Pedestrian Signal (APS). A yellow box, attached to a lamppost, makes a beep to let a person know where it is. When the pedestrian feels the large button on the APS and presses it, they will hear: "WAIT... WAIT... Fifth Avenue.... Walk sign is on to cross Fifth Avenue." A problem, however, with many sound devices in the environment is competition with the noise of the surrounding streetscape.

Most of these devices work well, but not all intersections have them. Thus the complete path to the destination is choppy. The devices also require maintenance. The Department of Transportation plans to add seventy-five new APS signal boxes a year in New York City. Frank states that APS boxes are especially helpful on an angled street like Broadway, because he can hear the beeping from the other side of the avenue and know that he will be crossing diagonal to the curb, instead of straight across as at most intersections.

A proposal to add a tactile diagram above each APS button is being developed by Steven Landau, president of Touch Graphics, and the NYC Department of Transportation (DOT). Through touch and sight, these diagrams will give additional information about the crossing: the width of the street, the number of lanes it has, the direction of traffic flow, and whether there is a mid-street island or bike lane. After testing these diagrams with users at the intersection of 23rd Street and 7th Avenue, DOT will consider implementing them at other street crossings.

West 23rd Street
You Are Here
push button for accessible signal

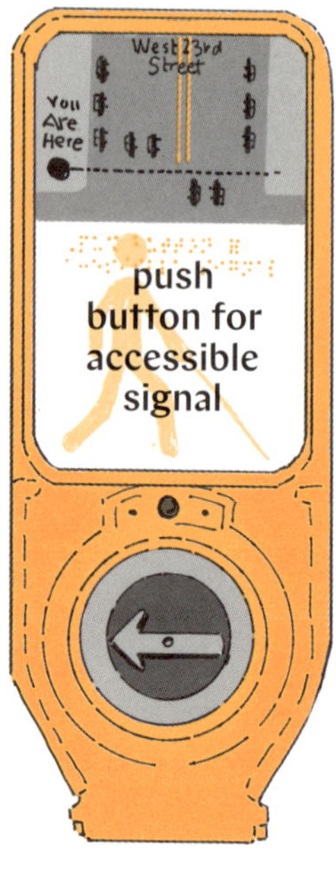

The drawing shows an accessible pedestrian signal, which has an arrow for triggering an audible crossing signal. Here, added to the standard crosswalk box is a tactile sign describing the direction of traffic at that intersection. These graphics would also help seniors, children, and anyone else who might need a moment to assess the layout of the intersection (as streetscapes have become more complex).

Another digital solution to navigation, developed by AIRA Visual Interpreter for the Blind, incorporates Google Glass. Users wear a special pair of glasses with a camera attached; the camera takes video images and screenshots of everything the user's head turns toward. These images are transmitted to a "live agent" sitting at a computer in a remote location. The agent talks with the user, letting him or her know how to get to a particular place. ("You are five feet from the entrance to the building...") The agent views a map of the user's location as well as the individual's profile on the screen, and the agent can inform them of options in the area that might be of interest. Frank observes that this system is especially helpful in open spaces such as parks. An agent can guide a user to a bench "on the right," to the entrance gate, "two feet away," and the like. Agents work for an hourly wage, and, much like today's taxi services, they are called upon when the need arises and when they are available. The project is still in beta, and may be expensive at this moment. Frank is one of the users testing the system. AIRA gives him confidence, plus detail and company. The fact that you have "realtime eyes with you" is reassuring.

Annie Leist would like to see facial recognition added to AIRA. When she's in a crowded restaurant or at a conference, she would like the live agent to be able to tell her who is there and that her friend from college is across the room. (Annie has low vision.) This she hopes could be done by data transmission of attendees at a conference, or by facial-recognition software.

Finding fixtures in the environment, and avoiding them when they are in the path of travel, is a design opportunity that architect Chris Downey has addressed. His proposal has two parts. First, he would create a planter strip bordering the edge of the sidewalk (stopping at the corner curb cut). In that plant-filled area, the bus stop, a bike rack, a trash can, and anything needed in a pedestrian's travels would be located. Pedestrians would always know where to find them. The planter strip would beautify the area—and walkers would enjoy the flowers for their scent, their sound in the wind, or their visual qualities. In between the planter strip and the buildings on that street travelers would circulate. As the planter strip would have on the ground a different texture from the circulation area, a person using a mobility cane could feel that difference and let that guide his or her movement. This technique of cane use, called "shorelining," helps one's path stay straight, or curved, as the landform necessitates.

A second part of Chris Downey's proposal is to place the amenities in the area close to the perimeter of the buildings (instead of, or in addition to, the interior of the planter strip). In the world of retail, the area around the building(s) is called the "pop-out zone." In this space, the business owner might set down clothing racks or tables with merchandise to expand the sales area. A bay window could project into that zone, and planters could enhance the area from that window as well. A bike rack, a bench, and/or a trash can would be found next to the building. Both of these solutions (the planter strip at the curb and the pop-out zone beside the building) keep necessary objects out of the path of travel. They beautify an area and leave an open circulation path either between the planter strip and the pop-out zone, or simply beside one or the other.

Inside buildings, wayfinding takes a different form. GPS does not penetrate the interiors of buildings, so "beacons" (or proximity sensors) can be posted at different points. Beacons placed at the reception desk, the café, the restroom, etc. can communicate via Bluetooth with the user's smartphone at some hotels and airports. They tell visitors where that facility is located, how to get there, and how near they are to it. An app at the San Francisco Airport can help one find a power outlet, an important tool in travel today.

A range of apps and simple, nontechnological solutions are options in the home as well, particularly the kitchen. Joan Reveyoso, a professional singer, roasts ham, lamb, and beef frequently in her oven. Her husband has marked key numbers (at 50-degree intervals) on the oven dial with hardened silicone dots that she reads by touch.

Christine Ha, a professional chef, uses technology regularly. For cooking in the oven or on the grill, she uses iGrill, from iDevice's line of accessible tools. iGrill sports a thermometer which she inserts into a roast before placing it in the oven. A wire from the thermometer exits the oven and connects to a device attached to her smartphone. On the phone, she can read and set the temperature via VoiceOver.

When pouring and measuring cold liquids, Christine uses a plastic Pyrex measuring cup to which her sighted husband has attached hardened silicone dots at the ½ cup and ¼ cup levels. For hot liquids, she recommends creating separate glass measuring cups, one for ¼ cup, one for ½ cup, and so on. On the rim of one measuring cup, she can set a Liquid Level Indicator that beeps when the cup is almost full, and changes tone when it is completely full. The measuring cups she has in mind would need to have space at the top to let the prongs of the Liquid Level Indicator device hang over the rim. Pourfect makes plastic cups of this type, but measuring hot liquids requires glass.

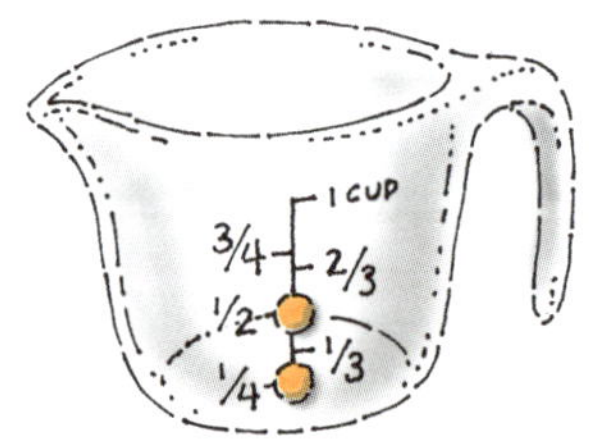

The image shows a measuring cup that has been customized with adhesive siliicone dots. The user presses her thumb on the outside of the measuring cup at the required level and puts her pointer finger inside the measurer, its tip matching up with the dot on the outside.

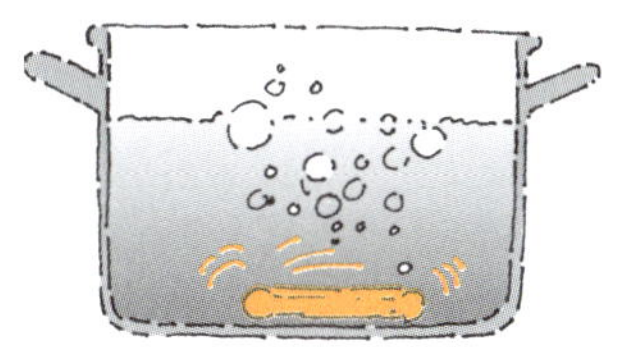

The image shows a boil alert placed in a cooking pot. When the water boils, the object rattles in the bottom.

Many people use their sense of hearing to know if water in a pot is boiling. Christine knows the sound of water boiling as well as when it simmers. Some people may not be able to hear this; in a noisy environment, when the guests are chatting before dinner is served, not many can. A "boil alert" is a filled-in doughnut-shaped slab of plastic that can be set in the bottom of a pot of water. It crackles when the water is boiling. One can also pull out the traditional whistling teakettle, which Barbara does; it lets her know when water, or soup, is ready. The boil alert or the whistling teakettle are handy for anyone who wants to know when the water is boiling, especially if they have to leave the kitchen when food is on the stove.

Sound thus plays an important role in the design of kitchen appliances, as do shape and texture. With the many features that kitchen appliances offer today—slow cook, yogurt, or rice—there is a need for universal controls. Print controls address only one portion of the population—those with sight—but other options are available. If one doesn't have a way of knowing the appliance's functions, one is forced to rely on another person. Or one must learn and memorize the layout of controls. Barbara uses an audio-enabled rice cooker: when she presses a button (labeled "porridge," perhaps), the rice cooker announces the option; if she wishes to use that setting she does nothing or presses the Start button to the right. If that is not her choice, she goes to the next button in the row and repeats these actions. Some users (such as Christine and Joan) prefer old-fashioned tools, such as the stovetop pressure cooker, which has virtually no controls. Barbara's choice is the decades-old coffee grinder, which has only one button. Sometimes users ask a relative or friend to attach braille labels, constructing their own interface.

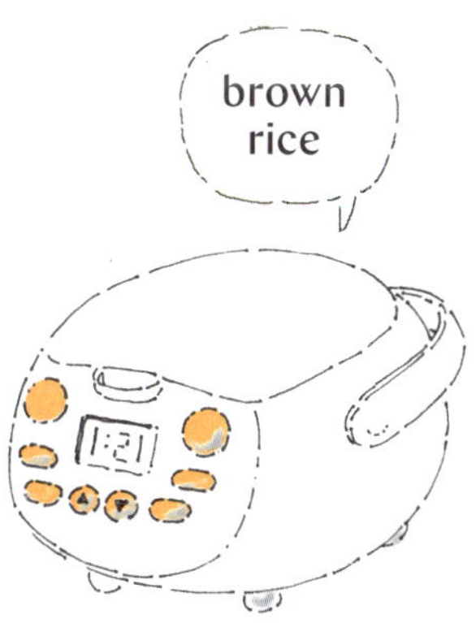

The image shows a rice cooker with spoken controls. Many appliances could be designed with this feature.

Christine suggests that appliances (such as rice makers and pressure cookers) be connected to one's tablet or smartphone by Bluetooth. Options could be spoken or visible, depending on the best mode for the user. Another concept is to design buttons with different shapes or textures. For example, a horizontal or vertical row of four buttons, each with a different shape, could be memorized more easily. An arrangement of buttons (all in a circle or a square) can work as well. Raised letters or braille letters on buttons can be helpful on a variety of appliances; for example one could place a raised *H* or *C* for hot or cold on the office water cooler handles. Thoughtful positioning of buttons, changes in shape or texture, and raised lettering or braille can make appliances and devices function successfully for all users.

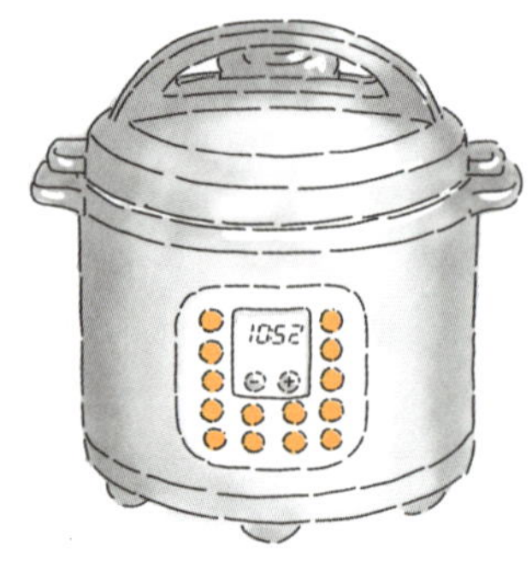

The drawing shows an Instant Pot Smart Multifunctional Pressure Cooker, which is an example of an appliance that has a simple arrangement of touch controls as well as Bluetooth connectivity.

This direction of design thinking could enhance many machines in daily life. When Joan took a taxi to my office, she had to ask the driver to process her credit card as the payment information and Enter button were solely in print, not audio. We thought about how universal symbols (such as a raised arrow, or a circle for Enter) could be placed on the plastic frame and direct her to a screen icon at the edge. However, I learned that there is indeed an audio mode, called VIP Mode, accessed by gently double- (or triple-) tapping the screen opposite the backseat. The basic system (there are slightly different versions) is composed of screens with a large rectangle on the left and a similar one on the right; below that there can be a row of three smaller rectangles—the bottom row. Audio instructions tell you to "tap left for cash, tap right for credit"; "tap the minus sign on the left to lower volume; tap the plus sign on the right to raise it," and so on. You must listen carefully to the audio instructions, which takes a bit of time, to know exactly where to tap. "Tap at the bottom in the center to repeat instructions," etc. Some people may feel a little unsure that they will tap the right area.

Chancey and others feel that VoiceOver technology (or TalkBack) is more efficient for taxi functions. Users of VoiceOver explore the whole screen with their hand and hear the names of the icons that their fingers touch; they double tap the one they wish to open. Using one of those screen readers, Chancey feels, would make the process of paying one's fare accessible to all. I would add that there could be an option to speak or not speak, and a simple double tap could serve those who preferred not to have a sound option. The screen could also invite users to listen to news or entertainment. In that way, the one screen would be useful for everybody: one could pay one's fare by auditory or visual cues; one could choose an option to listen to or view news or entertainment. Thus, Chancey suggests, one screen would be useful to many users; it would not single out one group of people as needing something different from others. Passengers would use the mode that suits them best.

An audio option has also made ATMs at banks accessible when one plugs in one's headphones. Voice directions tell the user what number on the keypad to press for Withdraw, Deposit, Transfer, etc. A raised dot on the 5 (middle key) enables one to infer by touch the positions of the other keys. My experience using my local ATM machine showed me that it worked well, but sometimes the voice commands did not fully coincide with what was on the screen. The mismatch wasn't enough to prevent me from making a transaction, but it was not quite in accord with our current digital prowess. Christine and Chancey would like to see VoiceOver on ATM screens as well, and any other machine with options; they prefer this to translating from voice to physical numbered keys. Clearly, the integration of computer technology with machine capabilities needs to be explored further with users.

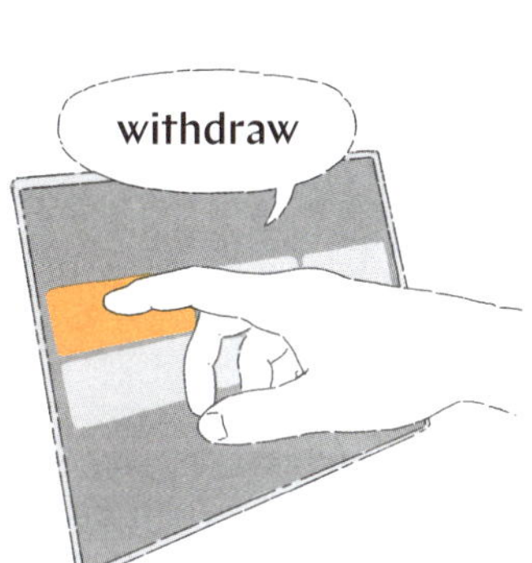

In the image, a user touches an ATM machine to hear options. Chancey Fleet suggests that this VoiceOver feature replace the keypad-based audio systems currently used in ATM machines.

Returning to the kitchen, and also considering the bathroom, we come to the design of packaging. Apps can help users read the text on the outside, but when you're in the bathroom, or even busy in the kitchen, that may not always be the best technique. When Joan gets ready to wash her hair, she lifts a bottle and does not know if it is shampoo or conditioner, because they are identical in shape. Sometimes she nicks the conditioner bottle cap or asks the salesperson to mark it with a piece of tape. Other times, she puts the bottles in different places—the conditioner on the sink, the shampoo on the tub.

One hotel she stayed in placed braille on the lids of the bottles. The Super 8 Motel in Lee, Massachusetts, uses a two-part wall-mounted dispenser with shampoo on the left, and conditioner on the right (from Dispenser Amenities).

The dispenser can always be found on the wall opposite the showerhead. For Joan, these solutions are excellent, as their positioning is consistent and it's easy to memorize "right" and "left." The general manager of the Super 8, Sam Patel, who installed them, chose them for other reasons as well. Dispensers are more economical and sustainable than small bottles. Additionally, it's easier in the shower to pump from the dispenser than to fumble with a tiny bottle. Christine encounters this situation in her travels. Hotels provide bottles of body lotion, soap, and shower gel as well as shampoo and conditioner on the shelf in the bathroom; but often they are packaged in bottles of the same size and shape. Designers could place a raised S and raised C, and/or braille, on the bottle for those who use touch (including people who take off their eyeglasses before bathing).

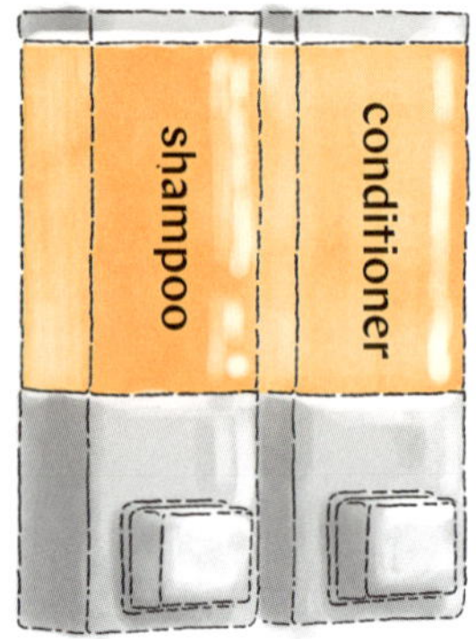

The drawing shows a shampoo dispenser used in hotels. The dispenser keeps shampoo on the left and conditioner on the right, making it easy for users to find each product by touch.

Getting dressed each day presents its own challenges. Sound and touch expand our range of options. When Joan goes shopping for shoes, she uses touch to identify a patent leather shoe and distinguish it from a leather shoe, and purchases a pair of each. (Tags don't stay in shoes.) Or she'll buy one pair with a buckle and one without. For clothing, when she gets home after purchasing a dress in different colors, she'll adjust the tag of each—the white one will have no tag (she'll cut it out), the green one will have only the top of the tag, and the fuchsia one will bear the existing tag. White or beige sweaters in her closet will never have a tag. Could we not have a system of differently textured or shaped tags to represent the color range? How about tags to identify clothes that fit me when I'm above my normal weight, and different ones to identify those that fit me when my weight is in the normal range?

Christine and Barbara have well-organized closets. Shopping allows Barbara to tap into her experience from her youth as a fashion model. She knows quite well what looks good on her. When she shops, she touches a dress to feel its construction. When she intuits cap sleeves, quarter-length sleeves, or full-length sleeves, she decides which to purchase. She asks

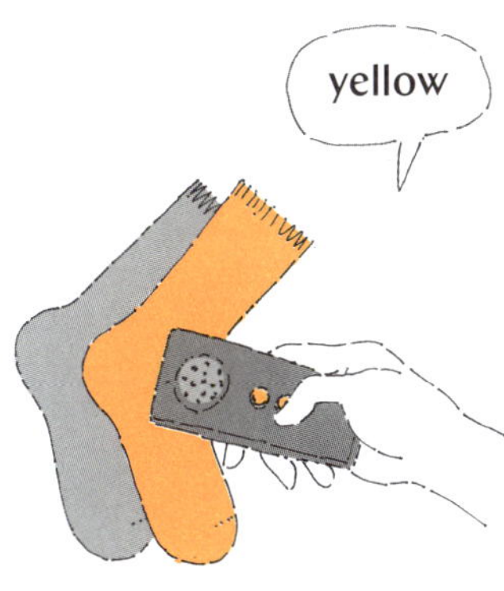

The image shows a device that scans colors and says their name. A tech-inclined user can place the gadget up against a garment, and it will say, "Yellow."

the salesperson, "Is it dark blue, light blue, or bright blue?" She uses this dialogue and her sense of touch to make a decision. With TapTapSee, an iPhone app, you can take a picture, and in a few seconds hear (from a volunteer), "Blue and black stripes." The more advanced app, Be My Eyes, can generate an extended conversation in real time—a volunteer can tell you not only the color of your shirt but also if there's a spot on it!

Joan selected her wedding dress by touching bride dolls and inferring their style and texture. She made her choice in a major NYC department store from this tactile information. Christine enjoys online shopping, but rues the descriptions of some products (read by her screen reader). Makeup described as the color of "LSD" or "Mildew" is tough to picture. It would be helpful, she suggests, if descriptions were more straightforward, more imaginable ("tree bark," "blue sky"). Christine reminds us that she, like all our interviewees, values fashion and its role in her daily life. She regularly consults InStyle and Refinery29 online.

Systems for managing money are also individually devised as well as tech-based. In the United States, coins can be distinguished from one another because of their size. However, bills are all the same rectangular size. Today, Frank folds his ten-dollar bills in half the long way, his five-dollar bills in half the short way, etc. (Twenty-dollar bills go in his right pocket, and singles in his left.) Joan uses a satchel with many pockets, with designated, and memorized, denominations. Wallets are available with several parallel pockets for organizing bills. For the tech user, apps such as Money Reader let you take a picture of the bill, followed by an announcement ("Twenty dollars").

Euros have a different system. One can feel short, parallel, tactile lines, spaced differently on each note, on the short edge of the 200- and 500-Euro banknotes. Coins are distinguishable by weight, thickness, and edge texture. The heavier the coin, the higher the value (excepting the one-Euro coin); the thicker the coin, the higher the value (with the exception of the 2 and 1 Euro coins). Some coins bear smooth edges, while others have scalloped or grooved perimeters. The European

Central Bank consulted on the design with the European Blind Union, knowing that "a good design for the blind and partially sighted (is) a good design for everybody."

Traveling presents a host of design opportunities; one that Christine notes is the availability of a restroom that is private so that her husband can assist her in finding the toilet, the hand-dryer, and other amenities. She uses the family, or accessible, restroom, as he cannot assist her in the public restroom designated for women. She suggests constructing a group of individual enclosed stalls surrounding a communal sink, available to everyone. An individual stall makes it possible for a family member or companion to provide assistance. When pressed for time in an airport, taking a picture of a hand-dryer and waiting for an app to identify it by name is not always possible. Attaching braille labels, or a map that is both tactile and sanitary, might be design concepts to explore.

I hope, as do the individuals who have generously shared their day-to-day lives with me, that designers will consider all users in their decision making. Our shared environment can be improved when consumers, designers, and manufacturers keep the diversity of users in mind. Making products and spaces universally accessible—adjustable, communicating through different senses, and fitting a variety of needs—can support everyone. We all have different abilities, and at different times of our lives we may call on different skills. Knowledge about diverse needs, through interviewing, is necessary for informed decisions. Certainly, these conversations should happen while the design process is happening... not after the mold has been cast. Whether one is an architect, a teacher, a chef, or a pedestrian enjoying a city, we all need to feel that the environment is an accessory to our success.

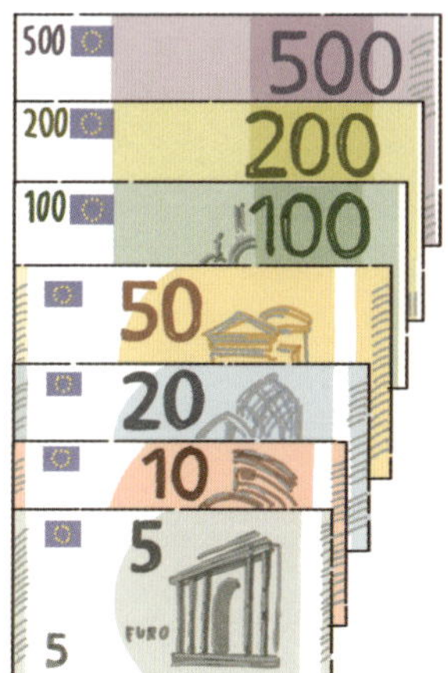

The image shows the design of Europa banknotes. The size of the banknote corresponds to the note's value (the higher the value, the larger the banknote). The notes differ in color as well: the 5 Euro banknote is gray and the 10 Euro is red, with neighboring denominations in contrasting colors. In addition, a raised image of a distinctive architectural landmark is printed on the face of each note. Sharp color differences and large numerals make neighboring denominations easy to differentiate.

New York City Department for the Aging

Aging in Place: Sensory Environments

Based on Aging in Place Guide for *Building Owners* (New York City Department for the Aging with AIA New York Design for Aging Committee, 2016, updated 2017).

In 2016, the NYC Department for the Aging collaborated with the American Institute of Architects New York Design for Aging Committee to publish guidelines that assist landlords and residents in upgrading multiunit residential buildings and apartments to support aging in place. Many of the recommendations are sensory, using color, light, and texture.

Tactility

- Use resilient floor coverings such as cork, rubber, and linoleum to provide comfort for walking and to make falls less dangerous.
- Employ non-glossy finishes on floor surfaces that require waxing.
- Use textured flooring to signal a level change.
- Use consistent floor surfaces to distinguish between a building's different functional areas, such as hallways and stairs.
- Mark circulation routes in shared or public areas of a building with handrails.
- Identify stair treads with slip-resistant textured strips in a contrasting color.
- Include braille in all signage.
- Use lever handles on doors, which are easier than knobs for many users to operate.
- Install lever-style hardware in sinks, showers, and baths as well as installing hand-held, adjustable showerheads.

Light

- Avoid creating glare (caused by strong contrast between a light source and its surroundings) by balancing natural and interior light sources.
- Use indirect light (directed against walls or ceilings) to avoid shining light directly into people's eyes.
- Install sun louvers or window blinds.
- Use even lighting to eliminate dark areas inside and outside a building.
- In apartments, illuminate hallways with motion-sensor night-lights.
- Install glow-in-the-dark light switches.
- Install doorbells that include a visible strobe as well as an adjustable audio signal.
- Ensure that all alarm systems are multisensory.

Color, Pattern, Line

- Make entrances stand out with contrasting colors as well as clear illumination.
- Use a change in floor color to signal a level change or threshold. Avoid concealing level changes with patterns or arbitrary color shifts.
- In hallways, apply contrasting wainscot trim to provide a visual and tactile point of reference.
- Use color contrast to make keyholes visible.
- Create a wayfinding system by using distinctive colors, patterns, and/or works of art to identify the different floors of a building.
- Employ light-colored numbers and letters on a dark background to create legible signage.
- Use different colors to identify different doorway functions, such as entrances to apartment units, trash areas, and stairwells.
- In bathrooms, change the color of tiles in the base row (where the wall meets to floor), to help residents perceive the edges of the room.

Smell

- Use plants to add fragrance as well as movement and life to public spaces.

UK Home Office

Accessible Service Design

Understanding accessibility helps us build services that work for everyone. Digital designers in the Home Office (a UK government department) created guidelines for making services accessible to people with different access needs. We're a small team of researchers and designers who study access needs in order to raise awareness about accessibility across our department and the UK government. We wanted to help our colleagues know more about accessibility so they can create government services that work for everyone. We wanted to engage them in a discussion about accessible services. Thus we developed a set of Do and Don't posters that provide simple guidance on how to design inclusive digital services.

We created a design aesthetic that has immediate impact, using illustrations to communicate and a clean, vivid style that unifies the posters as a set. The posters offer tips on how to design for low vision, screen readers, motor difficulties, the autism spectrum, deaf or hard of hearing, and dyslexia. A selection of posters is shown here.

Inclusive design is good design. The design principles used in these posters don't just benefit users with access needs—they help us make clear, usable services for everyone. The posters are publicly available on GitHub; with the help of people all over the world, the posters are now available in ten languages. We are now coding them to make them accessible in a responsive, online format.

UK HOME OFFICE, Access Needs Team, are the creators of these posters: Emily Ball, Oliver Beal, James Buller, Simon Castillo, Nick Cowan, Amy Everett, Charlotte Moore, Karwai Pun, Megan Rodgers, Bernard Tyers.

 Download the posters here: → accessibility.blog.gov.uk/2016/09/02/dos-and-donts-on-designing-for-accessibility

Designing for users of screen readers

Do...

describe images and provide transcripts for video

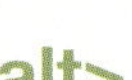

follow a linear, logical layout

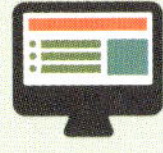

structure content using HTML5

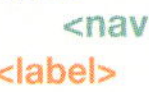

build for keyboard-only use

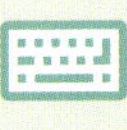

write descriptive links and headings

Contact us

Don't...

only show information in an image or video

spread content all over a page

rely on text size and placement for structure

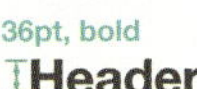

force mouse or screen use

write uninformative links and headings

Click here

Designing for users on the autistic spectrum

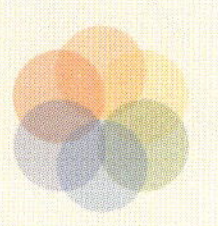

Do...

use simple colours

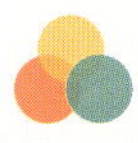

write in plain language

Do this.

use simple sentences and bullets

make buttons descriptive

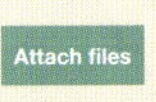

build simple and consistent layouts

Don't...

use bright contrasting colours

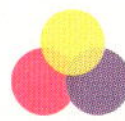

use figures of speech and idioms

create a wall of text

make buttons vague and unpredictable

build complex and cluttered layouts

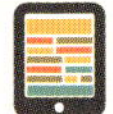

Designing for users with low vision

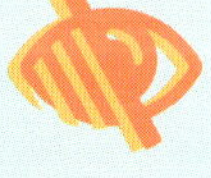

Do...

use good colour contrasts and a readable font size

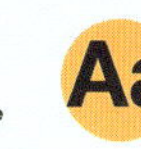

publish all information on web pages

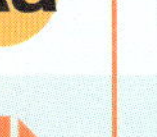

use a combination of colour, shapes and text

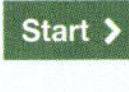

follow a linear, logical layout

200% magnification

put buttons and notifications in context

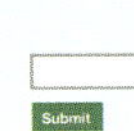

Don't...

use low colour contrasts and small font size

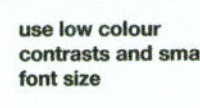

bury information in downloads

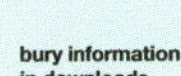

only use colour to convey meaning

spread content all over a page

200% magnification

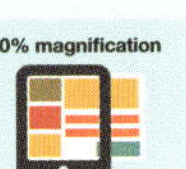

separate actions from their context

Designing for users who are D/deaf or hard of hearing

Do...

write in plain language

Do this.

use subtitles or provide transcripts for videos

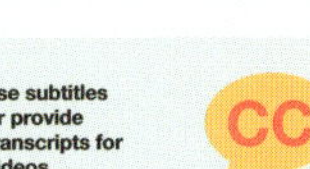
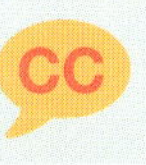

use a linear, logical layout

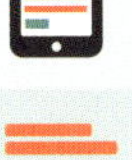

break up content with sub-headings, images and videos

let users ask for their preferred communication support when booking appointments

Don't...

use complicated words or figures of speech

put content in audio or video only

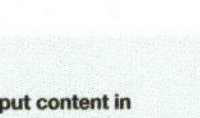

make complex layouts and menus

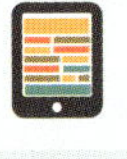

make users read long blocks of content

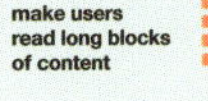

make telephone the only means of contact for users

Visualizing Sound

Capturing sound with graphic forms is an ancient human endeavor. Musical notation visualizes sound. So do alphabets and other phonetic writing systems, which translate speech into marks. Typographers have long sought to bring sound and voice to pages of print. Today, designers and musicians edit sound with visual software. Simple graphics—a jagged sound wave or a row of vertical bars—convey basic information about a track's loudness and frequency. Graphics pervade the interface of music production, and they also shape the experience of listening. Whether creating album covers, music posters, or code-driven data visualizations, designers use color, line, shape, motion, and texture to enrich the sonic landscape and create new graphic forms.

Look/Hear, 2016; Ran Zheng (Chinese, b. 1988); Typographic sound visualization, Multimedia, using Cinema 4D and other processing software; © Ran Zheng

Every place has its own ways of sounding. Graphic designer Ran Zheng created layers of sound to represent different environments—a café, an office, a park, a busy street. To visualize these sonic places, Zheng created modular letterforms spelling out the words "LOOK" and "HEAR" with a grid of shapes. Low-pitch sounds are visualized with round shapes (footsteps, a coffeemaker), and higher sounds are hard-edged and progressively sharper (wind chimes, a call bell, laughter). As the sounds become louder, the shapes get larger. Zheng's dynamic project plays with the tactility of sound—we tend to describe high-frequency sounds as bright or sharp, while low sounds are dull and round. The piece thus combines auditory, visual, and tactile experiences and associations.

Music visualizations are commonplace at clubs or concerts, where screen graphics pulse with frantic energy, translating soundtracks into spinning geometries or rhythmic bursts of color. Taking a more contemplative approach, Alexander Chen creates visualizations that are at once poetic and gently didactic. He wonders, "Could visual design help us hear better?"[1] His projects include a virtual string instrument based on the overlapping paths of New York City subway trains and depictions of piano music employing simple dots of color. According to Chen, assigning color to music has a long history. When Isaac Newton projected light through a prism and discovered the color spectrum around 1665, he chose to slice the rainbow (which occurs naturally as a gradient) into seven basic hues, believing that color must be structured like the musical scale.[2] Newton was so convinced that color and music were analogous, he added indigo to his color wheel to make his system a better match for music. (Indigo is tough to tell from blue).

Although mapping color to sound is an act of culture rather than a fact of physics, crafting such relationships takes many expressions. People with synesthesia may hear sound in color—high notes could appear in shades of pink, and low notes in purple or green. Such fusions result from a person's own exposure to certain stimuli (seeing Taylor Swift sing in a

System for typographic sound visualization, Look/Hear, 2016; Ran Zheng (Chinese, b. 1988); Multimedia, using Cinema 4D and Processing software; © Ran Zheng

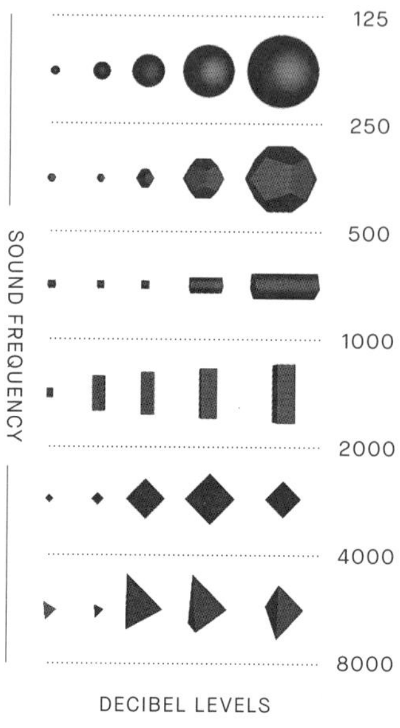

pink dress) combined with a neurological aptitude for bridging the senses.[3] Researchers at the University of California Berkeley found that people tend to associate lively music played in a major key with light, warm colors, while they associate low, slow music with hues of blue and gray.[4] Such associations are vaguer manifestations of the literal conjoining of color and sound experienced by people with synesthesia, a neurological condition.[5]

Chen's graphics visualize not the whole sound (all the water in a faucet) but rather its individual elements (each drop). He told us, "Many music visualizers use the entire recording. But I've been exploring how individual notes can be visualized." His subway piece, MTA.me, uses data from the subway system to generate simple musical compositions; the sound of a plucked string plays each time the paths of two trains intersect. The pitch depends on the location of the crossing. *Debussy Dots: Masques* visualizes a piano performance by Katsushiro Oguri. By playing the piece on a MIDI keyboard, Oguri created data with every note. Working with Oguri's data, Chen assigned a color to each note—Isaac Newton would have approved. When multiple notes play simultaneously, multiple

Digital Audio Map, *MTA.me* (still), 2011; Alexander Chen (American, b. 1981), music by Tim Kahn; Web Audio API; 3:23 minutes; Courtesy of Alexander Chen

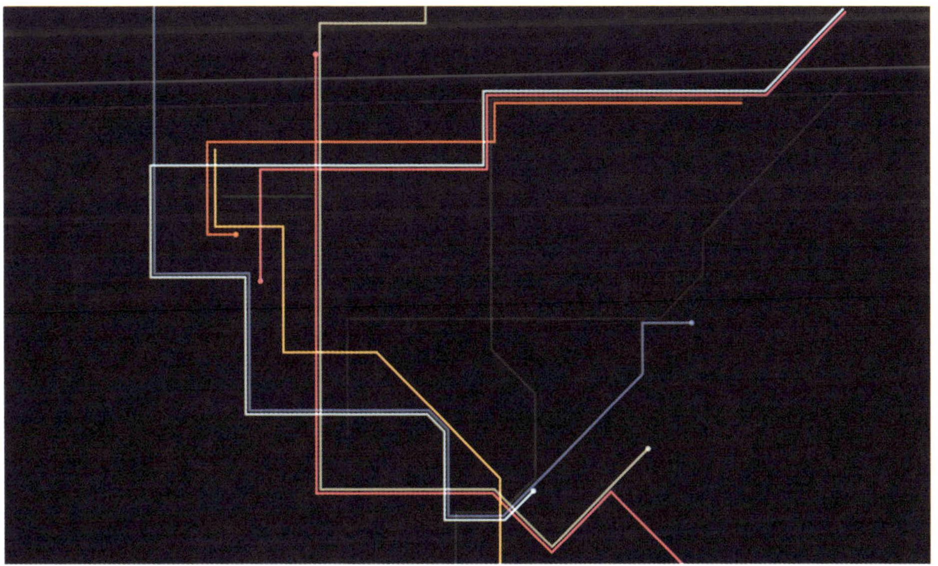

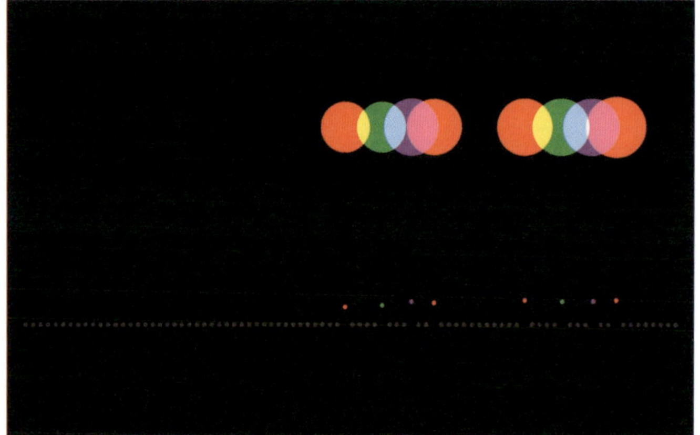

Still, Dot Piano, 2017; Alexander Chen (American, b. 1981) and Yotam Mann (American, b. 1987); Music visualization software; Courtesy of Alexander Chen

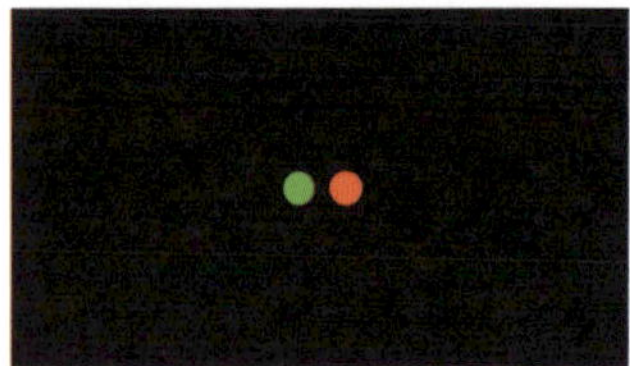

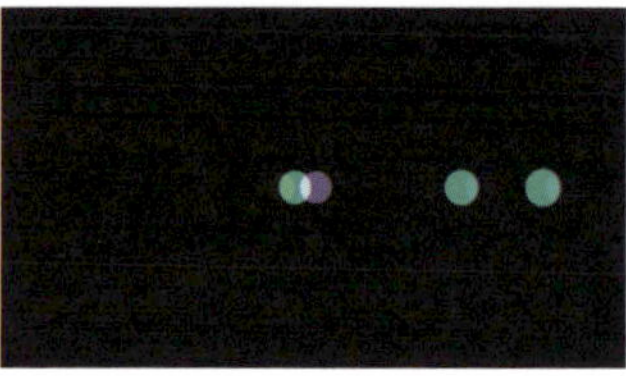

Stills, *Debussy Dots: Masques*, 2017; Alexander Chen (American, b. 1981), music by Katsushiro Oguri (Japanese, b. 1962); Digital Audio Map, Web Audio API, P5.js; 5:03 minutes; Courtesy of Alexander Chen

dots appear on-screen. Following the metaphor of light, the dots change color where they overlap. The dots change speed and intensity to reflect the structure and energy of the music. Taking this thinking further, Chen worked with Yotam Mann to create Dot Piano, a browser-based tool that users can connect to a MIDI controller to create their own dot-based visualizations of music and sound. "We care about how to make music more accessible to people through design and code," says Chen.

The Partners in London visualized music as gesture in their graphic identity for the London Symphony Orchestra's 2017/18 season. Sir Simon Rattle had recently joined the LSO as musical director. In a series of short animated films, the design team translated Rattle's movements while conducting the orchestra into digital constructions inspired by parts and pieces of musical instruments. The animations speak to haptic experience through their textured intensity and powerful movement. In a custom font, paths of motion sweep across sans serif letterforms to create a typographic identity.

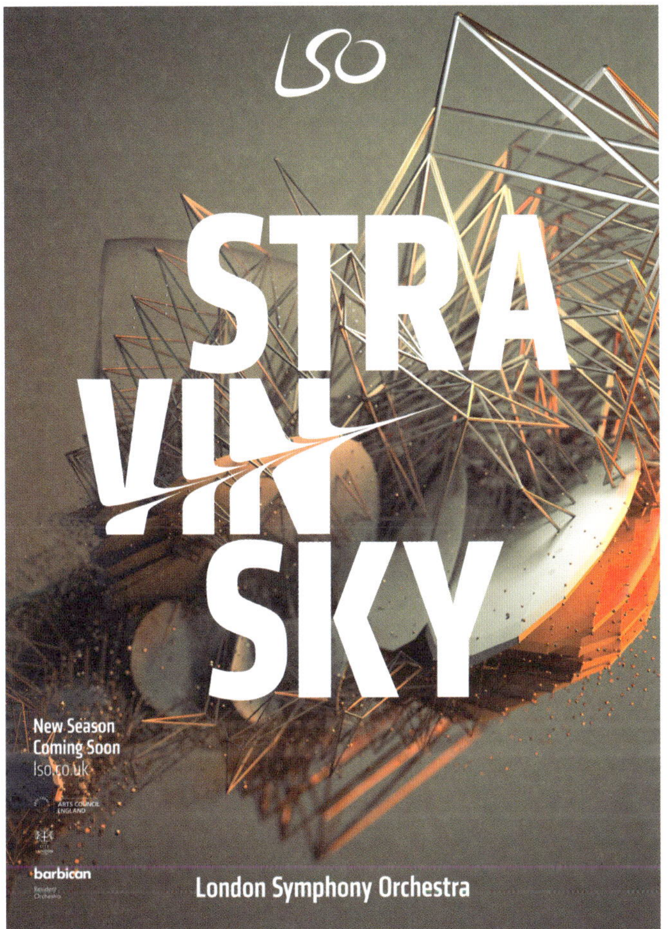

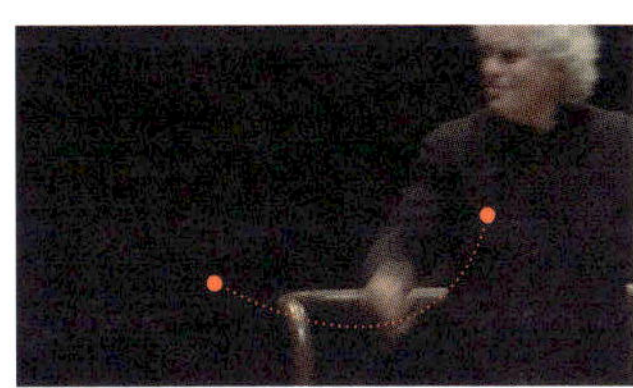

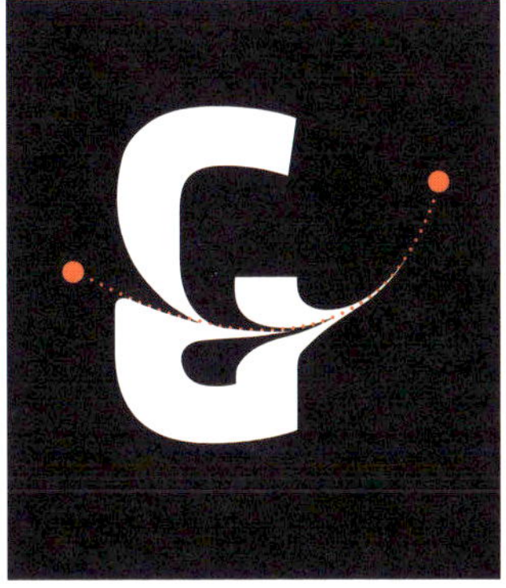

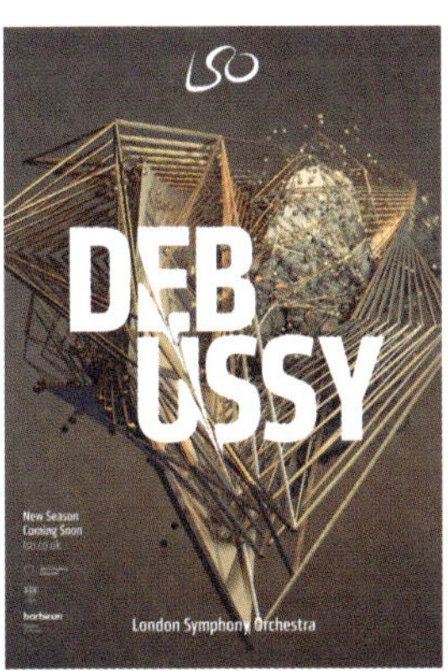

Stravinsky (TOP LEFT) and Debussy (BOTTOM) posters, and London Symphony Orchestra typography elements (RIGHT), 2017; The Partners (London, UK, founded 1983) for London Symphony Orchestra; Courtesy of The Partners

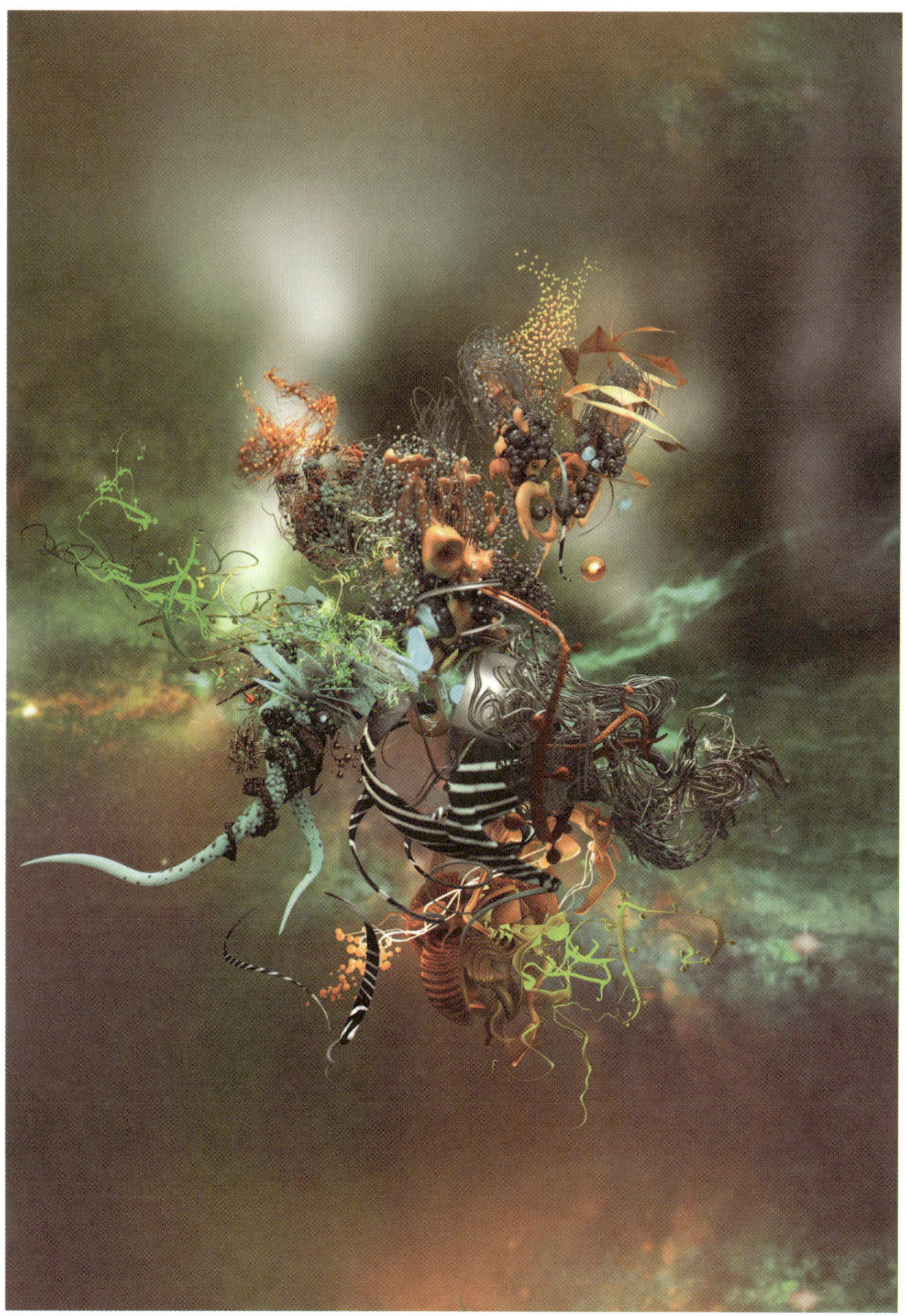

Nightingale & Canary: *Bird Sounds Visualized*, 2014; Andy Thomas (Australian, b. 1976); Digital audio, 3D particle effects software; Bird sounds from the archives of the Netherlands Institute for Sound and Vision; Courtesy of Andy Thomas

Andy Thomas creates animations inspired by the sounds of birds, whales, and other organisms. He is especially drawn to particle systems, an area of computer graphics that models the behavior of vast numbers of tiny discrete elements or "sprites." Each sprite moves independently yet responds to surrounding sprites. Game designers and digital effects artists use particle simulation to depict fuzzy or cloudy phenomena, such as a furry dog, a swarm of flies, or an exploding galaxy. In Thomas's piece *Bird Sounds Visualized*, recordings of tropical birds activate complex particle effects. Each unique birdcall creates its own graphic signature, bursting into life with sharp strands of color that fade into smoky reverb. The animations are artificial and abstract yet eerily alive. Contemporary designers remain fascinated by the cerebral abstractions of mid-century modernism.

Vinyl records, buoyed by a resurgent fan base, employ thoughtfully designed album art to underscore their status as objects. Brooklyn-based designer Mario Hugo started publishing "fake" album art online. He says, "I got kind of famous for a series of rejected Beck covers that got used for T-shirts and other stuff." Such projects led him to design real album covers

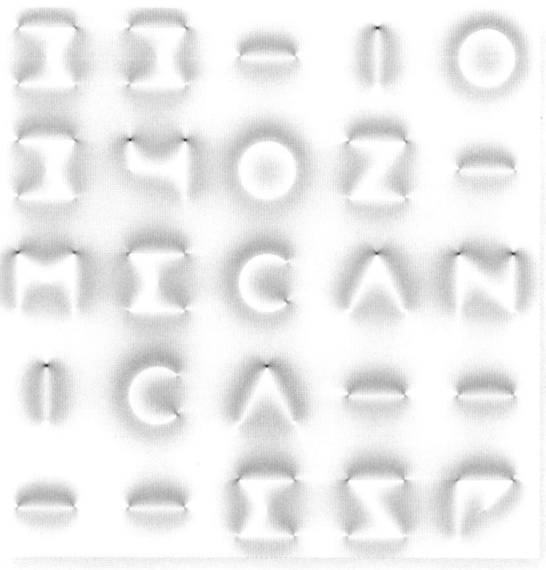

Record cover, 33103402—Mecanica, 2015; Mario Hugo (American, b. 1982); Design support, Sam Hodges and Andrew Hogge; Produced by Hugo & Marie; Offset lithograph; Published by ESP Institute (New York)

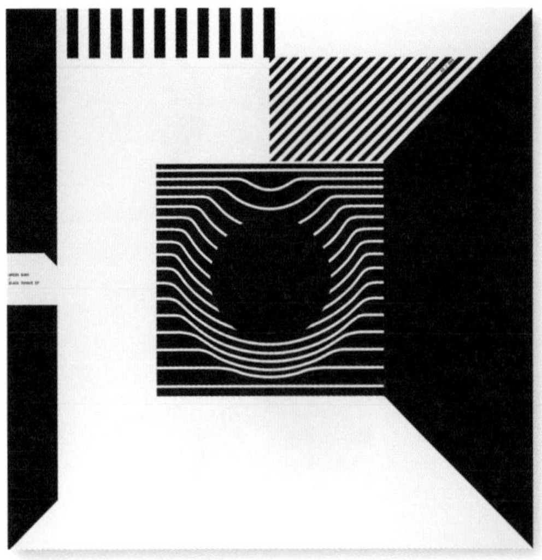

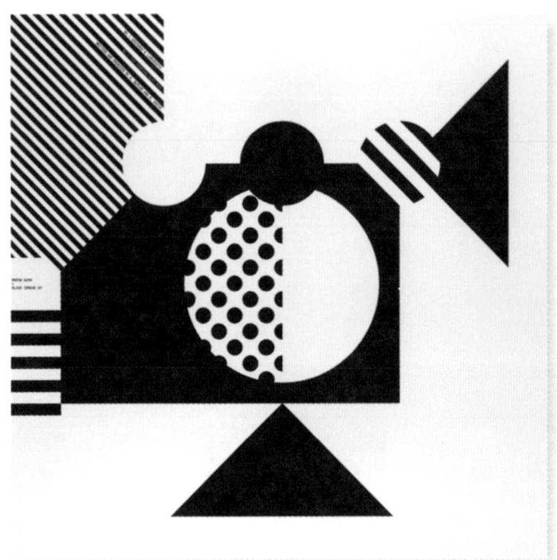

Green Gums: *Black Tongue* EP (DIAG020), 2015; Guy Featherstone (British, b. 1974) for Diagonal Records (London, UK, founded 2011); Courtesy of Guy Featherstone

for ESP Records, a small electronic music label, as well as for big acts like Rihanna and Alabama Shakes. When designing covers, Hugo chooses one or two tracks and listens to them repeatedly, "like a mantra." [6] His goal is "making things look like music sounds." [7] He uses a mix of digital and hand techniques to create a feeling of depth and materiality, and to suggest the texture of the music.

Diagonal Records in London produces sounds ranging from electronic dance tracks to post-punk and noise music. Creative director Guy Featherstone has crafted sensory counterparts to the music. Describing colors as tasting like toothpaste or biting like acid, he says, "I'd examine the music and try to work out, almost through a process of synesthesia really, what does that sound 'feel' like? What does it look like? And it's not just the sound, it's the 'experience' of listening to that music. How can I visualize that sonic terrain?" [8]

Russell Haswell: *37 Minute Workout* (DIAG007), 2014; Guy Featherstone (British, b. 1974) for Diagonal Records (London, UK, founded 2011); Courtesy of Guy Featherstone

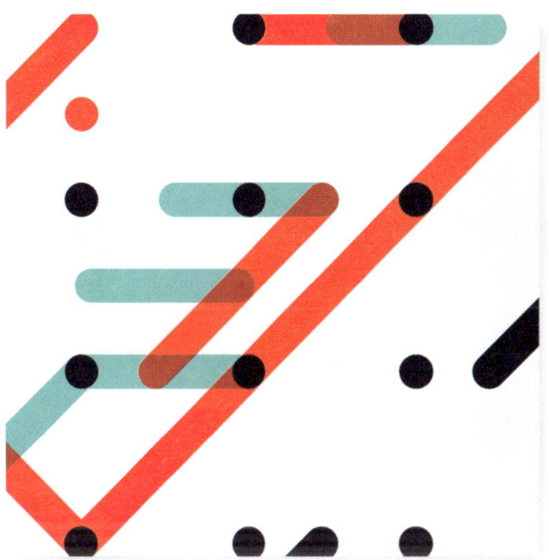

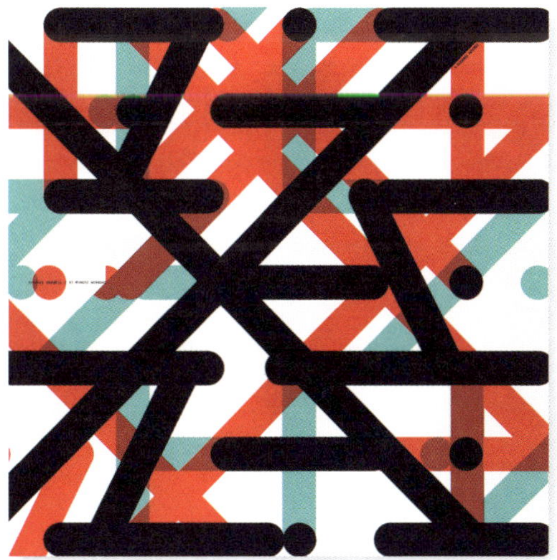

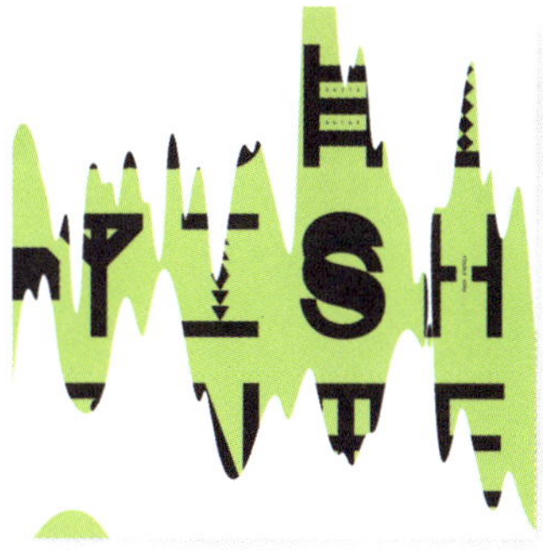

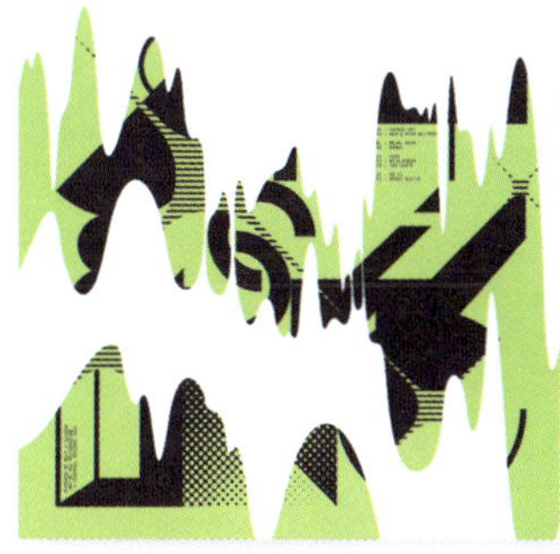

Shit and Shine: *Powder Horn* (DIAG012), 2014; Guy Featherstone (British, b. 1974) for Diagonal Records (London, UK, founded 2011); Courtesy of Guy Featherstone

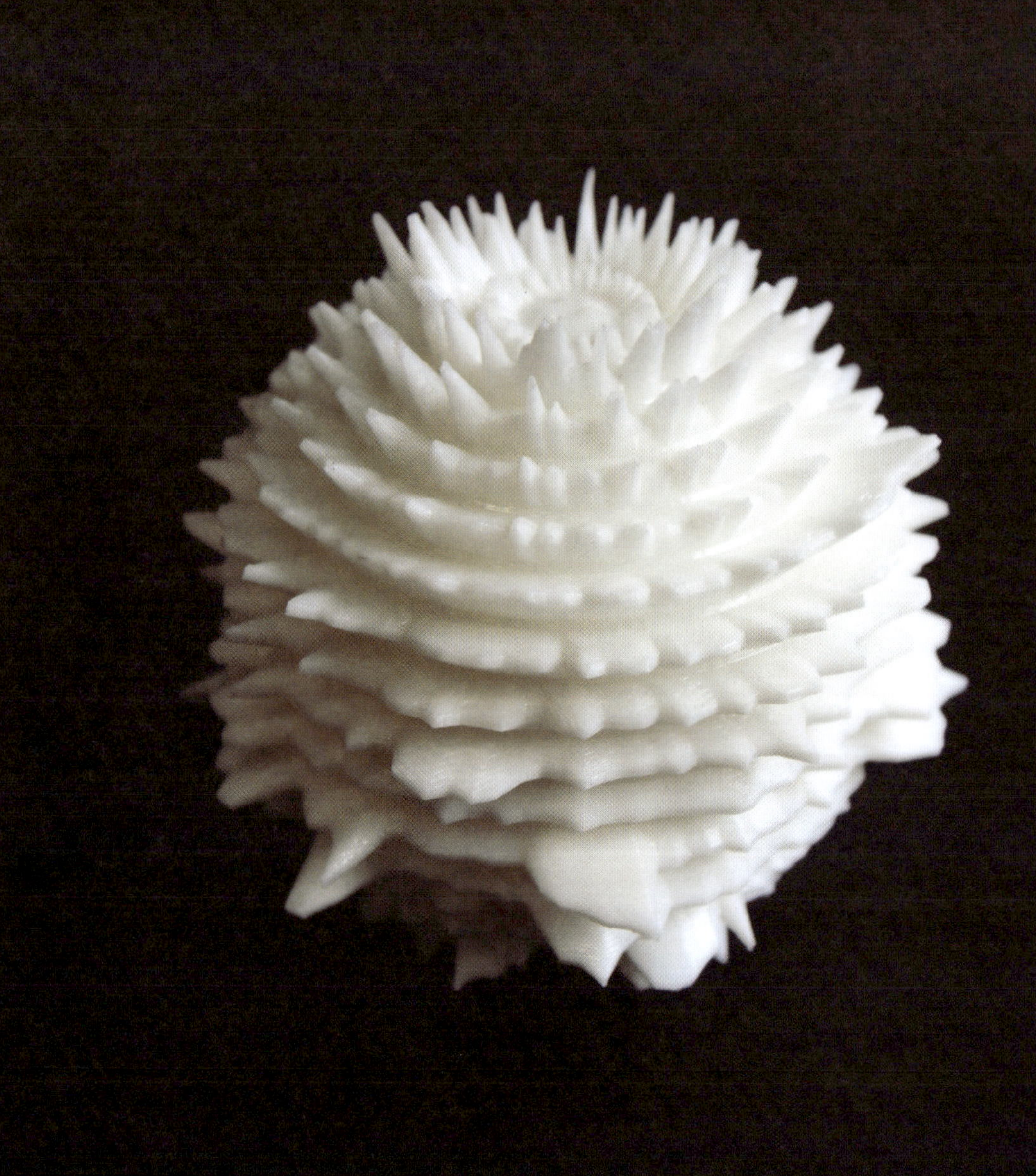

Swiss graphic designer Annik Troxler creates posters each year for the Jazz Festival Willisau, held in a small town in Switzerland. Her posters use fluid concoctions of line, texture, and color to express the improvised character of jazz. Many of her posters turn large-scale typography into a complex weave of patterned forms. Rather than attempt to visualize specific pieces of music, the posters anticipate the range of work presented in the festivals. “It’s good for graphic designers to be inspired by sources that come from somewhere else,” she says.[9] The Willisau Jazz Festival was founded in 1975 by Niklaus Troxler, Annik’s father, who designed the posters for thirty-five years. Cooper Hewitt acquired a set of Niklaus Troxler’s Willisau posters in 2009, courtesy of the artist.

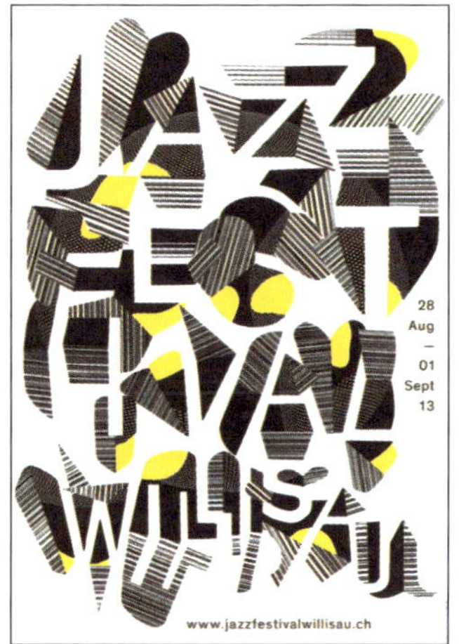

Poster, Jazz Festival Willisau 2013, 2013; Annik Troxler (Swiss, b. 1979) and Paula Troxler (Swiss, b. 1981) for Jazz Festival Willisau (Willisau, Switzerland); Screenprint on paper; 128.3 × 90.8 cm (50 ½ × 35 ¾ in.); Cooper Hewitt, Smithsonian Design Museum; Gift of Annik Troxler

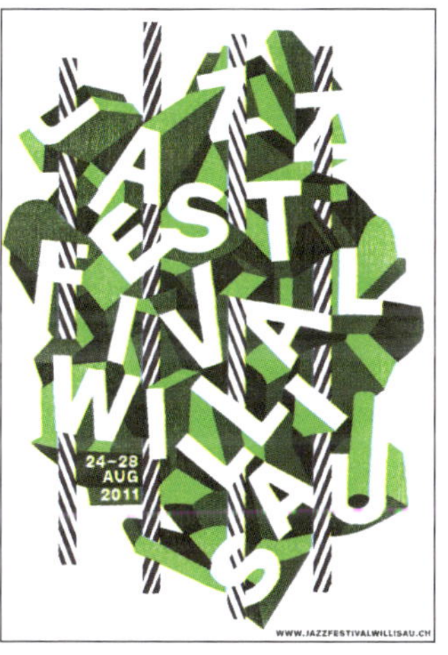

Poster, Jazz Festival Willisau 2011, 2011; Annik Troxler (Swiss, b. 1979) for Jazz Festival Willisau (Willisau, Switzerland); Screenprint on paper; 125.1 × 90.8 cm (49 ¼ × 35 ¾ in.); Cooper Hewitt, Smithsonian Design Museum; Gift of Annik Troxler

Sound can become physical as well as graphic. SoundScapes, a project that converts music into solid objects, was conceived at De Montfort University, UK, by designer Eujin Pei, music technology specialist Lorenzo Picinali, and PhD student Chris Feakes. The physical outcome of the team’s research is the Sound Sphere. The designers generated a script and software for printing 3D models of data derived from sound. In each sphere, lateral ridges represent the high, mid, and low tones of a piece of music. Low-frequency ridges occupy the bottom of the sphere (the south pole), and high-frequency

Sound Sphere, 2013; Eujin Pei (Singaporean, b. 1979), Lorenzo Picinali (Italian, b. 1981), and Chris Feakes (British, b. 1983), De Montfort University (Leicester, UK, founded 1969); 3D-printed plastic; Approx. 15 cm diam. (5 29/32 in.); Courtesy of Eujin Pei

ridges occupy the top (the north pole). Thus the location of each ridge indicates its band of frequency. The intensity or loudness of the sound at any moment is represented by the extent to which the ridge sticks out from the sphere. The higher the ridge, the louder the sound is in that frequency at that given time. The piece is a concrete representation of the physics of sound.

Human communication constantly mixes sound and vision. Typography is multisensory—it is audio and visual, sound and symbol. Speech is haptic and gestural as well as aural, felt in the muscles of the face, throat, and mouth. Writing is gesture. The sign languages created by deaf communities are fully functioning linguistic systems, designed for seeing not hearing. Helen Keller once said, "Blindness separates people from things; deafness separates people from people."[10] For the designers and artists explored here, studying sound through visual or tactile means is a powerful method of invention. Visualization offers a rich path for experiencing sound beyond the audible. Graphic interpretations of sound illuminate patterns and structure and generate new memories and associations. Communication that bridges our different senses helps connect us to each other and to the physical world.

Poster, Jazz Festival Willisau 2014, 2014; Annik Troxler (Swiss, b. 1979) for Jazz Festival Willisau (Willisau, Switzerland); Screenprint on paper; 125.1 × 90.8 cm (49 ¼ × 35 ¾ in.); Cooper Hewitt, Smithsonian Design Museum; Courtesy of Annik Troxler

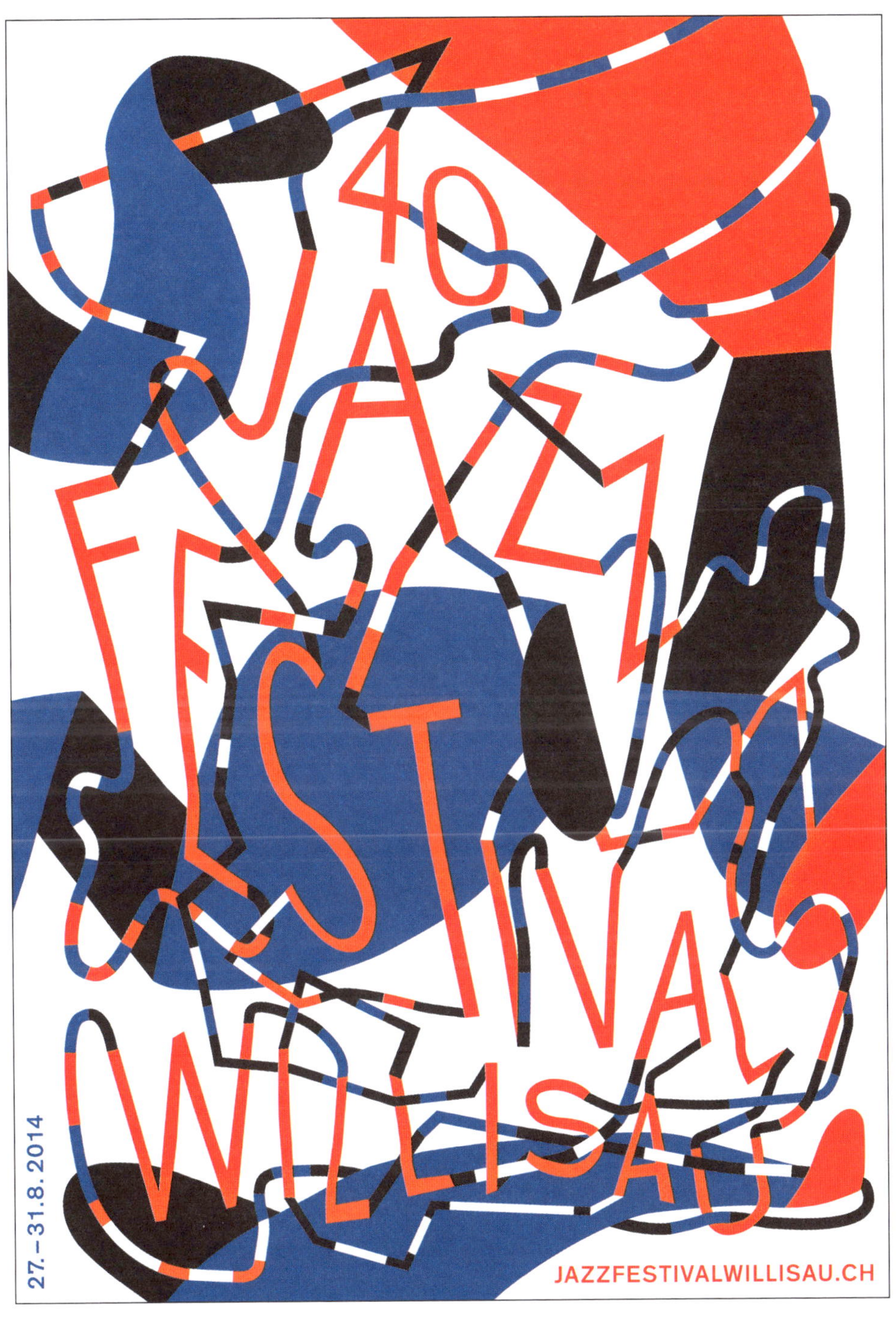
40
JAZZ
FESTIVAL
WILLISAU
27.–31.8.2014
JAZZFESTIVALWILLISAU.CH

Notes

WHY SENSORY DESIGN?

1 On perception as an active, purpose-driven, embodied process, see Andy Clark, *Supersizing the Mind: Embodiment, Action, and Cognitive Extension* (Oxford: Oxford University Press, 2011). Michael Haverkamp applies the principles of Gestalt psychology to sensory design in *Synesthetic Design: Handbook for a Multisensory Approach* (Basel: Birkhauser, 2013).

2 Richard E. Citowic, interview with Ellen Lupton, 23 February 2017. See also Richard E. Citowic, MD, and David M. Eagleman, PhD, *Wednesday Is Indigo Blue: Discovering the Brain of Synesthesia* (Cambridge, MA: MIT Press, 2009).

3 Cytowic, interview. See also Nicola Twilley, "Sight Unseen: Seeing with Your Tongue and Other Surprises of Sensory-Substitution Technology," *The New Yorker*, 15 May 2017, 38–42.

4 Juhani Pallasmaa, *The Eyes of the Skin: Architecture and the Senses* (West Sussex, England: Wiley, 2005). For an updated account of sensory architecture, see Sarah Williams Goldhagen, *How the Built Environment Shapes Our Lives* (New York: HarperCollins, 2017).

5 Mayor's Office for People with Disabilities, *Inclusive Design Guidelines*, 2nd ed. (New York City, 2017).

6 James J. Gibson, *The Senses Considered as Perceptual Systems* (Westport, CT: Greenwood Press, 1966, 1983); Jan Lauwereyns, *Brain and the Gaze: On the Active Boundaries of Vision* (Cambridge, MA: MIT Press, 2012).

7 David Abram, *The Spell of the Sensuous: Perception and Language in a More-Than-Human World* (New York: Vintage Books, 1997).

8 Joyce Monice Malnar and Frank Vodvarka, *Sensory Design* (Minneapolis: University of Minnesota Press, 2004).

9 Kate McLean, "Smellmap: Amsterdam—Olfactory Art and Smell Visualization," *Leonardo*, 50, no. 1 (2017): 92–93, doi.org/10.1162/LEON_a_01225.

10 Beatriz Colomina and Mark Wigley, *Are We Human? Notes on an Archaeology of Design* (Zürich: Lars Müller Publishers, 2016).

11 Museums did not always forbid sensory experience. See Constance Classen and David Howes, "The Museum as Sensescape: Western Sensibilities and Indigenous Artifacts," in *Sensible Objects: Colonialism, Museums and Material Culture*, ed. Elizabeth Edwards et al. (New York: Berg, 2006), 199–222.

12 Ellen Lupton, *Skin: Surface, Substance + Design* (New York: Cooper-Hewitt, National Design Museum and Princeton Architectural Press, 2012).

13 Quoted in Sarah Pink, *Doing Sensory Ethnography* (London: SAGE Publications, 2015).

NOTES ON TOUCH

1 David J. Linden, *Touch: The Science of Hand, Heart, and Mind* (New York: Viking, 2015).

2 Charles Spence and Alberto Gallace, "Multisensory Design: Reaching Out to Touch the Consumer," *Psychology & Marketing* 28, no. 3 (March 2011): 267–308, Doi.org/10.1002/mar.20392.

3 Jeremy D. Larson, "Letter of Recommendation: Hasbro Joy for All," *New York Times*, 24 March 2016, → nyti.ms/2k8LdFz, accessed 3 July 2017.

4 See Riitta Lahtinen Russ Palmer, "History of Social-Haptic Communication" (4th European Deafblind Conference, Espoo, Finland, 1996).

5 On haptics and the natural and artificial extensions of the body, see Gibson, *The Senses Considered as Perceptual Systems*, 99–104.

6 Mélina Gazsi, "An Easy Chair Can Be Hard to Make," *The Guardian*, 15 October 2013, → theguardian.com/artanddesign/2013/oct/15/tip-ton-chair-barber-osgerby-design, accessed 3 July 2017.

7 Edward Barber, quoted in Jaime Derringer, "Tipping Point: The Tip Ton Chair," *Design Milk*, 26 August 2013, → design-milk.com/tip-ton, accessed 3 July 2017.

8 Sarah Dweerdt, "Talking Sense: What Sensory Processing Disorder Says about Autism," *Spectrum*, 1 June 2016, → spectrumnews.org/features/talking-sense-what-sensory-processing-disorder-says-about-autism, accessed 3 July 2017.

9 For examples of compression clothing, see Kozie Clothes, → kozieclothes.com/compression-clothing, accessed 3 July 2017.

10 On kinesthetics, proprioception, and haptics, see James J. Gibson, *The Senses Considered as Perceptual Systems* (Westport, CT: Greenwood Press, 1966, 1983). See also R. S. Dahiy and M. Valle, "Tactile Sensing: Definitions and Classifications," in *Robotic Tactile Sensing*, DOI 10.1007/978-94-007-0579-1_2, (Dordrecht: Springer Science+Business Media, 2013), 13–17; and William Harris, "How Haptic Technology Works," HowStuffWorks, 30 June 2008, → electronics.howstuffworks.com/everyday-tech/haptic-technology.htm.**11** Josh Clark, *Designing for Touch* (New York: A Book Apart, 2015).

12 Elizabeth Cooney, "Gut Feelings: Sensory Neurons Detect Fullness and Nutrients in the GI Tract in Surprising Ways," *Harvard Medical School News*, 26 May 2016, → hms.harvard.edu/news/gut-feelings, accessed 3 July 2017.

13 Jennifer M. Barker, *The Tactile Eye: Touch and Cinematic Experience* (Berkeley: University of California Press, 2009).

14 Daniel Kahneman, *Thinking, Fast and Slow* (New York: Farrar, Straus, and Giroux, 2013).

15 Cellini, Cristiano, Lukas Kaim, and Knut Drewing, "Visual and Haptic Integration in the Estimation of Softness of Deformable Objects," *i-Perception* 4, no. 8 (2013): 516–31. PMC. Web. 15 April 2017.

NOTES ON SOUND

1 On the science of sound, see Andy Farnell, *Designing Sound* (Cambridge: MIT Press, 2010).

2 Conor O'Sullivan, "Sound and Picture" (lecture organized by AIGA NY, 9 March 2017).

3 Peter Otto, interview with Ellen Lupton, 11 May 2017.

4 Farnell, "Psychoacoustics," *Designing Sound*.

5 Cytowic et al., 104: 163–8.

6 Maija Kontukoski, Harri Luomala, Bruno Mesz, Mariano Sigman, Marcos Trevisan, Minna Rotola-Pukkila, Anu Inkeri Hopia, "Sweet and Sour: Music and Taste Associations," *Nutrition & Food Science* 45, no. 3 (2015): 357–76, → doi.org/10.1108/NFS-01-2015-0005 See also "Music Generates Taste of Sour, Salty, Sweet, and Bitter," MolecularRecipes.com, 8 August 2011,→ molecularrecipes.com/molecular-gastronomy/taste-music

7 Durand B. Begault, "Guidelines for NextGen Auditory Displays," *Journal of Audio Engineering Society* 60, no. 7/8 (July/August 2012): 519–30.

8 Joel Beckerman, interview with Ellen Lupton, 18 May 2016; Joel Beckerman, *Sonic Boom: How Sound Transforms the Way We Think, Feel, and Buy* (New York: Houghton Mifflin Harcourt, 2014).

NOTES ON FLAVOR

1 Quoted in Alla Katsnelson, "From the Tongue to the Brain," *Columbia Medicine* (Spring/Summer 2015). → columbiamedicinemagazine.org/features/spring-2015/tongue-brain, accessed 3 March 2017.

2 C. Bushdid, M. O. Magnasco, L. B. Vosshall, and A. Keller, "Humans Can Discriminate More than 1 Trillion Olfactory Stimuli," *Science* 343, no. 6177 (2014): 1370–72.

3 Gordon M. Shepherd, *Neurogastronomy: How the Brain Creates Flavor and Why It Matters* (New York: Columbia University Press, 2017).

4 Bevil R. Conway, "Processing," in *Experience: Culture, Cognition, and the Common Sense*, Caroline A. Jones, David Mather, and Rebecca Uchill, eds. (Cambridge, MA: MIT Press, 2016), 86–109.

5 Nicola Twiley, "Accounting for Taste: How Packaging Can Make Food More Flavorful," *The New Yorker*, 26 October 2015.

6 Brian Wansink, "Environmental Factors That Increase the Food Intake and Consumption Volume of Unknowing Consumers," *Annual Review of Nutrition* 24 (2004): 455–79, doi.org/ 10.1146/annurev.nutr.24.012003.132140.

7 Harold McGee, *On Food and Cooking: The Science and Lore of the Kitchen* (New York: Scribner, 2004), 364.

SENSORY MATERIALS

1 Tom Young and Stuart Taylor, PhysLink.com, accessed 14 September 2017, → physlink.com/education/askexperts/ae680.cfm.

2 Theo Richardson, interview with Ellen Lupton, 8 September 2017.

3 Peter Corboy, ed., "Johan Kappui Creates Sound Absorbing Furniture for Glimakra of Sweden," *Design Boom*, 29 January 2017, → designboom.com/design/johan-kauppi-wakufuru-glimakra-sweden-01-29-2017/.

4 Ronald Rael and Virginia San Fratello, *Printing Architecture: Innovative Recipes for 3D Printing* (New York: Princeton Architectural Press, 2018).

5 Sarah Scaturro, interview with Ellen Lupton, 2016.

6 Skylar Tibbits, interview with Andrea Lipps, 27 February 2017.

7 Roos Meerman, interview with Andrea Lipps, 20 March 2017.

THE SENSORY TABLE

1 Diane Ackerman, *A Natural History of the Senses* (New York: Vintage Books, 1990), 127.

2 Charles Zuker, "Symphony of the Senses" (lecture, Plaza Athénée, New York, NY, 22 March 2017).

3 Shepherd, *Neurogastronomy*, 3–16.

4 Jean Anthelme Brillat-Savarin, trans. M. F. K. Fisher, *The Physiology of Taste: Or, Meditations on Transcendental Gastronomy* (Washington, DC: Counterpoint Press, 1999), 39.

5 Charles Spence, "Sound: The Forgotten Flavor Sense," in *Multisensory Flavor Perception: From Fundamental Neuroscience through to the Marketplace*, ed. Betina Piqueras-Fiszman and Charles Spence (Cambridge, MA: Woodhead Publishing, 2016), 81–105, accessed 10 July 2017, doi.org/ 10.1016/B978-0-08-100350-3.00005-5; Carlos Velasco, Andy T. Woods, Lawrence E. Marks, Adrian David Cheok, and Charles Spence, "The Semantic Basis of Taste-Shape Associations," *Psychiatry and Psychology* 4 (2016), accessed 28 June 2016, doi.org/ 10.7717/peerj.1644; Betina Piqueras-Fiszmana, Vanessa Harrar, Jorge Alcaide, and Charles Spence, "Does the Weight of the Dish Influence Our Perception of Food?" *Food Quality and Preference* 22, no. 8 (2011): 753–56, accessed

10 July 2017, doi.org/ 10.1016/j.foodqual.2011.05.009; Charles Spence, Carmel A. Levitan, Maya U. Shankar, and Massimiliano Zampini, "Does Food Color Influence Taste and Flavor Perception in Humans?" *Chemosensory Perception* 3, no. 1 (2010): 68–84, accessed July 10, 2017, → doi.org/ 10.1007/s12078-010-9067-z.

6 Brillat-Savarin, *The Physiology of Taste.*

7 Jeffery Sobal and Brian Wansink, "Kitchenscapes, Tablescapes, Platescapes, and Foodscapes: Influences of Microscale Built Environments on Food Intake, Environment, and Behavior," *Environment and Behavior* 39, no. 1 (2007), 124–42, accessed 29 June 2017, → doi.org/ 10.1177/0013916506295574.

8 Charles Spence, Betina Piqueras-Fiszman, Charles Michel, and Ophelia Deroy, "Plating Manifesto (II): The Art and Science of Plating," *Flavour* 3, no. 4 (2014), accessed 20 June 2017, → doi.org/ 10.1186/2044-7248-3-4; Vanessa Harrar and Charles Spence, "The Taste of Cutlery: How the Taste of Food Is Affected by the Weight, Size, Shape, and Colour of the Cutlery Used to Eat It," *Flavour* 2, no. 21 (2013), accessed 7 June 2017, → doi.org/ 10.1186/2044-7248-2-21.

9 Oxford Dictionary Online, s.v. "hygge," accessed 10 June 2017, → en.oxforddictionaries.com/ definition/hygge.

10 Vanessa Harrar, Betina Piqueras-Fiszman, and Charles Spence, "There's More to Taste in a Coloured Bowl," *Perception* 40 (2011): 880–82, accessed 22 June 2016, → doi.org/ 10.1068/p7040; Betina Piqueras-Fiszman, Jorge Alcaide, Elena Roura, and Charles Spence, "Is It the Plate or Is It the Food? Assessing the Influence of the Color (Black or White) and Shape of the Plate on the Perception of the Food Placed on It," *Food Quality and Preference* 24 (2012): 205–8, accessed 22 June 2016, → doi.org/ 10.1016/j.foodqual.2011.08.011

SCENTSCAPES

1 Marcelo Roxo et al., "The Limbic System Conception and Its Historical Evolution," *Scientific World Journal* 11 (2011): 2428–41, → dx.doi.org/10.1100/2011/157150.

2 Vladimir Nabokov, *Mary* (New York: Vintage International, 1970), 60.

3 Christopher Brosius, interview with Ellen Lupton, 8 December 2016.

4 Christophe Laudamiel, interview with Ellen Lupton, 10 August 2016.

5 Ibid.

6 Megan Sullivan, "An Interview with Perfumer Christopher Laudamiel," National Science Teachers Association WebNews Digest, 23 December 2003, → nsta.org/publications/news/story.aspx?id=48898

7 Christophe Laudamiel, interview with Ellen Lupton, 10 August 2016.

8 Nsikan Akpan, "What a Smell Looks Like," *Scientific American*, 16 June 2016, → scientificamerican.com/article/what-a-smell-looks-like/?wt.mc_id=sa_fb_mb_news

9 Reiko Sakamoto et al., "Effectiveness of Aroma on Work Efficiency: Lavender Aroma during Recesses Prevents Deterioration of Work Performance," *Chemical Senses* 30, no. 8 (October 2005): 683–91, → doi.org/10.1093/chemse/bji061; Mark Ross et al., "Aromas of Rosemary and Lavender Essential Oils Differentially Affect Cognition and Mood in Healthy Adults," *International Journal of Neuroscience* 113, no. 1 (January 2003): 15–38, → doi.org/10.1016/j.ajme.2017.05.004; Susan C. Knasko, "Ambient Odor's Effect on Creativity, Mood, and Perceived Health," *Chemical Senses* 17, no. 1 (February 1992): 21–35, → doi.org/10.1093/chemse/17.1.27; H. Wayne Ludvigson and Theresa R. Rottman, "Effects of Ambient Odors of Lavender and Cloves on Cognition, Memory, Affect and Mood," *Chemical Senses* 14, no. 4 (August 1989): 525–36, → doi.org/10.1093/chemse/14.4.525

10 Brad Johnson, Rehan M. Khan, and Noam Sobel, "Human Olfactory Pyschophysics," *The Senses: A Comprehensive Reference* (Amsterdam: Elsevier Academic Press, 2008), 823–57.

11 Debra A. Zellner, "Color–Odor Interactions: A Review and Model," *Chemosensory Perception* 6, no. 4 (December 2013): 155–69, → link.springer.com/article/10.1007/s12078-013-9154-z

12 Debra A. Zellner, Angela M. Bartoli, and Robert Eckard, "Influence of Color on Odor Identification and Liking Ratings," *American Journal of Psychology* 104, no. 4 (Winter 1991): 547–61, → jstor.org/stable/1422940

13 Noah Browning, "Israeli 'Skunk' Fouls West Bank Protests," Reuters, 3 September 2012, → reuters.com/article/us-israel-palestinians-skunk/israeli-skunk-fouls-west-bank-protests-idusbre88208w20120903

14 "Who, What, Why: What Is Skunk Water?" *BBC News Magazine*, 12 September 2015, → bbc.com/news/magazine-34227609

15 Harold McGee, *On Food and Cooking: The Science and Lure of the Kitchen* (New York: Scribner, 2004).

16 Sharififard, Mona et al., "Evaluation of Some Plant Essential Oils against the Brown-Banded Cockroach, *Supella Longipalpa* (*Blattaria: Ectobiidae*): A Mechanical Vector of Human Pathogens." *Journal of Arthropod-Borne Diseases* 10, no. 4 (2016): 528–37.

17 John McQuaid, "The Mysteries of Chili Heat: Why People Love the Pain," *Salon*, 7 February 2015, → salon.com/2015/02/07/the_mysteries_of_chili_heat_why_people_love_the_pain/, cited September 29, 2017.

18 C. Bushdid et al., "Humans Can Discriminate More than 1 Trillion Olfactory Stimuli," *Science* 343, no. 6177 (21 March 2012): 1370–72, → science.sciencemag.org/content/343/6177/1370

SENSORY ENVIRONMENTS

1 H-Dirksen L. Bauman and Joseph J. Murray, "Reframing: From Hearing Loss to Deaf Gain," *Deaf Studies Digital Journal* 1 (Fall 2009): 1–10.

2 Hansel Bauman, interview with Ellen Lupton, 27 January 2017; Amanda Kolson Hurley, "How Gallaudet University's Architects Are Redefining Deaf Space," *Curbed*, 2 March 2016, → curbed.com/2016/3/2/11140210/gallaudet-deafspace-washington-dc; accessed 17 March 2017.

3 Stephen Gorman and Richard Cytowic, interview with Ellen Lupton, 23 February 2017.

4 Melinda Miller, "How Does Acoustical Absorption Work?" *Acoustics by Design*, 8 December 2011, → acousticsbydesign.com/acoustics-blog/how-does-acoustical-absorption-work.htm, accessed 11 March 2017; "The Laws of Sound Physics (Acoustics), or How Does It Work?" Sounds of Science, accessed 11 March 2017, → sofsci.com/some-info, "How Sound Works (in Rooms)," video, Acoustic Geometry, 1 August 2013, → youtu.be/JPYt1OzrclQ; accessed 11 March 2017.

5 Jonathan Hopkins, interview with Ellen Lupton, 4 April 2017.

6 David Byrne, *How Music Works* (San Francisco: McSweeney's, 2012).

7 Dhruv Khullar, MD, "Bad Hospital Design Is Making Us Sicker," *New York Times*, 22 February 2017. → nyti.ms/2lujQ76; accessed 11 March 2017.

8 "Sound Masking in Healthcare Environments," *Healthcare Design Magazine* (1 November 2005), → healthcaredesignmagazine.com/architecture/sound-masking-healthcare-environments/2; accessed 11 March 2017.

9 Chris Downey, interview with Ellen Lupton, 20 December 2016.

10 Chris Downey, interview with Ellen Lupton, 3 May 2017.

11 H. Sekiguchi and H. Nakayama, "On a History and a Present Circumstances of Walking for Persons with Visual Impairments in Japan" (5th International Conference on Civil Engineering, 29–31 August 2002, Manila, Philippines).

TACTILE SOUND

1 Irwin Stambler, *The World of Sounds* (New York: W. W. Norton, 1967), 29.

2 Peter V. Paul, *Toward a Psychology of Deafness: Theoretical and Empirical Perspectives* (MA: Allyn & Bacon, 1993), 24–25.

3 Rachel Kolb, "Sensations of Sound: On Deafness and Music," *New York Times*, 3 November 2017, → nyti.ms/2iYHCe4, accessed 3 November 2017; Aharona Ament, "Beyond Vibrations: The Deaf Experience in Music," *Gapers Block*, 22 July 2010, → gapersblock.com/transmission/2010/07/22/beyond_vibrations_the_deaf_musical_experience/, accessed 5 May 2017.

4 Riccardo Ferreira Bento, "Beethoven's Deafness, the Defiance of a Genius," *International Archives of Otorhinolaryngol* 13, no. 3 (2009): 317–21.

5 A. El Saddik et al., "Haptics: General Principles," in *Haptics Technologies* (Berlin: Springer-Verlag, 2011), 2.

6 Ibid., 3.

7 Ibid., 5.

8 "Leading Automotive Supplier Demonstrates Ultrahaptics' Midair Haptics in Concept Car at CES® 2017," *Ultrahaptics* (5 January 2017), → ultrahaptics.com/ces2017car Accessed 5 May 2017.

9 Stambler, *The World of Sounds*, 33.

TACTILE GRAPHICS

1 Wendell Jamieson, "The Crime of His Childhood," *New York Times*, 2 March 2013, → nytimes.com/2013/03/03/nyregion/40-years-after-an-acid-attack-a-life-well-lived.html, accessed 28 January 2017

2 "Tactile Maps for the Blind," LightHouse Case Study, 25 June 2017.

3 Ross Atkin, "Sight Line: Designing Better Streets for People with Low Vision," Royal College of Art Helen Hamlyn Centre, 2010.

4 Quoted in Merlin Coverley, *Psychogeography* (Harpendon, UK: Pocket Essentials, 2012).

5 Cari Romm, "How Sticks and Shell Charts Became a Sophisticated System for Navigation," Smithsonian.com, 26 January 2015, → smithsonianmag.com/smithsonian-institution/how-sticks-and-shell-charts-became-sophisticated-system-navigation-180954018; accessed 2 October 2017.

6 "Samuel Gridley Howe," American Printing House for the Blind Hall of Fame, accessed 21 June 2017, → aph.org/hall/inductees/howe.

7 Angela Reichers, "Comic Sans Just Might Be the Best Font for People with Dyslexia," *AIGA Eye on Design*, 23 August 2016, → eyeondesign.aiga.org/sad-but-true-comic-sans-might-just-be-the-best-font-for-dyslexics. Cited 20 November 2016.

8 David J. Linden, *Touch: The Science of Hand, Heart, and Mind* (New York: Viking, 2015), 51–54.

9 Chancey Fleet, interview with Ellen Lupton, 2017.

10 Ned Geeslin and S. Avery Brown, "With Her Mother's Eyesight Failing, Elia Chepaitis Creates a New, Simpler Alternative to Braille," *People*, 2 May 1988, → people.com/archive/with-her-mothers-eyesight-failing-elia-chepaitis-creates-a-new-simpler-alternative-to-braille-vol-29-no-17/, accessed 24 June 2017; Meg Miller, "The Complicated Quest to Redesign Braille," *Co.Design*, 28 September 2017, → fastcodesign.com/90136975/the-complicated-quest-to-redesign-braille, accessed 2 October 2017.

11 Andrew Chepaitis, interview with Ellen Lupton, 19 July 2017.

12 Kimon Nicolaides, *The Natural Way to Draw: A Working Plan for Art Study* (Boston: Houghton Mifflin Company, 1941), 6.

13 Ann Cunningham, interview with Ellen Lupton, 10 December 2016. Cunningham is a sighted artist and educator.

COLOR AND COGNITION

1 Annie Leist, artist statement, → local-artists.org/user/621/profile, accessed 1 July 2017.

2 Annie Leist, interview with Ellen Lupton, 9 June 2017.

3 "Feelipa Color Code—Color Is for Everyone," Indiegogo, accessed 14 April 2017, → indiegogo.com/projects/feelipa-color-code-color-is-for-everyone; Filipa Nogueira Pires, "Feelipa: Revolution in Learning Color," TEDxLisboaED, 12 October 2013, accessed 14 April 2017, → youtu.be/hWtFMTq9VTY.

4 Lawrence E. Marks, "The Unity of the Senses," in *The Unity of the Senses: Interrelations among the Modalities* (New York: Academic Press, 1978), 182.

5 Juhani Pallasmaa, *Eyes of the Skin: Architecture and Senses*, 10.

6 Ashley Montagu, *Touching: The Human Significance of the Skin* (New York: Harper & Row, 1986), 3.

7 Marks, "Unity of the Senses," 183.

8 Pallasmaa, *Eyes of the Skin*, 42.

9 Marie-Kathrin Zettl, "Interview with Simon Kinneir: The Leaven Range," *Form* 268 (2016), accessed 16 April 2017, → form.de/en/news/interview-mit-simon-kinneir-the-leaven-range.

10 Emma Tucker, "Simon Kinneir Creates Tilting Leaven Jug for Visually Impaired Users," *Dezeen*, 22 March 2016, → dezeen.com/2016/03/22/leaven-collection-simon-kinneir-kitchenware-homeware-visually-impaired-sight-loss-design, accessed 16 April 2017.

11 "What Is Alzheimer's Disease?" CNADC of the Northwestern University Feinberg School of Medicine, → brain.northwestern.edu/dementia/ad/index.html, accessed 19 April 2017.

12 Kathryn A. Bayles and Alfred W. Kaszniak, *Communication and Cognition in Normal Aging and Dementia* (Austin: PRO-ED, 1987), xiv, 251.

13 "Color and Function: Orientation through Contrast," HEWI, → hewi.com/en/accessibility/washbasin-dementia, accessed 19 April 2017.

14 Lee H. Wurm et al., "Color Improves Object Recognition in Normal and Low Vision," *Journal of Experimental Psychology: Human Perception and Performance* 19, no. 4 (1993): 899.

15 Ibid., 904–5.

16 Charles Spence and Alberto Gallace. "Multisensory Design: Reaching Out to Touch the Consumer," *Psychology & Marketing* 28, no. 3 (March 2011): 267–308, doi.org/10.1002/mar.20392

17 Bayles and Kaszniak, *Communication and Cognition in Normal Aging and Dementia*, 2.

18 Sha Yao, "Inspiration," Eatwell, accessed 19 April 2017, → eatwellset.com/inspiration-cqyc

19 Miranda Hitti, "Eating and Alzheimer's," *CBS News*, 28 September 2004, accessed 19 April 2017, → cbsnews.com/news/eating-and-alzheimers

VISUALIZING SOUND

1 Alexander Chen, interview with Ellen Lupton, 23 May, 2017.

2 Ashley P. Taylor, "Newton's Color Theory, ca. 1665," *The Scientist*, 1 March 2017, → the-scientist.com/?articles.view/articleNo/48584/title/Newton-s-Color-Theory--ca--1665, accessed 27 May 2017.

3 Richard E. Citowic, MD, and David M. Eagleman, PhD, *Wednesday Is Indigo Blue: Discovering the Brain of Synesthesia* (Cambridge, MA: MIT Press, 2009).

4 Yasmin Anwar, "Back to the Blues, Our Emotions Match Music to Colors," *Berkeley News*, 16 May 2013, → news.berkeley.edu/2013/05/16/musiccolors/, accessed 6 June 2017; Palmer, Stephen E. et al., "Music–Color Associations Are Mediated by Emotion," *Proceedings of the National Academy of Sciences of the United States of America* 110, no. 22 (2013): 8836–41, PMC, accessed 6 June 2017.

5 Citowic and Eagleman, *Wednesday Is Indigo Blue*.

6 Mario Hugo, interview with Ellen Lupton, 30 June 2017.

7 "Where Designers Work (Video): Hugo & Marie Is Actually 2 Design Businesses in 1," AIGA Eye on Design, 8 December 2016, → eyeondesign.aiga.org/where-designers-work-video-hugo-marie-actually-runs-2-design-businesses-cuz-yknow-why-not, accessed July 4, 2017.

8 Mark Sinclair, "Serious Fun with Diagonal Records," *Creative Review*, 13 January 2017, → creativereview.co.uk/design-diagonal-records, accessed 1 February 2017.

9 Annik Troxler, interview with Ellen Lupton, 15 June 2017.

10 Vona B. and Haaf T., eds., *Genetics of Deafness, Monographs in Human Genetics*, 20 (Basel: Karger, 2016), 30–39; Helen Keller quoted 31.

Index

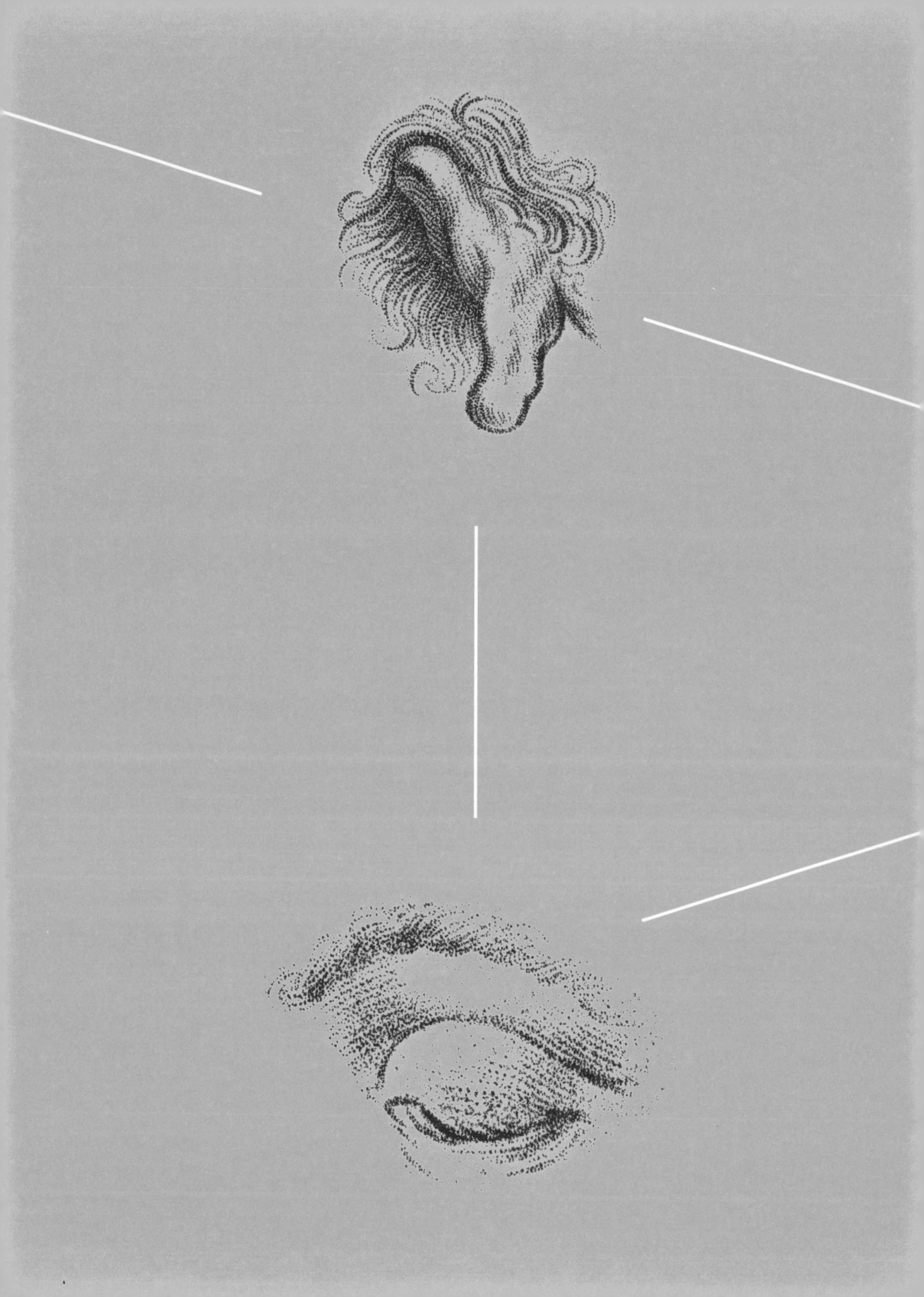